I0868579

Novel Carriers for Psoriasis Management and Pharmacotherapy

Edited by

Anjali Sharma
Department of Pharmaceutics
Guru Gobind Singh College of Pharmacy
Yamunanagar, Haryana
India

Prerna Sharma
Department of Pharmacognosy
Shri Krishna Ayush University
Kurukshetra, Haryana
India

Roy Rillera Marzo
Department of Public Health
Management and Science University
Malaysia

&

Ahmed A. Al Karmalawy
Department of Pharmaceutical Chemistry
College of Pharmacy
The University of Mashreq
Baghdad 10023
Iraq

Department of Pharmaceutical Chemistry
Faculty of Pharmacy
Horus University-Egypt
New Damietta 34518
Egypt

Novel Carriers for Psoriasis Management and Pharmacotherapy

Editors: Anjali Sharma, Prerna Sharma, Roy Rillera Marzo and Ahmed A. AI Karmalawy

ISBN (Online): 979-8-89881-273-7

ISBN (Print): 979-8-89881-274-4

ISBN (Paperback): 979-8-89881-275-1

Published by Bentham Science Publishers Pte. Ltd. Singapore,

in collaboration with Eureka Conferences, USA.

First published in 2026.

Bentham Science Publishers Pte. Ltd.
No. 9 Raffles Place
Office No. 26-01
Singapore 048619
Singapore
Email: subscriptions@benthamscience.net

BENTHAM
SCIENCE

CONTENTS

FOREWORD i

PREFACE ii

LIST OF CONTRIBUTORS iii

CHAPTER 1 UNDERSTANDING PSORIASIS: A CHRONIC SKIN CONDITION 1
Muskan Srivastava and *Deepika Sharma*
INTRODUCTION 2
Background 2
Epidemiology 3
CLINICAL TYPES OF PSORIASIS 4
Plaque Psoriasis 4
Guttate Psoriasis 4
Flexural (Inverse) Psoriasis 5
Erythroderma 5
Generalized Pustular Psoriasis 5
Palmoplantar Pustulosis 5
Psoriatic Nail Condition 6
Triggers 6
Pathophysiology 7
Diagnosis 8
Psoriasis Treatment 9
Methotrexate 9
Cyclosporine 9
Angiotensin Converting Enzyme Inhibitors (ACEI) 10
Phototherapy 10
CONCLUSION 10
REFERENCES 10

CHAPTER 2 PATHOPHYSIOLOGY AND MOLECULAR BASIS OF PSORIASIS 13
Kashish Wilson, Tanvi, Rajat Goyal, Sumeet Gupta, Chander Parkash Dora and Garima
INTRODUCTION 14
Epidemiology of Psoriasis 14
Prevalence and Age Distribution of Psoriasis 15
Prevalence 15
Age Distribution 15
Etiology of Psoriasis 16
PSORIASIS'S IMPACT ON LIFE QUALITY 16
PATHOGENESIS OF PSORIASIS 17
Uncontrolled Keratinocyte Proliferation 17
Genetic Factors 17
Cell Cycle Dysregulation 18
Immune Dysregulation and Cytokine Production 18
Angiogenesis and Neovascularization 18
Therapeutic Interventions 18
Dysregulation of the Immune System 18
Involvement of Innate Immunocytes 19
Initial Innate Immune Activation 19
Innate Immune Cells and the IL-23/Th17 Axis 20

Involvement of Acquired or Adaptive Immunocytes ... 20
T Cells ... 20
B Cells ... 20
T Regulatory Cells (Tregs) ... 21
Interplay between Adaptive and Innate Immune Systems ... 21
INFLAMMATION AND CLINICAL MANIFESTATIONS ... 21
Cellular and Molecular Mechanisms of Inflammation ... 21
Clinical Manifestations ... 22
BIOLOGICAL THERAPIES FOR PSORIASIS ... 22
CLINICAL TRIALS FOR PSORIASIS ... 22
FDA APPROVAL OF DRUGS IN PSORIASIS ... 23
REFERENCES ... 25

CHAPTER 3 COMBINATION APPROACH FOR THE MANAGEMENT OF PSORIASIS ... 29
Karan Goel, Sapna Rani, Rama Devi, Sarita Sharma and *Simran Saini*
INTRODUCTION TO PSORIASIS ... 29
Epidemiology and Clinical Presentation ... 30
Impact on Quality of Life ... 30
UNDERSTANDING THE PATHOPHYSIOLOGY ... 31
Immune Dysregulation and Inflammatory Cascade ... 31
Abnormal Keratinocyte Proliferation ... 31
Role of Genetic and Environmental Factors ... 32
CURRENT TREATMENT OPTIONS ... 32
Topical Therapies ... 33
Phototherapy [Light Therapy] ... 33
Systemic Medications ... 33
Biologic Agents ... 34
LIMITATIONS OF MONOTHERAPY ... 34
Efficacy Challenges ... 34
Variability in Response ... 34
Limited Disease Control ... 34
Partial Response ... 35
Side Effects and Safety Concerns ... 35
Topical Agents ... 35
Systemic Medications ... 35
Biologic Agents ... 35
Development of Treatment Resistance ... 35
Primary Resistance ... 35
Secondary Resistance ... 35
RATIONALE FOR COMBINATION APPROACH ... 36
Multifactorial Nature of Psoriasis ... 36
Targeting Multiple Pathogenic Pathways ... 36
Potential Synergistic Effects ... 37
CLINICAL EVIDENCE FOR COMBINATION THERAPY ... 37
Clinical Studies ... 37
Comparative Efficacy of Combination vs. Monotherapy ... 37
Safety and Tolerability Profiles ... 38
ADVANTAGES OF COMBINATION THERAPY ... 38
Enhanced Therapeutic Efficacy ... 38
Synergistic Effects ... 38
Complementary Mechanisms of Action ... 38

Improved Disease Control 38
Reduced Risk of Treatment Resistance 39
Mitigation of Resistance Development 39
Diverse Mechanisms of Action 39
Prevention of Flare-Ups 39
Improved Patient Outcomes and Quality of Life 39
Enhanced Symptom Relief 39
Longer Remission Periods 39
Greater Treatment Satisfaction 40
CHALLENGES AND CONSIDERATIONS 40
Treatment Complexity 40
Multimodal Approach 40
Individualized Treatment Plans 40
Treatment Adherence 40
Cost Considerations 40
Financial Burden 40
Cost-Effectiveness 41
Drug Interactions and Toxicities 41
Polypharmacy Risks 41
Toxicity Monitoring 41
Patient Monitoring and Management 41
Regular Follow-Up 41
Patient Education 41
FUTURE DIRECTIONS 42
Emerging Therapeutic Targets 42
Precision Medicine 42
Biologic Innovations 42
Personalized Treatment Approaches 42
Genomic Profiling 42
Precision Medicine Algorithms 42
Innovation in Combination Therapy 43
Optimized Combination Regimens 43
Integrated Treatment Platforms 43
CONCLUSION AND TAKEAWAYS 43
REFERENCES 44
CHAPTER 4 GENE THERAPIES IN THE MANAGEMENT OF PSORIASIS 48
Nidhi Gairola, Shalu Verma and *Bhawna*
INTRODUCTION 49
PREVALENCE 50
CLINICAL MANIFESTATIONS OF PSORIASIS 51
PATHOPHYSIOLOGY 52
DIAGNOSIS 54
CURRENT ARMAMENTARIUM 54
Biologics Available 55
Phototherapy 55
Topical Therapy 56
Advanced Drug Delivery System for Psoriasis 56
Gene Therapy 57
GENE THERAPY IN THE TREATMENT OF PSORIASIS 58

Gene Therapy for Psoriasis in the K14-VEGF Transgenic Mouse Model by Topical Transdermal Delivery of Interleukin-4 Using Ultra-Deformable Cationic Liposome 60
Halting Engiogenesis by Non-Viral Somatic Gene Therapy Alleviates Psoriasis and Murine Psoriasiform Skin Lesions 60
Pharmacogenomics 61
Anti-Tumour Necrosis Factor Drugs 62
Cytokine Inhibitors 64
CHALLENGES TO GENE THERAPY 65
CONCLUSION 66
REFERENCES 66

CHAPTER 5 CONVENTIONAL THERAPIES AND CHALLENGES IN THE TREATMENT OF PSORIASIS 72
Himani Bajaj, Seema B. Chauhan, Mayank Yadav and *Anjali Sharma*
INTRODUCTION 72
Current choices for Treatment 73
Topical Therapy 74
Oral therapy 74
Acitretin 74
Methotrexate 74
Cyclosporine 74
Apremilast 75
Fumaric Acid Esters 75
Mycophenolate Mofetil 75
Biological Therapy and Parenteral Therapy 75
Phototherapy 76
Marketed Formulations 77
Role of Traditional Medicine in Psoriasis: 78
Treatment Challenges 80
Profile of Patients 80
Pregnant Women 80
Obese Patients 81
Children 81
Skin Barrier 82
Patient's point of view 82
Compliance with Therapy 83
Psychological Impact 83
Compliance with Treatment 83
CONCLUSION 84
REFERENCES 84

CHAPTER 6 PHYTOPHARMACEUTICALS IN THE MANAGEMENT OF PSORIASIS 88
Bhawna Chopra, Ashwani Kumar Dhingra and *Priyanka Kriplani*
INTRODUCTION 88
SUBSTANCES OF NATURAL ORIGIN—PLANTS AND PHYTOCHEMICALS WITH POTENTIAL THERAPEUTIC SIGNIFICANCE 89
Vegetal Medicinal Plants 89
Aloe vera 89
Artemisia capillaris 90
Hypericum perforatum 90
Rehmannia glutinosa 90
Salvia miltiorrhiza 90

Psoralea corylifolia 91
Curcuma longa 91
Polyherbal formulations 91
Phytoconstituents 92
Capsaicin 92
Resveratrol 92
Curcumin 92
Rottlerin 93
Quercetin 93
Apigenin 93
Kaempferol 94
Genistein 94
Rutin 94
Naringenin 94
Naringin 94
Anthocyanidins 95
Lycopene 95
Emodin 95
EPIDEMIOLOGY AND PATHOPHYSIOLOGY OF PSORIASIS 95
CONCLUSION 96
REFERENCES 96

CHAPTER 7 LIPOSOME-BASED PHARMACOTHERAPY FOR THE MANAGEMENT OF PSORIASIS 103
Manish Kumar, Shubhi, Bhuwanendra Singh, Anuradha, Abhishek Tiwari and *Varsha Tiwari*
INTRODUCTION 104
TYPES OF PSORIASIS 105
Categorization According to Prevalence 106
Plaque Psoriasis 106
Guttate Psoriasis 106
Pustular Psoriasis 107
Erythrodermic Psoriasis 107
Categorization According to Anatomical Locations 107
Nail Psoriasis 107
Inverse Psoriasis 108
Palmoplantar 108
Scalp Psoriasis 108
PATHOGENESIS OF PSORIASIS 108
Histology, Keratinocytes, Proliferation and Abnormal Differentiation 109
Modifications in the Vascular System 109
Infiltration of Inflammatory Cells in Skin and Cytokine Production 110
Psoriasis Treatment Management 110
PHYSIOCHEMISTRY OF LIPOSOMES 111
Methodology for the Preparation of Liposomes 112
Thin Film Hydration Method 113
Ethanol Injection Method 114
Reverse Phase Evaporation Method 115
Preparation of Drug-Loaded Liposomes 115
Preparation of Drug-Loaded Liposomal Gels 115
Pharmacokinetics of Liposomes 115

PDI, Particle Size, and Zeta Potential ... 119
Entrapment Efficiency ... 119
Scanning Electron Microscopy ... 120
FTIR-ATR Interaction Study ... 120
Liposome Stability ... 120
A NEW MEDICATION DELIVERY SYSTEM FOR PSORIASIS TREATMENT ... 120
Possible Transporter for Topical Administration: Liposomes ... 121
Psoriasis Prodigy: Liposomal Drug Delivery Innovation ... 122
Future Potential Uses of Lipid-Based Liposomes in Pharmaceuticals ... 124
CONCLUSION ... 125
REFERENCES ... 126

CHAPTER 8 NIOSOMES-BASED PHARMACOTHERAPY FOR THE MANAGEMENT OF PSORIASIS ... 130
Vishnu Mittal, Anjali Sharma, Abhinav Singhal, Pushkar Upadhyay and *Devkant Sharma*
INTRODUCTION ... 131
PATHOPHYSIOLOGY OF PSORIASIS ... 132
Types of Psoriasis ... 133
Plaque Psoriasis ... 133
Flexural Psoriasis ... 133
Guttate Psoriasis ... 133
Nail Psoriasis ... 133
Psoriatic arthritis ... 134
Erythrodermic Psoriasis ... 134
Pustular Psoriasis ... 134
CONVENTIONAL TOPICAL TREATMENT ... 134
Coal Tar ... 135
Dithranol ... 135
Retinoids ... 135
Calcineurin Inhibitors ... 136
Salicylic Acid ... 136
Vitamin D Analogues ... 136
CHALLENGES IN TOPICAL FORMULATION ... 136
NANOTECHNOLOGY ... 137
CURRENT NANOTECHNOLOGY-BASED APPROACHES ... 137
NIOSOMES ... 138
Composition of Niosomes ... 139
Niosome in Psoriasis Management ... 140
EXPERT OPINION ... 143
FUTURE PERSPECTIVES AND CHALLENGES ... 144
CONCLUSION ... 144
REFERENCES ... 144

CHAPTER 9 NANOSTRUCTURED LIPID-BASED PHARMACOTHERAPY FOR THE MANAGEMENT OF PSORIASIS ... 151
Manish Kumar, Dev Kashyup, Nidhi Arora, Ajay Kumar and *Dileep Kumar*
INTRODUCTION ... 152
Types of Psoriasis ... 152
Pathogenesis of Psoriasis ... 153
Challenges in Psoriasis Treatment ... 154
Novel Carriers for Psoriasis Management and Pharmacotherapy ... 155

Lipid-BasedColloidalCarriers 156
Lipid-Vesicular Carriers 157
Microemulsions 160
Lipidic Particulate Carriers 160
CONCLUSION 166
REFERENCES 166

CHAPTER 10 NANOSPONGES AS DRUG CARRIERS FOR THE MANAGEMENT OF PSORIASIS 172
Rashmi Ghosh, Manish Kumar, Ankit Awasthi, Shubham Thakur and *Prabha Singh*
INTRODUCTION 172
Psoriasis: A Brief Overview 175
Psoriasis Pathophysiology 175
Current Challenges in Psoriasis Treatment 176
NANOSPONGES IN PSORIASIS MANAGEMENT 178
Advantages of Using Nanosponges for Psoriasis Management 179
Potential Applications and Benefits 179
METHOD OF PREPARATION OF NANOSPONGES 182
Solvent Method 182
Ultrasound-Assisted Method 182
Bubble Electrospinning 183
Synthesis by the Use of Microwave Radiation 183
Synthesis and Application of Beta-Cyclodextrin Nanosponges as Drug Transporters 184
Preparation of Naproxen Sodium Nanosponges by Solvent Diffusion Method 184
CHARACTERIZATION OF NANOSPONGES 185
Preparation of Drug-Loaded Nanosponges 185
Particle Size Determination 185
Pore Analysis of Nanosponges 186
Swelling and Water Uptake 186
In vitro Drug Release 186
Microscopic Study 187
CASE STUDIES 188
CONCLUSION AND FUTURE PROSPECTS 189
REFERENCES 190

CHAPTER 11 POLYMERIC NANOPARTICLES BASED PHARMACOTHERAPY FOR THE MANAGEMENT OF PSORIASIS 192
Prachi Saini, Kanika Mangla, Girish Kumar, Reshu Virmani and *Tarun Virmani*
INTRODUCTION 192
Conventional Treatment of Psoriasis 194
Advantages of Nanotechnology Over Conventional Treatment 195
Nanoparticles for the Pharmacotherapy of Psoriasis 195
Topical Applications of Polymers 196
Polymeric Nanocarriers Based Topical Delivery of Anti-Psoriatic Drugs 199
Advantages of Polymeric Nanoparticles 200
Marketed Formulation 202
CONCLUSION 203
REFERENCES 203

CHAPTER 12 METALLIC NANOPARTICLES-BASED PHARMACOTHERAPY FOR THE MANAGEMENT OF PSORIASIS 208

Anjali Mishra, Manisha Bhatia, Manish Kumar and *G.T. Kulkarni*
INTRODUCTION ... 208
Psoriasis: Overview and Burden ... 209
Current Psoriasis Treatments: Limitations and Challenges ... 209
Promise of Nanomedicine in Psoriasis Management ... 209
METALLIC NANOPARTICLES FOR PSORIASIS TREATMENT ... 210
Types of Metallic Nanoparticles for Psoriasis ... 210
Gold Nanoparticles (AuNPs) ... 210
Silver Nanoparticles (AgNPs) ... 211
Other Metallic Nanoparticles ... 212
Advantages of Metallic Nanoparticles for Psoriasis Therapy ... 214
MECHANISMS OF ACTION OF METALLIC NANOPARTICLES IN PSORIASIS ... 214
Interaction with Inflammatory Mediators ... 215
Modulation of Immune Response ... 216
Anti-proliferative Effects ... 216
Additional Mechanisms ... 216
Combination Effects ... 216
PRE-CLINICAL AND CLINICAL STUDIES ... 217
Pre-Clinical Studies ... 217
Exploring the Potential of Metallic NPs ... 220
Methods of Exploration ... 221
Benefits of Pre-clinical Studies ... 221
Clinical Trials: Current Status and Future Directions ... 221
Current Status ... 221
Challenges and Limitations ... 222
Future Directions ... 223
CHALLENGES AND FUTURE CONSIDERATIONS ... 223
Biocompatibility and Long-Term Toxicity ... 223
Scalability and Manufacturing Costs ... 224
Regulatory Landscape ... 224
Future Directions ... 224
CONCLUSION ... 224
REFERENCES ... 225

CHAPTER 13 ETHOSOMES – BASED PHARMACOTHERAPY FOR THE MANAGEMENT OF PSORIASIS ... 231
Ritika Saini, Jasmine Chaudhary, Akash Jain and *Bhawna Chopra*
INTRODUCTION ... 232
Mechanism of Action of Ethosomes ... 233
Ethosomal Delivery Systems ... 233
Classic Ethosomes ... 234
Transethosomes ... 234
Invasomes ... 234
Preparation of Ethosomes ... 235
Cold Method (Cold Approach) ... 235
Hot Method ... 235
Classic Method ... 235
Mechanical Dispersion Method ... 235
Vortex/sonication Method ... 236
Rotary Film Evaporation ... 236
Additives used in the Formulation of Ethosomes ... 236

Stability of Ethosomes ... 237
Characterisation of Ethosomes ... 237
Vesicle Shape ... 237
Particle size and Zeta Potential ... 237
Entrapment Efficiency ... 237
Entrapment Efficiency = De/Dt* 100 ... 237
Transition Temperature ... 238
Drug Content ... 238
Surface Tension Measurement ... 238
Skin Permeation Studies ... 238
EVALUATION OF ETHOSOMES [26, 27] ... 238
Filter Membrane-Vesicle Interaction Study ... 238
Skin Permeation ... 238
Stability Study ... 239
Vesicle-Skin Interaction Study ... 239
Drug Uptake Studies ... 239
HPLC Assay ... 239
APPLICATION OF ETHOSOMES ... 239
Therapeutic Applications ... 239
Cosmeceutical Applications ... 240
ETHOSOMES FOR THE MANAGEMENT OF PSORIASIS ... 240
PATHOPHYSIOLOGY AND PHARMACOTHERAPY OF PSORIASIS ... 241
ROLE OF MOLECULAR FACTORS RESPONSIBLE FOR PSORIASIS ... 241
T-Lymphocytes ... 241
NKT Cells ... 241
Other Leukocytes ... 241
Chemokines and Cytokines ... 242
Approaches for Treatment of Psoriasis ... 242
STRATEGIES BASED ON THE SOURCE ... 242
Phytotherapeutics ... 242
Aloe vera ... 242
Capsicum annum ... 242
Curcuma longa ... 242
Nigella sativa (Thymoquinone) ... 243
Punica granatum L ... 243
Wrightia tinctoria (Roxb) ... 243
Reseda luteola ... 244
Scutellaria lateriflora ... 244
Genistein ... 244
Synthetic Drugs ... 244
Infliximab, Adalimumab, and Etanercept (TNF-α Inhibitors) ... 244
Apilimod and Uztekinumab (IL-12/IL-23 p40 Inhibitors) ... 244
Alefacept (T-cell Inhibitors) ... 244
Adapalene, Tazarotene, Tazorac, and Zorac (Vitamin A Analogs) ... 245
Vitamin D3 Analogues ... 245
Strategies based on the mode of Administration ... 245
Topical Treatment ... 245
Systemic Treatment ... 245
Phototherapy Treatment ... 245
Limitations of the traditional (conventional) drug delivery method for psoriasis Treatment 246
NANOTECHNOLOGY-BASED DRUG DELIVERY SYSTEMS ... 246

Lipid-Based Nanocarriers [55] 246
Polymeric Nanoparticles 246
Solid Lipid Nanoparticles (SLN) 246
Nanostructured Lipid Carriers (NLC) 247
Liposomes 247
Nanoemulsions 247
Transferosomes 247
Niosomes 247
Ethosomes 247
POLYMER-BASED NANOCARRIER 248
Microspheres 248
Micelles 248
Nanocapsule 248
METALLIC NANOCARRIERS (MNPS) 248
Management of Psoriasis Using Ethosomes 249
Psoralen-Based Ethosomes 249
Acitretin-loaded nanoethosomal gel 249
Nigella sativa Linn loaded ethosomes and transethosomes gel 249
Curcumin and glycyrrhetinic acid-loaded ethosomes 250
Mangiferin-loaded glycethosomes 250
Diclofenac potassium-loaded ethosomes 250
Curcumin-Loaded Hyaluronan-Modified Ethosomes 250
Methotrexate-loaded ethosomal topical gel containing salicylic acid 251
Thymoquinone-loaded lipid vesicles 251
Anthralin-loaded ethosomes 251
Clobetasol-loaded ethosomal gel 251
Tacrolimus-loaded ethosomes 251
Resveratrol-loaded ethosomes 251
Advantages of Ethosomal Drug Delivery [81, 12] 252
CONCLUSION AND FUTURE PROSPECTS 252
REFERENCES 253

CHAPTER 14 TRANSFEROSOMES AS A DRUG CARRIER FOR THE MANAGEMENT OF PSORIASIS 259
Garima, Pankaj Popli, Kashish Wilson, Deepak Sharma and *Meenakshi Dhanawat*
INTRODUCTION 259
MECHANISM OF ACTION OF TRANSFEROSOMES 261
MATERIALS FOR TRANSFEROSOMES 262
METHODS OF PREPARATION OF TRANSFEROSOMES 263
Thin Film Hydration Technique/Rotary Evaporation-Sonication Method 263
Modified Handshaking Process 264
Vortexing-Sonication Method 264
Reverse-Phase Evaporation Method 264
Ethanol Injection Method 265
CHARACTERIZATION OF TRANSFEROSOMES 265
Vesicle Size Distribution, Zeta Potential, Morphology, Surface Charge, and its Density 265
Entrapment efficiency 265
Drug Content 265
Turbidity, Permeability Measurement, and Penetration Capacity 266
Sealing Effect 266
In-vitro Skin Permeation Studies 266

Stability of Formulation 266
APPLICATION OF TRANSFEROSOMES IN PSORIASIS 267
CONCLUSION 267
REFERENCES 268

CHAPTER 15 EMULSOMES-BASED PHARMACOTHERAPY FOR THE MANAGEMENT OF PSORIASIS 272
Vishnu Mittal, Devkant Sharma and *Anjali Sharma*
INTRODUCTION 273
Types of Psoriasis 273
Plaque Psoriasis 273
Pustular Psoriasis 274
Inverse Psoriasis 274
Guttate Psoriasis 274
Erythrodermic Psoriasis 274
Symptoms of Psoriasis 274
Causes of Psoriasis 275
CURRENT CHALLENGES IN PSORIASIS MANAGEMENT 275
Treatments for Mild Psoriasis 275
Treatments for Moderate-to-Severe 276
Phototherapy 276
Oral Systemic Treatments 276
Challenges in the Current Treatment of Psoriasis 277
Pathophysiology of Psoriasis 277
Epidemiology 278
Use of Nanomedicines in Psoriasis Medication Treatment 278
EMULSOMES: CONCEPT AND CHARACTERISTICS 279
Emulsomes 279
Structure of Emulsomes 281
Phospholipids 281
Cholesterol 281
Solid Lipids 281
Charge Inducers 282
Methods of Preparation of Emulsomes 282
Lipid Film Formation (Hand Shaking Method) 282
Reserve Phase Evaporation 282
High-Pressure Extrusion Technique 282
Sonication Method 283
Cast Film Method 283
Ethanol Injection 284
Detergent Removal Technique 284
Applications of Emulsomes in Various Medical Fields 284
Drug Targeting 284
Anti-Fungal Therapy 285
Anti-Inflammatory Action 285
Anti-Neoplastic Therapy 285
Anti-viral Therapy 285
Autoimmunity 286
Biotechnology 286
Dermal Therapy 286
MECHANISMS OF ACTION OF EMULSOMES IN PSORIASIS MANAGEMENT 286

EXPERT OPINION 287
FUTURE PERSPECTIVES AND CHALLENGES 287
CONCLUSION 288
REFERENCES 289

CHAPTER 16 NANOEMULSIONS-BASED SYSTEM FOR THE MANAGEMENT OF PSORIASIS 294
Minky Mukhija, Sonia Kamboj, Monga Jyoti, Prabhjot Singh Bajwa and *Bhuwan Chandra Joshi*
INTRODUCTION 295
Pathogenesis of Psoriasis 295
TREATMENT STRATEGIES FOR PSORIASIS 297
Modern System of Medicine (Allopathy) 297
Alternative Systems of Medicine (ASM) 299
PSORIASIS TREATMENT WITH NANOEMULSIONS: A NEW COLLOIDAL DRUG DELIVERY METHOD 301
METHODS OF PREPARATION OF NANOEMULSION 302
High Pressure Homogenization 302
Microfluidisation 302
Sonication 302
Phase Inversion Temperature Technique 302
Solvent Displacement Method 302
Spontaneous Emulsification 303
COMPONENTS IN THE TOPICAL NANOEMULSION FORMULATIONS FOR ANTIPSORIATIC DRUGS 303
Oil Phase 303
Surfactant 303
Co-surfactant 303
Other Excipients 303
CHARACTERIZATION OF NANOEMULSION 304
EXAMPLES OF ANTIPSORIATIC DRUGS LOADED INTO NANOEMULSION 305
CONCLUSION 312
REFERENCES 313

CHAPTER 17 FUTURE PROSPECTS OF NOVEL CARRIER-BASED PHARMACOTHERAPY 319
Esha Vatsa, Nidhi Chaudhary and *Shipra Gautam*
INTRODUCTION 319
Classification of Disease on the Basis of Severity of Psoriasis 321
Accustomed Combination of Drugs for the Treatment of Psoriasis 322
Phase 1 324
Phase 2 324
Phase 3 324
Lipid-based Nano carriers 325
Polymer-based nanocarriers 327
CONCLUDING REMARKS 328
REFERENCES 329

CHAPTER 18 PSORIASIS IN THE MODERN WORLD: LIFESTYLE, DIET AND HOLISTIC APPROACHES 331
Geeta Mahlawat, Tarun Virmani, Ashwani Sharma, Girish Kumar, Reshu Virmani, Prachi Saini and *Kanika Mangla*

INTRODUCTION 331
Overview of Psoriasis 331
Types of Psoriasis 332
Causes and Triggers 333
Mechanical Stress 333
Air Pollutants and Exposure to the Sun 333
Drugs 334
Vaccinations 334
Infections 335
Lifestyles 335
Imtrinsic Factors 335
Obesity 335
Diabetes Mellitus 335
Dyslipidemia 336
Hypertension 336
Mental Stress 336
Pathophysiology 337
MEDICAL APPROACHES 337
Conventional Treatments [Topical Treatments, Phototherapy, Systemic Medications and Biological] 337
Topical Therapy 339
Systemic Therapies and Phototherapy 340
Biological Therapy 340
Potential Side Effects 340
LIFESTYLE MODIFICATIONS 342
Stress Management 342
Importance of Regular Exercise 343
Adequate Sleep and its Impact on Psoriasis 344
DIETARY CONSIDERATION 345
Anti-Inflammatory Diet 345
Hydration and Supplements 347
Hydration 347
Supplements 348
HOLISTIC APPROACHES 349
Herbal Remedies 349
Aloevera 349
Artemisia Capillaris 349
Curcumin 349
Feverfew 350
Acupuncture and alternative therapies 350
Essential oil 350
MIND-BODY CONNECTION 351
Mental Health and Psoriasis 351
Mindfulness Techniques 352
Meditation 352
Cognitive Behavioral Therapy 352
Aromatherapy 353
PRACTICAL DAILY LIVING TIPS 353
Choosing Psoriasis-Friendly Products 353
Clothing and Sun Protection 353
CONCLUSION 354

REFERNCES 354
SUBJECT INDEX 362

FOREWORD

The treatment landscape for psoriasis has undergone significant evolution over the past few decades, yet the quest for more effective and targeted therapies remains ongoing. Traditional topical treatments, systemic medications, and biologics have provided relief to many patients, but challenges such as limited efficacy, side effects, and patient adherence persist. The advent of novel drug delivery systems offers a promising avenue to overcome these hurdles and enhance the therapeutic outcomes for psoriasis patients.

"Novel Carriers for Psoriasis Management and Pharmacotherapy" is a timely and essential contribution to the field of dermatological pharmacotherapy. This book meticulously explores the potential of innovative carriers in improving drug delivery, ensuring better penetration, controlled release, and reduced systemic exposure. It sheds light on the transformative impact that these advanced delivery systems can have on treating psoriasis.

The authors and contributors to this book are distinguished experts who bring a wealth of knowledge and experience in pharmaceutical sciences, dermatology, and drug delivery technologies. Their collective insights provide a thorough understanding of the current state and prospects of novel carriers in psoriasis management.

As we look forward to the next generation of psoriasis treatments, this book stands as a testament to the relentless pursuit of excellence in research and clinical practice. It is an invaluable resource for anyone dedicated to advancing the field of psoriasis therapy and improving patient care.

I commend the authors for their outstanding work and dedication in bringing this comprehensive and insightful book to fruition. It is a must-read for researchers, healthcare professionals, and students eager to stay abreast of the latest developments in psoriasis management and pharmacotherapy.

Ajmer Singh Grewal
Guru Gobind Singh College of Pharmacy
Yamuna Nagar, Haryana
India

PREFACE

Psoriasis is a chronic, inflammatory skin disease affecting millions of people worldwide. Despite numerous advancements in understanding its pathogenesis and the development of therapeutic strategies, psoriasis remains a challenging condition to manage effectively. The need for novel and efficient delivery systems to enhance the therapeutic efficacy of existing and new drugs is paramount.

"Novel Carriers for Psoriasis Management and Pharmacotherapy" aims to bridge the gap between current treatment limitations and emerging innovations in drug delivery systems. This book provides a comprehensive overview of the latest advancements in carrier technologies, including nanostructured lipid carriers, liposomes, ethosomes, and other cutting-edge formulations designed to optimize the delivery of therapeutic agents to psoriatic lesions.

Through detailed chapters contributed by leading researchers and experts in the field, readers will gain insights into the principles of carrier design, the mechanisms of action, and the therapeutic potential of various novel carriers. Additionally, the book discusses the challenges and future directions in the development and clinical application of these advanced delivery systems.

We hope this book serves as a valuable resource for researchers, clinicians, and students interested in dermatology, pharmaceutical sciences, and drug delivery technologies. By exploring the intersection of psoriasis management and innovative drug delivery systems, we aim to inspire further research and development, ultimately improving the quality of life for patients suffering from this debilitating condition.

Anjali Sharma
Department of Pharmaceutics
Guru Gobind Singh College of Pharmacy
Yamunanagar, Haryana, India

Prerna Sharma
Department of Pharmacognosy
Shri Krishna Ayush University
Kurukshetra, Haryana, India

Roy Rillera Marzo
Department of Public Health
Management and Science University, Malaysia

&

Ahmed A. Al Karmalawy
Department of Pharmaceutical Chemistry
College of Pharmacy, The University of Mashreq
Baghdad 10023, Iraq
Department of Pharmaceutical Chemistry
Faculty of Pharmacy, Horus University-Egypt
New Damietta 34518, Egypt

List of Contributors

Abhinav Singhal	Department of Pharmaceutics, Guru Gobind Singh College of Pharmacy, Yamunanagar 135001, Haryana, India
Abhishek Kumar	Pharmacy Academy, IFTM University, Lodhipur-Rajput, Delhi Road, Moradabad 244102, Uttar Pradesh, India
Abhishek Tiwari	Pharmacy Academy, IFTM University, Lodhipur-Rajput, Delhi Road, Moradabad 244102, Uttar Pradesh, India
Ajay Kumar	Department of Pharmacology, Sardar Patel College of Pharmacy, Gorakhpur, Uttar Pradesh 273013, India
Anjali Mishra	M.M. College of Pharmacy, Maharishi Markandeshwar (Deemed to be University), Mullana, Ambala 133207, Haryana, India
Anjali Sharma	Department of Pharmaceutics, Guru Gobind Singh College of Pharmacy, Yamunanagar 135001, Haryana, India
Ankit Awasthi	Department of Pharmaceutics, ISF College of Pharmacy, Moga 142001, Punjab, India
Anuradha	Bharat Institute of Technology, NH58 Bypass, Partapur, Meerut, Mahroli 250103, Uttar Pradesh, India
Ashwani Sharma	Department of Pharmaceutics, Delhi Institute of Pharmaceutical Sciences and Research, New Delhi, India
Bhawna Chopra	Department of Pharmaceutical Chemistry, Guru Gobind Singh College of Pharmacy, Yamuna Nagar 135001, Haryana, India
Bhuwan Chandra Joshi	Faculty of Pharmacy, Maharaja Agrasen Himalayan Garhwal University, Pauri Garhwal, Uttarakhand 246169, India
Bhuwanendra Singh	Department of Pharmacognosy, S.D College of Pharmacy & Vocational Studies, Muzaffarnagar 251001, Uttar Pradesh, India
Chander Parkash Dora	Department of Pharmaceutics, Chitkara College of Pharmacy, Chitkara University, Rajpura, Punjab, India
Deepak Sharma	Institute of Pharmacy, Assam Don Bosco University, Tapesi 782402, Assam, India
Dev Kashyup	Department of Pharmaceutics, ISF College of Pharmacy, Moga 142001, Punjab, India
Devkant Sharma	Department of Pharmaceutics, Ch. DeviLal College of Pharmacy, Jagadhai 135003, Haryana, India
Dileep Kumar	Department of Pharmaceutics, , ISF College of Pharmacy, Moga 142001, Punjab, India
Esha Vatsa	School of Pharmaceutical Sciences, Jigyasa University (Formerly Himgiri Zee University), Dehradun, Uttarakhand, India
Kulkarni G.T.	Faculty of Pharmacy, DIT University, Dehradun, Uttarakhand, India
Garima	Department of Pharmaceutics, Chitkara College of Pharmacy, Chitkara University, Rajpura, Punjab, Indiaii

Geeta Mahlawat	School of Pharmaceutical Sciences, MVN University, Palwal, Haryana, India
Girish Kumar	Amity Institute of Pharmacy, Amity University, Greater Noida, Uttar Pradesh, India
Himani Bajaj	Adarsh Vijendra Institute of Pharmaceutical Sciences, Shobhit University, Gangoh, Saharanpur, India
Kanika Mangla	School of Pharmaceutical Sciences, MVN University, Palwal, Haryana, India
Kashish Wilson	Department of Pharmaceutics, M. M. College of Pharmacy, Maharishi Markandeshwar (Deemed to be University), Ambala, Haryana, India
Manish Kumar	Department of Pharmaceutics, ISF College of Pharmacy, Moga 142001, Punjab, India
Manisha Bhatia	M.M. College of Pharmacy, Maharishi Markandeshwar (Deemed to be University), Mullana, Ambala 133207, Haryana, India
Mayank Yadav	Adarsh Vijendra Institute of Pharmaceutical Sciences, Shobhit University, Gangoh, Saharanpur, India
Meenakshi Dhanawat	Amity Institute of Pharmacy, Amity University Haryana, Amity Education Valley, Panchgaon, Manesar, Gurugram 122413, Haryana, India
Minky Mukhija	Department of Pharmacognosy, Ch. Devi Lal College of Pharmacy, Jagadhri, Haryana, India
Monga Jyoti	Department of Pharmaceutical Chemistry, Ch. Devi Lal College of Pharmacy, Jagadhri, Haryana, India
Muskan Srivastava	Department of Pharmacology, Chandigarh College of Pharmacy, Landran, Mohali 140307, India
Nidhi Arora	Department of Pharmacy, Chandigarh Pharmacy College, Chandigarh Group of Colleges, Jhanjeri 140307, Punjab, India
Nidhi Chaudhary	School of Pharmaceutical Sciences, Jigyasa University (Formerly Himgiri Zee University), Dehradun, Uttarakhand, India
Pankaj Popli	Department of Pharmaceutics, Chitkara College of Pharmacy, Chitkara University, Rajpura, Punjab, India
Prachi Saini	School of Pharmaceutical Sciences, MVN University, Palwal, Haryana, India
Prabha Singh	Department of Pharmaceutics, Sanjay College of Pharmacy, Mathura-Delhi Road, Mathura 281406, Uttar Pradesh, India
Prabhjot Singh Bajwa	Department of Pharmaceutics, Ch. Devi Lal College of Pharmacy, Jagadhri, Haryana, India
Priyanka Kriplani	Department of Pharmaceutics, Guru Gobind Singh College of Pharmacy, Yamuna Nagar 135001, Haryana, India
Pushkar Upadhyay	Department of Pharmaceutics, Guru Gobind Singh College of Pharmacy, Yamunanagar 135001, Haryana, India
Rama Devi	Department of Pharmacology, Chitkara College of Pharmacy, Chitkara University, Rajpura 140401, Punjab, India
Rashmi Ghosh	Department of Pharmaceutics, ISF College of Pharmacy, Moga 142001, Punjab, India

Rajat Goyal	MM College of Pharmacy, Maharishi Markandeshwar (Deemed to be University), Mullana, Ambala 133207, India
Reshu Virmani	School of Pharmaceutical Sciences, MVN University, Palwal, Haryana, India
Sapna Rani	Department of Pharmacology, Maharishi Markandeshwar College of Pharmacy, Maharishi Markandeshwar (Deemed to be University), Mullana, Ambala 133207, Haryana, India
Sarita Sharma	Department of Pharmacology, Maharishi Markandeshwar College of Pharmacy, Maharishi Markandeshwar (Deemed to be University), Mullana, Ambala 133207, Haryana, India
Seema B. Chauhan	Adarsh Vijendra Institute of Pharmaceutical Sciences, Shobhit University, Gangoh, Saharanpur, India
Shalu Verma	Uttaranchal Institute of Pharmaceutical Sciences, Uttaranchal University, Dehradun 248001, Uttarakhand, India
Shipra Gautam	Department of Pharmacy, Himachal institute of Pharmacy, Paonta sahib, Himachal Pradesh, India
Shubhi	Department of Quality Assurance, ISF College of Pharmacy, Moga 142001, Punjab, India
Shubham Thakur	Department of Pharmaceutics, ISF College of Pharmacy, Moga 142001, Punjab, India
Simran Saini	Department of Pharmacology, Maharishi Markandeshwar College of Pharmacy, Mullana, Ambala 133207, Haryana, India
Sonia Kamboj	Department of Pharmacognosy, Ch. Devi Lal College of Pharmacy, Jagadhri, Haryana, India
Tanvi	MM College of Pharmacy, Maharishi Markandeshwar (Deemed to be University), Mullana, Ambala 133207, India
Sumeet Gupta	Department of Pharmacology, M. M. College of Pharmacy, Maharishi Markandeshwar (Deemed to be University), Mullana, Ambala 133207, Haryana, India
Tarun Virmani	Amity Institute of Pharmacy, Amity University, Greater Noida Campus, Uttar Pradesh, India
Varsha Tiwari	Pharmacy Academy, IFTM University, Lodhipur-Rajput, Delhi Road, Moradabad 244102, Uttar Pradesh, India
Vishnu Mittal	Adesh Institute of Pharmacy and Biomedical Sciences, Adesh University, Bathinda 151101, Punjab, India

CHAPTER 1

Understanding Psoriasis: A Chronic Skin Condition

Muskan Srivastava[1] and **Deepika Sharma**[1,*]

[1] *Department of Pharmacology, Chandigarh College of Pharmacy, Landran, Mohali 140307, India*

Abstract: The ancestral form of immune-mediated ailments, psoriasis, can affect the joints, the skin, or both. An interdisciplinary team of professionals with diverse expertise is often necessary to effectively treat the disease. Several challenges are associated with psoriasis, including its high frequency, chronicity, disability, and the coexisting medical disorders that often accompany it. Understanding the importance of immune regulation in psoriasis, along with the interactions between the innate and adaptive branches of the immune system, has been instrumental in controlling the progression of this multifaceted disease, which affects individuals in ways that go beyond skin involvement. Psoriasis is a widespread skin condition that causes both emotional and physical suffering. Like other dermatoses, visible disfigurement may cause an increasingly undesirable response in others, which can account for a large portion of the disease's noticeable psychological stress. The present day disease demand has been exacerbated by several coexisting issues and including the syndrome of metabolism and cardiovascular conditions brought on by the syndrome. Certain environmental risk factors, including trauma (*e.g.*, the Koebner phenomenon), infection, and medication, have been linked to the development of this inflammatory skin disorder. Psoriasis of the plaque type is distinguished by itchy plaques covered with silvery scales. Both adaptive and innate immune responses can contribute to psoriatic inflammation; however, innate immune responses appear to be more prevalent in psoriasis, regardless of plaque type. Comorbid diseases comprise psoriatic arthritis, the metabolic syndrome or its components, cardiovascular issues, and a host of additional conditions, including depression and anxiety, nonalcoholic fatty liver, Crohn's disease, and cancer.

Keywords: Inflammatory skin disease, IL-17 inhibitors, IL-23 inhibitors, Koebner phenomenon, Psoriasis, Psoriatic arthritis, Skin lesions, TNF-inhibitors.

* **Corresponding author Deepika Sharma:** Department of Pharmacology, Chandigarh College of Pharmacy, Landran, Mohali 140307, India; E-mail: Deepika.sharma.nahan@gmail.com

Anjali Sharma, Prerna Sharma, Roy Rillera Marzo & Ahmed A. Al Karmalawy (Eds.)

INTRODUCTION

Background

Since the inception of human existence, psoriasis has been a prevalent condition. These days, it has become recognized as a distinct skin condition influenced by both immunological and environmental factors. Even considering its prevalence, chronicity, and outward manifestations, historical accounts of psoriasis in the manuscripts of ancient physicians are scarce. As dermatologists began to appear around the latter part of the century, the field of skin care developed into a distinct field. Psoriasis became acknowledged as a disease over time. Many intellectuals across different civilizations — both well-known and lesser-known — have documented the existence of psoriasis-like skin sores. Hippocrates (460–377 BCE) was an Ancient Greek physician who used the terms "psora" (itchiness) and "lopoi" (scaly skin) to refer to inflammatory skin diseases, such as psoriasis. A landed gentry by the name of Cornelius Celsus (25 BCE–50 CE) described a skin ailment that afflicted both the skin and the nails generations afterward during the Roman Empire. During antiquity and the medieval era, there was a limited written record of skin diseases, which sometimes led to misconceptions in discourse. This tendency endured for centuries, most notably in the Middle Ages, when psoriasis sufferers and leprosy sufferers were subject to similar social exclusion. This convergence underscores the persistent challenge of accurately understanding and treating cutaneous disorders, shedding light on the significant advances in contemporary dermatology that have enabled a deeper differentiation and classification of these conditions [1]. The shadowy past illuminates today's specialist knowledge, yet it took a while for various skin illnesses to be understood rather than mysterious. English physician Robert Willan, who greatly advanced the science of dermatology in the late nineteenth century, described psoriasis and other skin disorders in great detail, providing doctors with clear diagnostic standards. His groundbreaking study methodically classified distinct forms of psoriasis, including guttate, which involves tiny patches; scalp-centric; and palm, which affects the hands. When Dr. Willan referred to psoriasis as "lepra vulgaris," he was reflecting on the inadequate understanding of the condition at the time. His groundbreaking work laid down the foundation for contemporary dermatology and profoundly influenced our understanding of skin ailments. His thorough documentation remains a valuable source of knowledge for medical experts. Throughout the course of the century, medical professionals and scholars amassed a vast amount of knowledge about psoriasis, including detailed descriptions of its various forms. John M. Moll and Verna Wright made a significant discovery in 1973 when they published research demonstrating that psoriasis or psoriatic arthritis is a distinct condition, setting it apart from rheumatoid arthritis. Scientists now acknowledge that psoriasis is more than just a skin ailment; it is an autoimmune disease that endures and causes inflammation throughout the whole organism. Modern therapeutic strategies have been significantly influenced by this evolving understanding, particularly through the application of biologics that target specific components of the immune system [2].

Epidemiology

Millions of individuals worldwide suffer from a persistent inflammatory skin condition each year. The red, itchy, scaly lesions of this autoimmune illness affect approximately 3.2% of adults and 0.13% of children in the United States alone. According to certain demographic estimates, there are approximately 80 new cases per 100,000 people each year. Location has a significant effect on prevalence, with estimates indicating rates as low as 0.5% in some parts of Asia and as high as 8% in Norway. The most intriguing aspect is that psoriasis affects men and women with nearly equal incidence across a wide range of populations. Although the illness may develop at any stage of life, there is a unique doubling chance of developing it initially in the years 18 to 39 and again in the years 50 to 69. Psoriasis presents enduring challenges regardless of when it manifests; nevertheless, new insights and innovative therapies offer renewed hope. The stage in life at which psoriasis first appears can vary depending on whether inherited or environmental factors cause it. For instance, having the human leukocyte antigen (HLA)-C*06 variants, a genetic element that influences one's propensity, has been linked to an earlier onset of psoriasis. Especially those who are prone, external cues such as stress or recent trauma may accelerate their symptoms. The complex interplay of biological and lifestyle elements introduces heterogeneity into the typical course of disease onset and progression across [3].

There were no restrictions on the area, ethnicity, or period that were taken into account. Seventy-six suitable empirical findings have been incorporated in the aforementioned systematic review after fulfilling all eligibility requirements. Estimates for the prevalence of psoriasis in individuals ranged from 0.5% to 11.4%, although estimates for children varied from 0% to 1.3%. A few prevalent conditions that are known to worsen with age are psoriasis. There is little information available concerning the epidemiology of psoriasis. The degree of data now obtainable is not accessible to everyone due to its origins in only twenty countries, most of which belong to wealthy portions of the world. There are geographical imperfections, especially about economically disadvantaged regions where there has not been much research into epidemiology [4].

CLINICAL TYPES OF PSORIASIS

Plaque Psoriasis

Approximately 80% to 90% of cases of psoriasis include plaque psoriasis. Sharply identified, erythematous, flaky regions are known as plaques in psoriasis. Plaque psoriasis frequently affects the hair follicles, trunk, gluteal fold, and extensor surfaces, including the knees and elbows. Plaque psoriasis may appear as little erythematous as well as scaly papules or as massive, thick plaque lesions. The impacted regions are typically bilaterally symmetrical and have distinct borders. In the Koebner phenomenon, trauma, such as scratches, wounds, or pressure, can result in the development of new psoriasis lesions. Whenever the coating of scale is eliminated from the plaque, this causes pinpoint bleeding, which results in the Auspitz sign. In moderately to severely affected cases, or during flare-ups, they may also experience intense itching. Plaques are capable of taking on a wide range of shapes, especially when they extend to the edge:

- Psoriasis gyrata, or arcing as well as straightening lines.
- Annular psoriasis: As a result of central clearance, the lesions take the form of an irregular ring.
- Psoriasis folliculitis: tiny scaly papules near the apertures of hair follicles [5].

Lesions attributed to plaque psoriasis can be observed on the extensor surfaces of the scalp, the buttocks, trunk, arms, and legs. Though they are not common in body folds that include the perineal, inframammary, axillary, inguinal, or intergluteal areas, these forms of psoriasis are nonetheless scarier than plaques. Thermal harm or infection may be the root cause of inflammation [6].

Guttate Psoriasis

The acronym guttate psoriasis, originating from the Greek word gutta, referring to a droplet, describes the appearance of many tiny psoriasis lesions which range in dimension from 2 to 10 mm. These typically spread in a converging pattern, although guttate lesions may also affect the head and limbs. Traditionally, guttate psoriasis appears soon after an acute pharyngeal or tonsillar infection caused by group B hemolytic streptococcal infection. It may be the first episode of psoriasis in children or, in rare cases, adults. The quantity of lesions could range from five to ten to more than one hundred. Perhaps more than 2% of all instances of psoriasis are guttate. Short-term manifestations of guttate psoriasis in children typically resolve on their own; in adulthood, guttate flare-ups can exacerbate persistent plaque disease, making it more difficult to treat. 33% of the people with acute guttate psoriasis went on to acquire chronic plaque illness, despite the fact that little research has assessed the prognosis for the future of children exhibiting this condition.

Flexural (Inverse) Psoriasis

Inverse psoriasis, frequently designated as flexural psoriasis, strikes intertriginous areas and is distinguished by erythematous plaques and patches of skin that are gradually disintegrating [7]. Psoriasis afflicts the flexures, primarily the axillary, perineal, and inframammary areas; therefore, it differs anatomically from the normal plaques on the rest of the body. Lacking scales, flexural patches appear as red, glossy, well-defined plaques that can be routinely misdiagnosed as intertrigo, candidal, or dermatophyte infections.

Erythroderma

Erythroderma is a devastating and possibly lethal form of psoriasis; nevertheless, it frequently occurs in 2–3% of adults who suffer from the skin condition. It typically presents as combined erythema, rashes, or peeling covering more than 75% of the body's total surface area. This level of skin commitment can be associated with skin pain, pruritus, high-output heart failure, hypothermia, and an imbalance in electrolyte levels. Having erythrodermic psoriasis, over ninety per cent of the body's surface is red and irritated. This constitutes an extremely serious illness. Any form of psoriasis may trigger erythroderma, which also demands emergency therapy [8].

Generalized Pustular Psoriasis

Clean pustules that coalesce in multitude are the characteristic features of generalized pustular psoriasis. Psoriasis causing acne may be isolated or widespread. Two unique local phenotypes, acrodermatitis continua of Hallopeau and psoriasis pustulosa palmoplantaris (PPP), have been recently elucidated. Both of them have consequences on the hands and feet; PPP has a limited impact on the hands and soles, though ACS is broader in reach and affects the nail device in addition to the tips of both fingers and toes. Subcorneal pustules and diffuse inflammation characterized the grave as well as rapidly developing manifestations of generalized pustular psoriasis, which is frequently accompanied by systemic symptoms [9].

Palmoplantar Pustulosis

The next subgroup, palmoplantar pustulosis, tends to appear as sterile, clean yellow pustules on the hands and soles that gradually resolve down to reddish-brownish macules over a period of weeks. Women who smoke cigarettes and are between the ages of thirty and sixty are more likely to develop palmoplantar pustulosis; 20% of patients additionally suffer from secondary chronic plaque psoriasis. Hallopeau is a rare disorder that causes crodermatitis, characterized by pustules around the distal portions of the fingers and, rarely, the toes, which can cause the nail plate to drop. Approximately 40% of these patients have underlying persistent plaque psoriasis [10].

Psoriatic Nail Condition

When compared to nails, toenails frequently sustain far less recurrent damage. One of the most widely recognized indications of nail plate irregularities is the presence of damaged nail growth in the vicinity of the nail matrix. Whenever the nail splits from its surrounding tissue, particularly at its distal or lateral edges, it is referred to as onycholysis. Orange-yellow patches" are found beneath the nail plate. Moreover, the nail plate may become larger, dystrophic, and discolored. Subungual hyperkeratosis is a collection of keratinous, yellow material beneath the nail plate. Different types and body site manifestations of psoriasis are shown in Fig. (**1**).

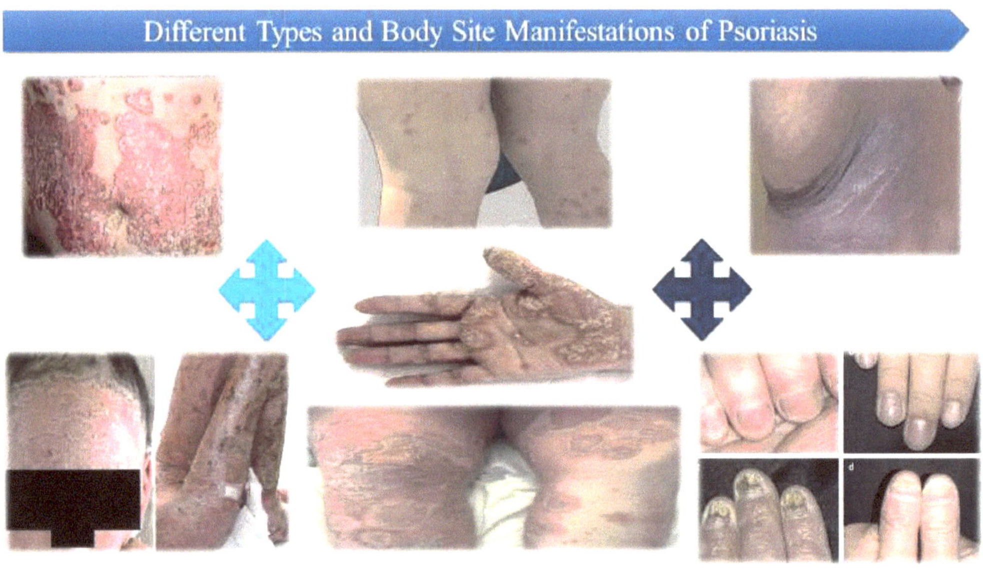

Fig. (1). Different types and body site manifestations of psoriasis.

Triggers

Expression about psoriasis is contingent on gene-environment interaction because the disorder fails to get better even though there is an ecological trigger, such as stress, alcohol consumption, smoking, exposure to medications (such as nonsteroidal anti-inflammatory agents and lithium antimalarial), natural light, or tension illnesses (particularly streptococcal infections). Obtaining or maintaining too much weight poses a problem and can have a joint effect on managing psoriasis.

Pathophysiology

T cell activation, as well as migration into the epidermal layer, are the primary pathophysiological mechanisms of the disorder. The following leads to the production of cytokines, particularly the production of tumor necrosis factor-alpha, or TNF-alpha, that triggers inflammation and speeds up the rapid growth of skin cells. Psoriasis has an intricate pathophysiology that is of unknown origin. The most significant assumption regarding the onset of psoriasis is that excessive stimulation of specific components of the adaptive immune system occurs. During the early stages of psoriasis pathogenesis, a variety of cell types, including macrophages, keratinocytes, and naturally occurring killer T cells, such as plasmacytoid dendritic cells, release cytokines that may motivate myeloid dendritic cells. Despite psoriasis being a condition mediated by the immune system with a hereditary predisposition, no particular immunogenic factor has been identified as its etiology. The identification of T lymphocytes, dendritic cells, and cytokines in psoriatic lesions has sparked an era of biologic medications. Skin and immune cells play a part in the pathological process of psoriasis. Aggressive skin with surface scales, thickening of the skin's epidermis (acanthosis; diminished or missing granular layer), and parakeratosis—caused by aberrant maturation and hyperproliferation of the keratinocytes that line the epidermis in the SC—are characteristic signs of psoriasis [11].

Multiple studies in academia claim that nitric oxide (NO), which keratinocytes produce in large amounts, is a key catalyst of cell differentiation and an inhibitor of cell proliferation *in vitro*. The high-output NO synthesis within psoriasis lesions is demonstrated by the expression of mRNA, proteins, and inducible NO synthase (iNOS); however, the pronounced increase in proliferation of psoriatic keratinocytes may suggest that iNOS activity is insufficient to supply antiproliferative NO concentrations. Thus, the impairment of corneocyte differentiation, which includes an impaired generation with secretion of lamellar body components and an impaired processing of lamellar lipid contents into lamellar bilayers, reduces the function of the psoriatic skin barrier [12].

Furthermore, skin barrier difficulties such as psoriasis can be triggered by aberrant differentiation and excessive growth of corneocytes, a deficiency of normal moisturizing factors (NMFs), an imbalance in skin lipids (a boost in cholesterol accompanied by decreased ceramide levels), and dry, sensitive skin. In addition, the immune system, along with its intricate connections between leukocytes and cytokines, was discussed in relation to the pathophysiology of disease [13]. Psoriatic lesions exhibit high infiltration of immune cells, particularly CD3+ T cells and CD11c+ dendritic cells. These cells secrete proinflammatory cytokines, including tumor necrosis factor-alpha (TNF-α), interferon-γ (IFN-γ), interleukin-17 (IL-17), IL-20, IL-22, IL-23, IL-12, and IL-1β. Because they cause keratinocytes to hyperproliferate, these messenger molecules have been linked to the genesis of psoriasis. Additionally, it suggests that IFN-γ and IL-15 enhance the ability of keratinocytes to resist apoptosis [14].

Moreover, it has been recommended that growth factors and genetic factors, among which are mutations in transforming growth factor (TGF)-β, toll-like receptor (TLR)-2, signaling molecules, and activators of transcription (STAT-3), coiled-coil alpha-helical rod protein 1 (CCHCR1), steroidogenic acute regulatory protein (StAR), and vitamin D receptor (VDR), are the primary factors influencing the exacerbation of psoriasis. The fundamental transcription factor in psoriasis, nuclear factor kappa B (NF-κB), is an essential regulatory component in several autoimmune and inflammation-related processes, including cellular proliferation, particularly differentiation, and cell death. It has been demonstrated that psoriatic lesions undergo differentiation and hyperproliferation, in contrast to normal cells, due to a discrepancy in the proapoptotic and antiapoptotic effects of NF-κB proteins [15].

Diagnosis

This corresponds to how psoriasis is typically diagnosed by examining the skin's appearance. There are no specific blood tests or diagnostic techniques for psoriasis. In certain cases, a biopsy of the skin or skin infusion may be necessary in addition to other diagnostic tests to confirm the diagnosis. Through the epidermis, if the biopsy is positive for chronic psoriasis, clubbed rete pegs should be seen. Pink blood is seen when coverings are cleaned, which is another sign of psoriasis. The outermost layer is underlying. A medical examination can quickly recognize psoriasis. In general, no testing is carried out. Recognition of psoriasis is crucial, but additional disorders remain ignored. Issues include screening for blood, urine, and imaging [16].

These undergo inquiry frequently. On rare occasions, a biopsy might be required. It needed to be differentiated from fungal diseases. Total levels, ESSR, RA factor, ASO titers, serum uric acid levels, T-cells, and other characteristics are measured in blood tests. An increase in T-cells and leukocytosis is often noticed. The microscopic investigation. The abscess or discharge exclusively depicts lymphocytes. The equipment's installation. Diagnostic procedures, including bone scans and X-rays, can help determine the source of joint discomfort. Examine the historical records of infections caused by streptococci. It will be critical to pay close attention and avoid being far away from stressors. It serves to ascertain the extent of metabolic disruption in erythrodermic illnesses using the appropriate assays [17, 18].

Radiography should be used when appropriate for determining the degree and extent of joint damage. Accelerated epidermal cell division may trigger high nucleic acid turnover, which in turn can lead to excessive blood uric acid levels. Often asymptomatic, this illness barely necessitates medical attention. Assessing the degree of emotional and social impairment resulting from the abnormality is crucial. For a few individuals, treatment for psychological anguish is additionally required [19].

Psoriasis Treatment

The improvement of joint, skin, and nail lesions alongside an increase in quality of life are the primary objectives of treatment. Internally delivered pills or injectables are administered to treat psoriasis that is not susceptible to topical treatments or phototherapy. We refer to this as systemic treatment.

Methotrexate

A well-liked and efficacious anti-metabolite for the treatment of severe psoriasis. Usually, a weekly or, on occasion, fortnightly pulse dose of 15 mg is administered. It is also conceivable to administer an equivalent dosage intramuscularly or intravenously. Methotrexate is also effective for treating psoriatic arthritis. Before stopping the medication, ongoing therapy may be started on a low dose for a while. Methotrexate is a medication that is exceptionally well tolerated. Standard adverse reactions include nausea, anorexia, and pain in the epigastric area [20].

Cyclosporine

Cyclosporine is a cyclic polypeptide molecule widely used in organ transplantation as an immunosuppressive therapy. It restricts T-cells, which is how it works in psoriasis. Only those with severe psoriasis should use cyclosporine. Two split doses of 3–5 mg/kg are the conventional oral dosage. Hypertension and nephrotoxicity are the main adverse effects. The risk of cancer may rise as a result. This medical care, like oral retinoid, should only be used by dermatologists with experience in treating renal failure, hypertension, prior or current cancers, pregnancy, lactation, and concurrent therapy using immunosuppressive as well as nephrotoxic agents.

Angiotensin Converting Enzyme Inhibitors (ACEI)

ACEIs are frequently recommended as a first-choice therapy for diabetic patients and are used intensively to manage hypertension. Over five decades ago, ACEI had been associated with psoriasis in patients. However, as of this point, no informal relationship has been investigated. Based on recent studies, there may be a hereditary component to psoriasis that is associated with ACEI-induced [21].

Phototherapy

On a local level, ultraviolet (UV) radiation suppresses the immune system. It directly impacts Langerhans' cells, decreases angiogenesis and epidermal hyperproliferation, and suppresses cutaneous T cells selectively mediated apoptosis.109A number of phototherapy modalities consist of targeted phototherapy, broadband (280–320 nm) and narrowband (311–313 nm) UVB radiation, as well as oral psoralen UVA (photo chemotherapy), which is currently less common in some regions of globally due to the significant cumulative hazards associated with skin cancer [22].

Natural sources for treating psoriasis: Several possible natural sources, along with their distinct phytoconstituents, have been examined for their potential use in managing psoriasis.

CONCLUSION

Psoriasis is a chronic skin condition characterized by an overactive immune system, leading to the rapid proliferation of skin cells. This leads to the formation of scales, inflammation, and red patches on the skin. Despite its complex nature and the various symptoms and triggers it presents, advancements in medical research have greatly enhanced our understanding and management of this disease. Treatment options for psoriasis include topical creams, light therapy, systemic medications, and biologic drugs, all of which provide relief and improve the quality of life for patients. Effectively managing psoriasis requires a comprehensive approach that encompasses lifestyle modifications, stress management, and ongoing medical treatment. With continued research and personalized treatment plans, we can look forward to even better outcomes in the future, aiming to reduce the burden of psoriasis and improve the overall well-being of those affected.

REFERENCES

[1] Brajac I, Gruber F. History of Psoriasis. 2012 Mar 16. [http://dx.doi.org/10.5772/27640]

[2] Farber EM, Nall L. The natural history of psoriasis in 5,600 patients. Dermatology 1974; 148(1): 1-18.

[http://dx.doi.org/10.1159/000251595] [PMID: 4831963]

[3] Armstrong AW, Read C. Pathophysiology, clinical presentation, and treatment of psoriasis. JAMA 2020; 323(19): 1945-60. Available from: https://jamanetwork.com/journals/jama/article-abstract/2766169
[http://dx.doi.org/10.1001/jama.2020.4006] [PMID: 32427307]

[4] Michalek IM, Loring B, John SM. A systematic review of worldwide epidemiology of psoriasis. J Eur Acad Dermatol Venereol 2017; 31(2): 205-12.
[http://dx.doi.org/10.1111/jdv.13854] [PMID: 27573025]

[5] Langley RGB, Krueger GG, Griffiths CEM. Psoriasis: epidemiology, clinical features, and quality of life. Ann Rheum Dis 2005; 64(Suppl 2) (Suppl. 2): ii18-23. Available from: https://ard.bmj.com/content/64/suppl_2/ii18
[http://dx.doi.org/10.1136/ard.2004.033217] [PMID: 15708928]

[6] Weigle N, McBane S. Psoriasis. Am Fam Physician 2013; 87(9): 626-33.
[PMID: 23668525]

[7] Rendon A, Schäkel K. Psoriasis pathogenesis and treatment. Int J Mol Sci 2019; 20(6): 1475.
[http://dx.doi.org/10.3390/ijms20061475] [PMID: 30909615]

[8] Griffiths CEM, Armstrong AW, Gudjonsson JE, Barker JNWN. Psoriasis. Lancet 2021; 397(10281): 1301-15.
[http://dx.doi.org/10.1016/S0140-6736(20)32549-6] [PMID: 33812489]

[9] Herman A, Herman A. Topically used herbal products for the treatment of psoriasis – Mechanism of action, drug delivery, clinical studies. Planta Med 2016; 82(17): 1447-55.
[http://dx.doi.org/10.1055/s-0042-115177] [PMID: 27574899]

[10] Chalakanti S, Malothu N. Development and *in vitro* evaluation of solid lipid nano particles loaded topical gel containing combination of drugs used in the better therapy of psoriasis. Int J Life Sci Pharma Res 2022.

[11] Handa S, Mahajan R. Pathophysiology of psoriasis. Indian J Dermatol Venereol Leprol 2013; 79(7) (Suppl. 7): 1.
[http://dx.doi.org/10.4103/0378-6323.115505] [PMID: 23974689]

[12] Singh KK, Tripathy S. Natural treatment alternative for psoriasis: A review on herbal resources. Journal of Applied Pharmaceutical Science. 2014 Nov 27;4(11):114-21.
[http://dx.doi.org/10.1002/ptr.6973] [PMID: 33277958]

[13] De Oliveira M de FSP, Rocha B de O, Duarte GV. Psoriasis: classical and emerging comorbidities. Anais Brasileiros de Dermatologia [Internet]. 2015; 90(1): 9–20. Available from: https://www.ncbi.nlm.nih.gov/pmc/articles/PMC4323693/
[http://dx.doi.org/10.1590/abd1806-4841.20153038] [PMID: 25672294]

[14] Dabholkar N, Rapalli VK, Singhvi G. Potential herbal constituents for psoriasis treatment as protective and effective therapy. Phytother Res 2021; 35(5): 2429-44.
[http://dx.doi.org/10.1002/ptr.6973] [PMID: 33277958]

[15] Kamiya K, Kishimoto M, Sugai J, Komine M, Ohtsuki M. Risk Factors for the Development of Psoriasis. Int J Mol Sci 2019; 20(18): 4347.
[http://dx.doi.org/10.3390/ijms20184347] [PMID: 31491865]

[16] Tripathi P, Bhardwaj P. Psoriasis: An autoimmune disorder. J Drug Deliv Ther 2020; 10(5): 316-24.
[http://dx.doi.org/10.22270/jddt.v10i5.4327]

[17] Russomando M. Guttate psoriasis post-hand, foot and mouth disease. Eur. J. Pediat. Dermatol. [Internet]. 2019 Mar. 12 [cited 2024 Aug.23]; 29(1): 60. Available from: https://ejpd.com/index.php/journal/article/view/1954

[18] Syed ZU, Khachemoune A. Inverse psoriasis. Am J Clin Dermatol 2011; 12(2): 143-6.

[http://dx.doi.org/10.2165/11532060-000000000-00000] [PMID: 21184623]

[19] Teran CG, Teran-Escalera CN, Balderrama C. A severe case of erythrodermic psoriasis associated with advanced nail and joint manifestations: a case report. J Med Case Reports 2010; 4(1): 179. [http://dx.doi.org/10.1186/1752-1947-4-179] [PMID: 20550707]

[20] Sussman M, Napodano A, Huang S, Are A, Hsu S, Motaparthi K. Pustular psoriasis and acute generalized exanthematous pustulosis. Medicina (Kaunas) 2021; 57(10): 1004. [http://dx.doi.org/10.3390/medicina57101004] [PMID: 34684041]

[21] Ji C, Wang H, Bao C, *et al.* Challenge of nail psoriasis: An update review. Clin Rev Allergy Immunol 2021; 61(3): 377-402. [http://dx.doi.org/10.1007/s12016-021-08896-9] [PMID: 34478047]

[22] Michelucci A, Manzo Margiotta F, Panduri S, *et al.* A real-life experience as a proof of Guselkumab effectiveness and safety in patients with moderate to severe psoriasis. Dermatol Ther 2022; 35(4): e15339. [http://dx.doi.org/10.1111/dth.15339] [PMID: 35088508]

CHAPTER 2

Pathophysiology and Molecular Basis of Psoriasis

Kashish Wilson[1], **Tanvi**[2], **Rajat Goyal**[2], **Sumeet Gupta**[3,*], **Chander Parkash Dora**[4] and **Garima**[4]

[1] *Department of Pharmaceutics, M. M. College of Pharmacy, Maharishi Markandeshwar (Deemed to be University), Mullana, Ambala 133207, Haryana, India*

[2] *MM College of Pharmacy, Maharishi Markandeshwar (Deemed to be University), Mullana, Ambala 133207, India*

[3] *Department of Pharmacology, M. M. College of Pharmacy, Maharishi Markandeshwar (Deemed to be University), Mullana, Ambala 133207, Haryana, India*

[4] *Department of Pharmaceutics, Chitkara College of Pharmacy, Chitkara University, Rajpura, Punjab, India*

Abstract: Psoriasis, a papulosquamous skin disease, is estimated to affect 2% of the global population. Traditionally believed to be a problem largely affecting keratinocytes in the epidermis, psoriasis has recently been identified as one of the most common immune-related diseases. Though this condition may manifest at any life stage, a dual distribution of age was observed, having a peak occurring between the ages of 20 and 30 as well as 50 and 60. Psoriasis possesses a complicated etiology that includes immunologic, hereditary, and systemic/local factors. Psoriasis shows an immense negative impact on human life quality, probably equivalent in comparison to coronary artery disease, type 2 diabetes, depressive disorders, and carcinoma, regardless of the fact that it usually possesses a minor influence on survival. The unregulated development of keratinocytes is the main constraint behind psoriasis, and improper regulation of the immune system serves as a pathophysiological factor. The pathogenesis generally includes the cooperation among several populations for immunocytes along with corresponding transmitting molecules that are: (1) innate immunocytes, which are mediated by antigenic-displaying cells, such as neutrophils, the cells of Langerhans, and natural-killing T lymphoid cells (2) acquired or adaptable immunocytes, which are facilitated by developed CD^{4+} and CD^{8+} T lymphocyte residing in the epidermis. The result of such immunological dysfunction leads to inflammation, which causes clinical lesions as well as histopathological inflammation, diagnostic of psoriasis development and perpetuation. The standard of lifestyle in patients has increased with biologic treatments, which focus on the cytokine-mediated pathophysiology of psoriasis. This book chapter will cover the molecular basis and primary pathophysiology of psoriasis.

* **Corresponding author Sumeet Gupta:** Department of Pharmacology, M. M. College of Pharmacy, Maharishi Markandeshwar (Deemed to be University), Mullana, Ambala 133207, Haryana, India; E-mail: sumeetgupta25@gmail.com

Keywords: Molecular targets, Mechanism of action, Psoriasis, Pathophysiology, Skin disorder.

INTRODUCTION

The human body's largest organ, the skin, acts as armor to shield our bodies from the outside world. It is made up of the dermis, epidermis, and hypodermis as its three primary layers [1]. The topmost part of the skin, termed the epidermis, is mostly composed of keratinocytes, which provide waterproofing and protection against UV radiation [2]. Underneath the skin's outer layer, the dermis provides a home to numerous glands, including sebaceous glands and sweat glands, vessels for blood, and nerve fibers [3]. Through mechanisms like perspiration, the skin is essential in controlling the body's temperature [4]. The skin plays a significant role in the synthesis of vitamin D when exposed to sunlight [5]. The skin's appearance and health may be subjected to a number of variables, such as genetics, age, diet, and environmental exposures [6]. A persistent inflammatory skin condition caused by the immune system, psoriasis is characterized by distinctive, colored, scaly patches. It is among the most common autoimmune diseases, affecting approximately 2% of people worldwide [7]. This disease is known for its relapsing and remitting nature, causing a significant physical and psychological burden on affected individuals [8]. Many comorbidities, such as psoriatic arthritis, diabetes, heart disease, and a condition called metabolic syndrome, are linked to psoriasis and psychological disorders, further impacting the overall health and well-being of patients [9].

Environmental factors, impaired immune system responses, and genetic susceptibility interact intricately in the pathogenesis of psoriasis [10]. The development of psoriasis is significantly influenced by genetic factors, with strong familial aggregation observed in affected individuals [11]. Psoriasis has an important detrimental effect on people's quality of daily life, frequently equal to the effects associated with other persistent illnesses like depressive disorders, diabetes, and carcinoma [12]. Due to the obvious form of skin rashes and the discomfort and irritation they cause, stigmatization in society and emotional distress may result, which can negatively impact various aspects of daily life [13].

Epidemiology of Psoriasis

A common persistent inflammatory skin condition, psoriasis affects about 2% of people globally [14]. This psoriasis prevalence varies across different geographic regions and ethnic groups, with higher rates observed in certain populations [15]. Psoriasis may develop at any age; however, there are two distinct stages of its onset, typically occurring within the age ranges of 20-30 and 50-60 [16]. Studies have shown that the prevalence of psoriasis is transformed by genetic, environmental issues, and lifestyle variables, contributing to variability in its occurrence [17]. Psoriasis is associated with a substantial financial burden on individuals and healthcare systems. It has been connected to several medical conditions, such as psychological problems, a condition called metabolic syndrome, coronary artery disease, and arthritis caused by psoriasis, further impacting the overall health and well-being of patients [18]. Furthermore, the economic burden of psoriasis is substantial, with the total cost of the illness being increased by both immediate healthcare expenses and additional expenses related to disability and reduced productivity [19].

Prevalence and Age Distribution of Psoriasis

Prevalence

The prevalence of psoriasis varies significantly across populations, with estimates ranging from 0.27% to 11.4% in adults, depending on factors such as:

Geography: Prevalence varies based on location, with higher rates observed in certain regions like northern Europe and lower rates in Southeast Asia.

Ethnicity: Genetic predisposition plays a role, with higher rates among certain ethnic groups like Caucasians.

Age: Any person of any age can develop psoriasis; however, it typically manifests in two stages: early development (20–30 years) and late onset (50–60 years).

Here are some specific prevalence estimates:

- Global: 2.7% (lifetime prevalence)
- Italy: 3.5% at age 60-64 years
- United States: 1.6%
- North India: 0.44% to 2.8%
- Taiwan: 0.30% [20 - 24].

Age Distribution

The age distribution of psoriasis demonstrates a bimodal trend that includes two age-related groups:

Initiation very early: between the ages of 20 and 30

Delayed initiation, aged 50 to 60

This suggests that there are two distinct genetic as well as environmental variables contributing to psoriasis development at different stages of life.

Here are some specific observations regarding age distribution:

- The early-onset peak is more prominent in men, while the late-onset peak is similar in both sexes.
- The lifetime prevalence of psoriasis increases with age, reaching 3.5% among individuals aged 60-64 years before declining slightly in older age groups.
- Psoriasis incidence also shows a bimodal distribution, with peaks corresponding to the early-onset and late-onset groups [21].

Etiology of Psoriasis

This complex disorder psoriasis, has a complicated etiology that includes environmental variables, dysregulated immune responses, and genetic susceptibility [25]. The prevalence of psoriasis is significantly influenced by genetic factors, with a strong familial aggregation observed in affected individuals [26]. Numerous susceptibility loci and genetic variations associated with psoriasis have been identified through genome-wide association studies, underscoring the genetic complexity of the condition. The dysregulation of immune responses, particularly involving T lymphocytes and cytokines, leads to an impactful role in psoriasis pathogenesis [27]. Aberrant activation of T cells, particularly Th1 and Th17 cells, causes the release of pro-inflammatory cytokines, including interleukin-17 (IL-17), the alpha form of tumor necrosis factor (TNF-α), and interleukin-23 (IL-23), which contributes to the hyperproliferation of keratinocytes and the formation of psoriatic plaques [28].

Environmental factors, including stress, infections, and certain medications, can trigger or exacerbate psoriasis in genetically predisposed individuals [24]. The interaction among genetic susceptibility, immune dysregulation, and environmental triggers contributes to the growth and advancement of psoriasis. Understanding the multifaceted etiology of psoriasis is essential for the development of targeted treatments and personalized therapy approaches tailored to the underlying pathogenic mechanisms.

PSORIASIS'S IMPACT ON LIFE QUALITY

The effects of psoriasis on quality of life are significant, affecting various aspects of both physical and mental well-being. Studies have shown that individuals with psoriasis often experience diminished quality of life due to the visible nature of the condition, the discomfort it causes physically, and the emotional burden of enduring a chronic skin disease [16]. Moreover, psoriasis has been linked to the higher incidence of depressive disorders, anxiety, and stigma in society, each of which decreases the standard of living [29].

PATHOGENESIS OF PSORIASIS

Psoriasis is a chronic inflammatory skin condition characterized by inflammatory processes, immune-mediated imbalances, and excessive keratinocyte proliferation. Psoriasis is caused by a complex interaction of immune-mediated, environmental, and genetic factors, as shown in Fig. (**1**).

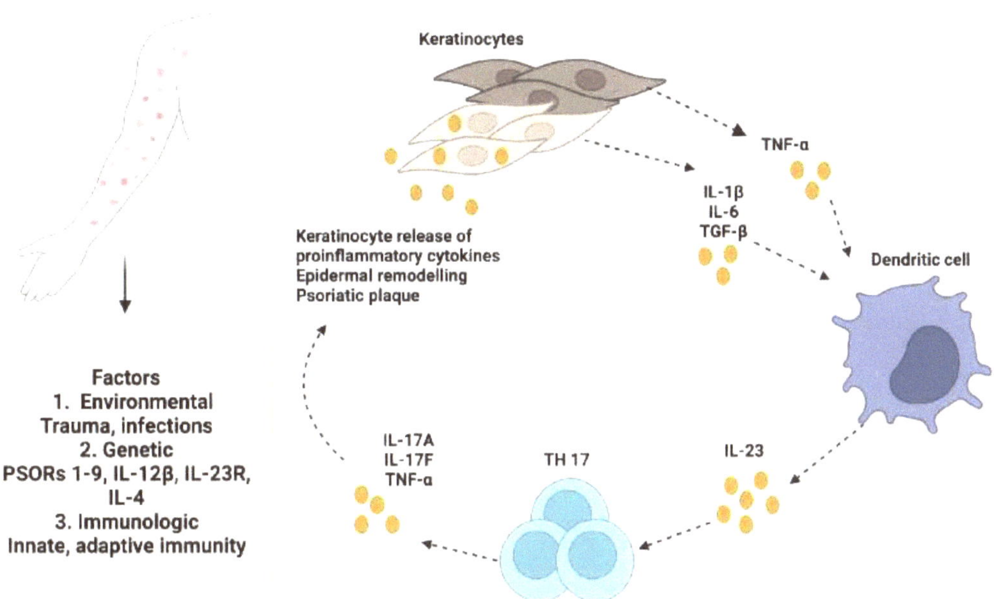

Fig. (1). Pathogenesis of psoriasis.

Uncontrolled Keratinocyte Proliferation

Keratinocytes, the primary cell type found within the epidermis, proliferate rapidly and uncontrollably in psoriasis, a chronic inflammatory skin disease [30]. This excessive cell turnover leads to the production of characteristic red, scaly lesions on the epidermis.

Genetic Factors

There is a significant genetic component in the onset of psoriasis. Specific susceptibility genes have been recently identified, with human leukocyte antigen (HLA) genes, particularly HLA-Cw6, being strongly associated with psoriasis susceptibility [31]. These genetic factors contribute to the dysregulation of immune responses and keratinocyte proliferation.

Cell Cycle Dysregulation

At the cellular level, the uncontrolled proliferation of keratinocytes is associated with dysregulation of the cell cycle. Psoriatic keratinocytes exhibit a shortened cell cycle, with an accelerated transition from the G1 to the S phase [32]. This abnormal cell cycle regulation results in an increased number of keratinocytes entering the DNA synthesis phase, contributing to the hyperplasia observed in psoriatic lesions.

Immune Dysregulation and Cytokine Production

In the psoriasis pathophysiology, the immune system is significant. Dysregulation of immune responses, particularly involving T cells, participates in sustained inflammation of psoriatic lesions. Pro-inflammatory cytokines such as interleukin-17 (IL-17), interleukin-23 (IL-23), and tumor necrosis factor-alpha (TNF-α), are released by activated T cells [33]. By relying on keratinocytes, these cytokines encourage continuing atypical growth and aid in the preservation of the psoriatic phenotype.

Angiogenesis and Neovascularization

Psoriatic lesions are characterized by increased angiogenesis and neovascularization, further supporting the uncontrolled keratinocyte proliferation. The development of new blood vessels inside the dermis provides an enhanced nutrient supply to rapidly dividing keratinocytes, sustaining the hyper proliferative state [34].

Therapeutic Interventions

Understanding the mechanisms of uncontrolled keratinocyte proliferation has paved the way for targeted therapies. Biologic agents, including IL-17 blockers and TNF-α inhibitors, show efficacy in reducing keratinocyte hyperproliferation and alleviating psoriatic symptoms [35]. Topical treatments, phototherapy, and systemic medications also aim to modulate immune responses and normalize keratinocyte proliferation.

Dysregulation of the Immune System

Psoriasis is a skin condition that also involves immune system dysfunction. The immune system misinterprets healthy cells in the skin for invading intruders, leading to chronic inflammation. Several immune cell types are involved in this inflammatory response, including:

Dendritic cells: These cells start the immunological response by associating T cells with antigens. In psoriasis, dendritic cells are activated by various stimuli, leading to the production of pro-inflammatory cytokines and the activation of T cells [36].

T cells: T lymphocytes are essential for the immunological response. In psoriasis, there is an imbalance between regulatory T cells (Tregs) and pro-inflammatory T cells (Th17 and Th22). Th17 and Th22 cells lead to the production of pro-inflammatory cytokines that promote keratinocyte proliferation and skin inflammation, while Tregs suppress the immune response [37].

Neutrophils: When psoriasis develops, these immune cells infiltrate the dermis, and produce proteases and reactive oxygen species, which lead to the breakdown of tissues [38].

Involvement of Innate Immunocytes

The inflammatory skin disease psoriasis is a result of a complex interaction among innate and adaptive immune systems. While the precise trigger for this interaction remains elusive, mounting evidence suggests a crucial role for innate immune cells in establishing and sustaining the inflammatory cascade characteristic of psoriasis.

Initial Innate Immune Activation

Keratinocytes: These epidermal cells act as the first line of defense, expressing pattern recognition receptors (PRRs) that recognize danger signals, such as microbial components or self-derived molecules released from damaged cells. PRR activation triggers keratinocytes to secrete chemokines and pro-inflammatory cytokines (TNF-α, IL-1β, IL-6), initiating an inflammatory response [39].

Dendritic cells (DCs): Resident skin DCs capture and process antigens, presenting them to T lymphocytes. This antigen presentation, coupled with the production of pro-inflammatory cytokines by DCs, activates T cells, especially Th17 cells, which are essential to psoriasis [40].

Natural Killer (NK) cells: These innate lymphocytes exhibit cytotoxic activity against infected or stressed cells. In psoriasis, NK cells are activated and contribute to psoriatic inflammation through the release of pro-inflammatory cytokines and perforin-mediated lysis of keratinocytes [41].

NKT cells: These innate T cells act as a link between adaptive and innate immunity by recognizing glycolipids that are provided by CD1d molecules. In psoriatic scars, NKT cells are abundant, contributing to disease development by promoting Th17 cell differentiation and inflammation [42].

Innate Immune Cells and the IL-23/Th17 Axis

IL-23: Macrophages and DCs that have been activated generate this key cytokine. IL-23 tends to promote both the limitation and expansion of pathogenic Th17 cells, which in turn amplify inflammation through the production of IL-17A and IL-17F [43].

IL-17A/F: These cytokines are deemed to be crucial mediators of psoriatic inflammation. They stimulate keratinocyte proliferation, induce the generation of chemokines and pro-inflammatory cytokines, and promote neutrophil recruitment for skin [44].

Involvement of Acquired or Adaptive Immunocytes

Chronic inflammation skin condition psoriasis is caused by a complicated interaction between several immune cell types as well as pathways. While innate immune cells are essential for initiating inflammatory cascade, the immune system, either acquired or adaptive is essential for perpetuating and amplifying the disease process.

T Cells

Th17 cells: These CD^{4+} T helper cells are considered to be key players in psoriasis. Th17 cells undergo activation by IL-23, generated by dendritic cells along with macrophages, and differentiate into pro-inflammatory effector cells. They secrete IL-17A, IL-17F, as well as other cytokines, which promote the proliferation of keratinocytes, neutrophil recruitment, and angiogenesis, all contributing to psoriatic inflammation [45].

Th1 cells: These CD4+ T helper cells are also associated with psoriasis through the generation of IFN-γ, a potent pro-inflammatory cytokine that further amplifies the inflammatory response. Th1 cells are recruited to the skin by chemokines and interact with other immune cells to perpetuate inflammation [46].

B Cells

Autoreactive B cells: These B cells produce autoantibodies that target healthy skin components. While the specific autoantigens remain elusive, autoantibodies against keratinocytes and other skin proteins have been detected in psoriatic lesions [40].

Plasma cells: The generation of antibodies is carried out by these substantially developed B cells. In psoriasis, plasma cells infiltrate the skin and contribute to inflammation by secreting large amounts of autoantibodies [41].

T Regulatory Cells (Tregs)

Functional Tregs: These CD4+ T cells are essential for preserving immunological tolerance as well as suppressing inflammatory responses. However, in psoriasis, Tregs are dysfunctional or depleted, leading to uncontrolled immune activation and persistent inflammation [42].

Interplay between Adaptive and Innate Immune Systems

Antigen presentation: T cells receive antigens from dendritic cells, which starts the process of adaptive immunity. In psoriasis, DCs are activated by pro-inflammatory cytokines and present antigens that drive the differentiation of Th17 cells [39].

INFLAMMATION AND CLINICAL MANIFESTATIONS

An improper and accelerated multiplication of skin cells causes psoriasis, a chronic inflammatory skin disorder that results in the creation of firm, colored, rough spots known as plaques. An inflammatory reaction in the epidermis is caused by a complex interaction between genetic and environmental factors, which leads to an overproduction of skin cells.

Cellular and Molecular Mechanisms of Inflammation

T cell activation: Th17 cells, in particular, autoreactive T cells, are essential for the inflammatory process. Pro-inflammatory cytokines, including IL-17 and IL-23, are released by these T cells, which activate immune cells and keratinocytes (skin cells).

Neutrophil infiltration: Neutrophils, another type of immune cell, travel to impacted skin and aid in inflammation by releasing reactive oxygen species and proteolytic enzymes.

Dendritic cell activation: T cells receive antigens from dendritic cells, which promotes their activation and perpetuates the inflammatory cycle.

Cytokine signaling: A complex network of pro- and anti-inflammatory cytokines (IL-10, TGF-β) and pro-inflammatory cytokines (IL-17, IL-23, TNF-α) regulates the inflammatory response.

Keratinocyte proliferation and differentiation: The inflammatory milieu stimulates keratinocytes to proliferate rapidly and lose their normal differentiation program, leading to the formation of psoriatic plaques [47].

Clinical Manifestations

Plaques: Psoriasis is characterized by thick, red, scaly plaques that are coated with silver-white scales. Though they can occur anywhere on the human body, the elbows, knees, the crown of the head, the trunk, the palms, and the soles of the feet are the most prevalent places.

Itching and burning: Psoriatic plaques can be itchy and burning, leading to discomfort and scratching that can worsen the lesions.

Nail changes: Psoriasis can affect the nails, causing pitting, discoloration, thickening, and crumbling [2].

Psoriatic arthritis: In some cases, psoriasis can be associated with joint inflammation and pain, known as psoriatic arthritis [48].

BIOLOGICAL THERAPIES FOR PSORIASIS

Biological therapies for psoriasis, also known as biologics, are a class of medications that target particular immune system components implicated in the development of psoriasis. Tumor necrosis factor (TNF), interleukin 17A (IL-17A), interleukin 23 (IL-23), and other specific proteins in the immune system are the targets of biologics. Biological therapies have proven to be highly effective for treating psoriasis, with many patients experiencing significant improvement in their symptoms. One example of a biologic used to treat psoriasis is adalimumab, which targets TNF. Another example is secukinumab, which targets IL-17A [49]. Typically, these medications are reserved for moderate-to-severe psoriasis that has not responded to conventional therapies. By doing so, they tend to decrease inflammation and overproduction of skin cells, which leads to the development of psoriatic plaques. These medications are typically administered *via* injection or intravenous infusion and are often given at specific intervals, such as once every few weeks. However, they also come with potential adverse consequences, such as a heightened risk of infections and specific cancer types [50].

CLINICAL TRIALS FOR PSORIASIS

Clinical research plays a crucial role in advancing Psoriasis treatment, bringing hope for improved management and potential cures. Here is a glimpse into several exciting clinical trials,

Roflumilast (ARQ-151): Recently FDA-approved (July 2022), this topical PDE4 inhibitor showed promising results among several phase III trials (DERMIS-1 & 2) for plaque psoriasis in adults [51].

Deucravacitinib (BMS-986165, Sotyktu): Another recent FDA approval (September 2022), this oral TYK2 inhibitor, administered once daily, demonstrated efficacy in the POETYK PSO-1 trial regarding mild to severe plaque psoriasis [52].

Types of Clinical Trials for Psoriasis:

Phase I: These small-scale studies (encompassing 20-100 participants) assess the safety and dosage range of a new treatment.

Phase II: These mid-size studies (100-300 participants) evaluate the effectiveness of the treatment for specific symptoms or endpoints.

Phase III: These large-scale studies (300+ participants) compare the new treatment to existing ones or a placebo to confirm its efficacy and safety for broader use.

Phase IV: These post-marketing studies monitor the authorized treatment's long-term safety and efficacy in an actual situation [53].

FDA APPROVAL OF DRUGS IN PSORIASIS

The Food and Drug Administration (FDA) approves a wide range of drugs in psoriasis therapy, targeting different types and severities of the condition. Here is a table summarizing the main categories and some examples (Table **1**):

Table 1. List of FDA-approved drugs used in psoriasis.

Category	Drug Name(s)	Mechanism of Action	References
Topical Corticosteroids	Hydrocortisone, Clobetasol, Triamcinolone	Reduce inflammation and itching	[54]
Retinoids	Tazarotene, Alitretinoin	Inhibit abnormal skin cell growth	[54]
Vitamin D Analogs	Calcipotriene, Tacalcitol	Modulate cell growth and differentiation	[55]
Biologics	Adalimumab, Etanercept, Ustekinumab, Brodalumab, Ixekizumab, Secukinumab, Bimekizumab	Target-specific inflammatory pathways	[55]

(Table 1) cont.....

Category	Drug Name(s)	Mechanism of Action	References
Aryl Hydrocarbon Receptor (AhR) Modulating Agents	Tapinarof	Regulate skin cell proliferation and differentiation	[56]
Small Molecules	Apremilast, Deucravacitinib (Sotyktu™)	Target specific inflammatory pathways through oral administration	[56]
Phosphodiesterase-4 (PDE4) Inhibitors	Roflumilast	Reduce inflammation by Inhibiting the PDE4 enzyme	[57]
Interleukin-36 Receptor Antagonists	Spesolimab-sbzo (Spevigo™)	Specifically for generalized pustular psoriasis	[57]

The formation of red, rough plaques is the hallmark of psoriasis, a chronic inflammatory skin illness mediated by the immune system. The pathophysiology of psoriasis is complex and involves dysregulation of the immune system, aberrant growth of keratinocytes, and a network of chemokines and pro-inflammatory cytokines. The discovery of targeted medicines has transformed the treatment of psoriasis, thanks to our growing understanding of the molecular basis of this disorder. At the molecular level, psoriasis is associated with a dysregulated immune response, particularly involving T cells. Tumor necrosis factor-alpha (TNF-α), interleukin-17 (IL-17), and interleukin-23 (IL-23) are among the pro-inflammatory cytokines released as a result of the activation of T cells and infiltration into the dermis. These cytokines are crucial to the pathophysiology of psoriasis, as they promote keratinocyte proliferation and induce a sustained inflammatory response. Moreover, genetic factors also contribute to the development of psoriasis. Many susceptibility loci have been identified through genome-wide association studies, underscoring the polygenic nature of the disease. The pathophysiology of psoriasis has been linked to variations in immune system genes, including HLA-C and genes involved in the IL-23/Th17 pathway.

Normal skin homeostasis is disrupted by the dysfunctional immune response and genetic susceptibility associated with psoriasis, resulting in the characteristic features of the disease, including epidermal hyperplasia, altered keratinocyte differentiation, and the formation of inflammatory infiltrates in the skin. In conclusion, the pathophysiology and molecular basis of psoriasis involve a complex interplay of immune dysregulation, genetic predisposition, and aberrant cytokine signaling. Advances in our understanding of these mechanisms have led to the development of specific biological treatments that alter psoriasis-related immunological pathways. This has significantly improved the management of psoriasis, offering hope for more effective and personalized treatment strategies in the future.

REFERENCES

[1] Hoffman M. The skin (human anatomy): Picture, definition, function, and skin conditions.

[2] Odom RB, James WD, Berger TG. Andrews' diseases of the skin: clinical dermatology. Philadelphia: WB Saunders Company; 2000 Mar.

[3] Proksch E, Nissen HP, Bremgartner M, Urquhart C. Bathing in a magnesium-rich Dead Sea salt solution improves skin barrier function, enhances skin hydration, and reduces inflammation in atopic dry skin. Int J Dermatol 2005; 44(2): 151-7.
[http://dx.doi.org/10.1111/j.1365-4632.2005.02079.x] [PMID: 15689218]

[4] Montagna W. Structure and function of skin. Apocrine Glands 1974; 11: 332-63.

[5] Holick MF, Vitamin D. Vitamin D: A millenium perspective. J Cell Biochem 2003; 88(2): 296-307.
[http://dx.doi.org/10.1002/jcb.10338] [PMID: 12520530]

[6] Mukherjee S, Date A, Patravale V, Korting HC, Roeder A, Weindl G. Retinoids in the treatment of skin aging: an overview of clinical efficacy and safety. Clin Interv Aging 2006; 1(4): 327-48.
[http://dx.doi.org/10.2147/ciia.2006.1.4.327] [PMID: 18046911]

[7] Parisi R, Symmons DPM, Griffiths CEM, Ashcroft DM. Global epidemiology of psoriasis: a systematic review of incidence and prevalence. J Invest Dermatol 2013; 133(2): 377-85.
[http://dx.doi.org/10.1038/jid.2012.339] [PMID: 23014338]

[8] Rapp SR, Feldman SR, Exum ML, Fleischer AB Jr, Reboussin DM. Psoriasis causes as much disability as other major medical diseases. J Am Acad Dermatol 1999; 41(3): 401-7.
[http://dx.doi.org/10.1016/S0190-9622(99)70112-X] [PMID: 10459113]

[9] Takeshita J, Grewal S, Langan SM, *et al.* Psoriasis and comorbid diseases. J Am Acad Dermatol 2017; 76(3): 377-90.
[http://dx.doi.org/10.1016/j.jaad.2016.07.064] [PMID: 28212759]

[10] Nograles KE, Davidovici B, Krueger JG. New insights in the immunologic basis of psoriasis. In Seminars in cutaneous medicine and surgery 2010 Mar; 29(1); 3.

[11] Zhang XJ, Huang W, Yang S, *et al.* Psoriasis genome-wide association study identifies susceptibility variants within LCE gene cluster at 1q21. Nat Genet 2009; 41(2): 205-10.
[http://dx.doi.org/10.1038/ng.310] [PMID: 19169255]

[12] Kimball AB, Jacobson C, Weiss S, Vreeland MG, Wu Y. The psychosocial burden of psoriasis. Am J Clin Dermatol 2005; 6(6): 383-92.
[http://dx.doi.org/10.2165/00128071-200506060-00005] [PMID: 16343026]

[13] Sampogna F, Tabolli S, Abeni D. Impact of different skin conditions on quality of life. Giornale Italiano di Dermatologia e Venereologia: Organo Ufficiale. Societa Italiana di Dermatologia e Sifilografia 2013; 148(3): 255-61.

[14] Michalek IM, Loring B, John SM. A systematic review of worldwide epidemiology of psoriasis. Journal of the European Academy of Dermatology and Venereology. 2017 Feb;31(2):205-12.

[15] Rachakonda TD, Schupp CW, Armstrong AW. Psoriasis prevalence among adults in the United States. J Am Acad Dermatol 2014; 70(3): 512-6.
[http://dx.doi.org/10.1016/j.jaad.2013.11.013] [PMID: 24388724]

[16] Kurd SK, Gelfand JM. The prevalence of previously diagnosed and undiagnosed psoriasis in US adults: Results from NHANES 2003-2004. J Am Acad Dermatol 2009; 60(2): 218-24.
[http://dx.doi.org/10.1016/j.jaad.2008.09.022] [PMID: 19022533]

[17] Tsoi LC, Stuart PE, Tian C, *et al.* Large scale meta-analysis characterizes genetic architecture for common psoriasis associated variants. Nat Commun 2017; 8(1): 15382.
[http://dx.doi.org/10.1038/ncomms15382] [PMID: 28537254]

[18] Ni C, Chiu MW. Psoriasis and comorbidities: links and risks. Clinical, cosmetic and investigational

dermatology. 2014 Apr 17:119-32.

[19] Feldman SR, Malakouti M, Koo JYM. Social impact of the burden of psoriasis: effects on patients and practice. Dermatol Online J 2014; 20(8): 13030/qt48r4w8h2. [http://dx.doi.org/10.5070/D3208023523] [PMID: 25148272]

[20] Dogra S, Mahajan R. Psoriasis: Epidemiology, clinical features, co-morbidities, and clinical scoring. Indian Dermatol Online J 2016; 7(6): 471-80. [http://dx.doi.org/10.4103/2229-5178.193906] [PMID: 27990381]

[21] Pezzolo E, Cazzaniga S, Colombo P, Chatenoud L, Naldi L. Psoriasis incidence and lifetime prevalence: suggestion for a higher mortality rate in older age-classes among psoriatic patients compared to the general population in Italy. Acta Derm Venereol 2019; 99(4): 400-3. [http://dx.doi.org/10.2340/00015555-3130] [PMID: 30673108]

[22] Armstrong AW, Mehta MD, Schupp CW, Gondo GC, Bell SJ, Griffiths CEM. Psoriasis prevalence in adults in the United States. JAMA Dermatol 2021; 157(8): 940-6. [http://dx.doi.org/10.1001/jamadermatol.2021.2007] [PMID: 34190957]

[23] Mohaidat ZM, Saleh AA. OBEIDAT AA, AL-OMARI MH, Khasawneh RA. Osteochondroma in Jordanian Patients: Clinical Manifestations and Management. J Clin Diagn Res 2018; 12(9)

[24] Parisi R, Iskandar IYK, Kontopantelis E, Augustin M, Griffiths CEM, Ashcroft DM. National, regional, and worldwide epidemiology of psoriasis: systematic analysis and modelling study. BMJ 2020; 369: m1590. [http://dx.doi.org/10.1136/bmj.m1590] [PMID: 32467098]

[25] Lowes MA, Suárez-Fariñas M, Krueger JG. Immunology of Psoriasis. Annu Rev Immunol 2014; 32(1): 227-55. [http://dx.doi.org/10.1146/annurev-immunol-032713-120225] [PMID: 24655295]

[26] Tang H, Jin X, Li Y, Jiang H, Tang X, Yang X, Cheng H, Qiu Y, Chen G, Mei J, Zhou F. A large-scale screen for coding variants predisposing to psoriasis. Nature Genetics. 2014 Jan;46(1):45-50.

[27] Mak RK, Hundhausen C, Nestle FO. Progress in understanding the immunopathogenesis of psoriasis. Actas dermo-sifiliograficas. 2009 Dec 1; 100: 2-13. [http://dx.doi.org/10.1016/S0001-7310(09)73372-1]

[28] Hawkes JE, Chan TC, Krueger JG. Psoriasis pathogenesis and the development of novel targeted immune therapies. J Allergy Clin Immunol 2017; 140(3): 645-53. [http://dx.doi.org/10.1016/j.jaci.2017.07.004] [PMID: 28887948]

[29] Kurd SK, Troxel AB, Crits-Christoph P, Gelfand JM. The risk of depression, anxiety, and suicidality in patients with psoriasis: a population-based cohort study. Arch Dermatol 2010; 146(8): 891-5. [PMID: 20713823]

[30] Griffiths CEM, Barker JNWN. Pathogenesis and clinical features of psoriasis. Lancet 2007; 370(9583): 263-71. [http://dx.doi.org/10.1016/S0140-6736(07)61128-3] [PMID: 17658397]

[31] Nair RP, Duffin KC, Helms C, *et al.* Genome-wide scan reveals association of psoriasis with IL-23 and NF-κB pathways. Nat Genet 2009; 41(2): 199-204. [http://dx.doi.org/10.1038/ng.311] [PMID: 19169254]

[32] Bowcock AM, Shannon W, Du F, *et al.* Insights into psoriasis and other inflammatory diseases from large-scale gene expression studies. Hum Mol Genet 2001; 10(17): 1793-805. [http://dx.doi.org/10.1093/hmg/10.17.1793] [PMID: 11532989]

[33] Lowes MA, Kikuchi T, Fuentes-Duculan J, *et al.* Psoriasis vulgaris lesions contain discrete populations of Th1 and Th17 T cells. J Invest Dermatol 2008; 128(5): 1207-11. [http://dx.doi.org/10.1038/sj.jid.5701213] [PMID: 18200064]

[34] Arbiser JL, Bonner MY, Ward N, Elsey J, Rao S. Selenium unmasks protective iron armor: A possible

defense against cutaneous inflammation and cancer. Biochim Biophys Acta, Gen Subj 2018; 1862(11): 2518-27.
[http://dx.doi.org/10.1016/j.bbagen.2018.05.018] [PMID: 29852199]

[35] Gough OJ, Rane SS, Saunders A, Priestley M, Ray-Jones H, Shi C, Warren RB, Adamson A, Eyre S. Dissection of a non-coding risk locus at 1p36. 23 identifies ERRFI1 as a novel gene in the pathogenesis of psoriasis and psoriatic arthritis. BioRxiv. 2023: 2023-12.
[http://dx.doi.org/10.1101/2023.12.04.569945]

[36] Mihu C, Neag MA, Bocşan IC, *et al.* Novel concepts in psoriasis: histopathology and markers related to modern treatment approaches. Rom J Morphol Embryol 2022; 62(4): 897-906.
[http://dx.doi.org/10.47162/RJME.62.4.02] [PMID: 35673809]

[37] Magina S, Filipe P. Pathophysiology of moderate to severe plaque psoriasis: anti-IL-17 towards disease modification. Drugs of Today (Barcelona, Spain: 1998). 2021 May 1; 57(5): 347-57.
[http://dx.doi.org/10.1358/dot.2021.57.5.3266244]

[38] Wang WM, Jin HZ. Role of neutrophils in psoriasis. J Immunol Res. 2020 Jun 5; 2020: 3709749.
[http://dx.doi.org/10.1155/2020/3709749] [PMID: 32587871] [PMCID: PMC7293746]

[39] Palla G, Derényi I, Farkas I, Vicsek T. Uncovering the overlapping community structure of complex networks in nature and society. Nature. 2005 Jun 9; 435(7043): 814-8.

[40] Nestle FO, Conrad C, Tun-Kyi A, *et al.* Plasmacytoid predendritic cells initiate psoriasis through interferon-α production. J Exp Med 2005; 202(1): 135-43.
[http://dx.doi.org/10.1084/jem.20050500] [PMID: 15998792]

[41] McKee CS, Hill DS, Redfern CPF, Armstrong JL, Lovat PE. Oncogenic BRAF signalling increases M cl-1 expression in cutaneous metastatic melanoma. Exp Dermatol 2013; 22(11): 767-9.
[http://dx.doi.org/10.1111/exd.12254] [PMID: 24118207]

[42] Raphael I, Joern RR, Forsthuber TG. Memory CD4+ T cells in immunity and autoimmune diseases. Cells 2020; 9(3): 531.
[http://dx.doi.org/10.3390/cells9030531] [PMID: 32106536]

[43] Krueger JG. The immunologic basis for the treatment of psoriasis with new biologic agents. J Am Acad Dermatol 2002; 46(1): 1-26.
[http://dx.doi.org/10.1067/mjd.2002.120568] [PMID: 11756941]

[44] Bronin A, Phelps R. Beyond JAAD July 2015: Articles of interest from the nondermatologic literature. J Am Acad Dermatol 2015; 73(1): 177-9.
[http://dx.doi.org/10.1016/j.jaad.2015.04.007]

[45] Onuora S. Steroidal nano-drug suppresses murine lupus. Nat Rev Rheumatol 2016; 12(5): 252.
[PMID: 27052485]

[46] Reich K, Iversen L, Puig L, *et al.* Long-term efficacy and safety of brodalumab in moderate-to-severe plaque psoriasis: a post hoc pooled analysis of AMAGINE-2 and -3. J Eur Acad Dermatol Venereol 2022; 36(8): 1275-83.
[http://dx.doi.org/10.1111/jdv.18068] [PMID: 35279890]

[47] Nickoloff BJ, Nestle FO. Recent insights into the immunopathogenesis of psoriasis provide new therapeutic opportunities. J Clin Invest 2004; 113(12): 1664-75.
[http://dx.doi.org/10.1172/JCI200422147] [PMID: 15199399]

[48] Armstrong AW, Read C. Pathophysiology, clinical presentation, and treatment of psoriasis: a review. JAMA 2020; 323(19): 1945-60.
[http://dx.doi.org/10.1001/jama.2020.4006] [PMID: 32427307]

[49] Mease PJ, Armstrong AW. Managing patients with psoriatic disease: the diagnosis and pharmacologic treatment of psoriatic arthritis in patients with psoriasis. Drugs 2014; 74(4): 423-41.
[http://dx.doi.org/10.1007/s40265-014-0191-y] [PMID: 24566842]

[50] Menter A, Strober BE, Kaplan DH, *et al.* Joint AAD-NPF guidelines of care for the management and treatment of psoriasis with biologics. J Am Acad Dermatol 2019; 80(4): 1029-72. [http://dx.doi.org/10.1016/j.jaad.2018.11.057] [PMID: 30772098]

[51] Lebwohl MG, Kircik LH, Moore AY, *et al.* Effect of roflumilast cream *vs* vehicle cream on chronic plaque psoriasis: the DERMIS-1 and DERMIS-2 randomized clinical trials. JAMA 2022; 328(11): 1073-84. [http://dx.doi.org/10.1001/jama.2022.15632] [PMID: 36125472]

[52] Vu A, Maloney V, Gordon KB. Deucravacitinib in moderate-to-severe psoriasis. Immunotherapy 2022; 14(16): 1279-90. [http://dx.doi.org/10.2217/imt-2022-0109] [PMID: 36373503]

[53] Food US. Drug Administration Drug Development and Drug Interactions: Table of Substrates, Inhibitors and Inducers. FDA. Available online: https://www. fda. gov/drugs/drug-interactionslabeling/drug-development-and-drug-interactions-table-substrates-inhibitors-and-inducers

[54] Gharge R, Phadatare S, Shinde S, Chogale E, Patil S, Pujare P. Psoriasis: Causes, diagnosis and management. Small 2021; 3: 4.

[55] Pershadsingh HA, Sproul JA, Benjamin E, Finnegan J, Amin NM. Treatment of psoriasis with troglitazone therapy. Arch Dermatol 1998; 134(10): 1304-5. [http://dx.doi.org/10.1001/archderm.134.10.1304] [PMID: 9801703]

[56] Nogueira S, Rodrigues MA, Vender R, Torres T. Tapinarof for the treatment of psoriasis. Dermatol Ther 2022; 35(12): e15931. [http://dx.doi.org/10.1111/dth.15931] [PMID: 36226669]

[57] Pixley JN, Schaetzle T, Feldman SR. A review of topical roflumilast for the treatment of plaque psoriasis. Ann Pharmacother 2023; 57(8): 966-9. [http://dx.doi.org/10.1177/10600280221137750] [PMID: 36420929]

CHAPTER 3

Combination Approach for the Management of Psoriasis

Karan Goel[1,*], **Sapna Rani**[2], **Rama Devi**[1], **Sarita Sharma**[2] and **Simran Saini**[2]

[1] *Department of Pharmacology, Chitkara College of Pharmacy, Chitkara University, Rajpura 140401, Punjab, India*

[2] *Department of Pharmacology, Maharishi Markandeshwar College of Pharmacy, Maharishi Markandeshwar (Deemed to be University), Mullana, Ambala 133207, Haryana, India*

Abstract: Psoriasis is a prominent autoimmune condition characterized by an abnormal increase in the production of skin cells, leading to the formation of thick, red, and scaly patches on the skin. Comprehending the intricate pathophysiology of this condition, which involves the deregulation of the immune system and inflammatory processes, is essential for the development of efficacious treatments. Existing treatment modalities, such as monotherapy, have inherent constraints in effectively managing psoriasis of moderate to severe intensity, resulting in persistent symptoms and reduced responsiveness to treatment. Therefore, using a combination strategy that focuses on various disease-causing pathways provides improved effectiveness in treatment, decreases the development of resistance, and improves patient outcomes. Nevertheless, it is crucial to carefully evaluate issues such as personalized treatment regimens, adherence to therapy, economic factors, and the handling of medication interactions and toxicities. Customized treatment methods, novel combination medications, and integrated therapy platforms have the potential to maximize psoriasis control. Thorough and personalized combination approaches hold great promise for improving the quality of life for individuals with psoriasis.

Keywords: Adherence therapy, Monotherapy, Psoriasis, Personalized combination approaches.

INTRODUCTION TO PSORIASIS

Psoriasis is a persistent autoimmune disorder marked by the rapid regeneration of skin cells, leading to the development of thick, red, scaly regions called plaques. This polygenic illness impacts about 2-3% of the worldwide population, establishing it as one of the most widespread persistent skin conditions globally. Psoriasis mainly appears on the skin but may also affect the nails, joints, and other

* **Corresponding author Karan Goel:** Department of Pharmacology, Chitkara College of Pharmacy, Chitkara University, Rajpura 140401, Punjab, India; E-mail: karangoelji@gmail.com

organs, resulting in various clinical presentations and problems. Psoriasis manifests in several forms, with plaque psoriasis being the predominant subtype, representing about 80-90% of cases [1, 2]. Additional variations of psoriasis include (i) guttate psoriasis, which is defined by tiny, droplet-shaped lesions, (ii) pustular psoriasis, which is characterized by blisters filled with pus, and (iii) erythrodermic psoriasis, which involves extensive inflammation and shedding of the skin. Psoriasis may vary significantly in its severity and extent across people, ranging from isolated, moderate lesions to severe, widespread involvement that affects huge regions of the body surface [1, 2].

Epidemiology and Clinical Presentation

Psoriasis can affect individuals of various age groups, races, and ethnic backgrounds; however, it is most often seen in adults aged 15 to 35 years. Psoriasis is influenced by both hereditary and environmental factors, and having a family history of the illness raises the likelihood of experiencing it. Psoriasis symptoms may worsen or cause disease flares due to environmental stressors such as stress, infections, trauma, and certain drugs [3].

From a clinical perspective, psoriasis often appears as distinct, red patches on the skin that are covered with white scales. These plaques often manifest on areas of the body with extended surfaces, such as the elbows, knees, scalp, and lower back, but they may emerge on any part of the body. Psoriasis not only affects the skin but may also cause problems with the nails, such as pitting, thickness, and discoloration. It can also impact the joints, resulting in psoriatic arthritis in about 30% of patients [2, 3].

Impact on Quality of Life

In addition to its visible symptoms, psoriasis significantly impacts the overall well-being of patients, including their emotional state, social relationships, and ability to carry out everyday activities. The observable characteristics of psoriatic lesions may cause individuals to experience emotions of shame, self-awareness, and social seclusion, resulting in psychological anguish and diminished self-worth. Furthermore, the persistent and recurring characteristics of psoriasis, along with the uncertain progression of the condition, may lead to emotions of frustration, worry, and sadness in those afflicted [4].

Psoriasis not only causes psychological and social difficulties, but also raises the likelihood of other health problems, such as cardiovascular disease, metabolic syndrome, and psoriatic arthritis. These additional conditions further harm the overall health and well-being of sufferers. It is crucial to consider and meet the comprehensive requirements of patients with psoriasis, including their physical, mental, and social aspects, to enhance treatment results and improve their overall well-being [1, 4].

UNDERSTANDING THE PATHOPHYSIOLOGY

Psoriasis is a multifaceted inflammatory condition characterized by disrupted immune responses, aberrant growth of skin cells called keratinocytes, and the interplay of genetic and environmental factors. Comprehending the fundamental pathophysiology is crucial for formulating effective therapy approaches to control this persistent illness.

Immune Dysregulation and Inflammatory Cascade

The dysregulation of immunological responses, namely involving T lymphocytes and dendritic cells, is a key factor in the development of psoriasis. Psoriatic lesions are characterized by the infiltration of activated T cells, mostly belonging to the Th1 and Th17 subsets. These T cells produce pro-inflammatory cytokines, including Tumor Necrosis Factor-alpha [TNF-α], Interleukin-17 [IL-17], and Interleukin-23 [IL-23], into the skin, all steps are illustrated in Figures 1-4. These cytokines activate keratinocytes and other immune cells, triggering a continuous process of inflammation and tissue damage. In addition, the deregulation of the innate immune system, which involves aberrant activation of dendritic cells and alterations in cytokine signaling pathways, plays a role in the inflammatory process of psoriasis.

Abnormal Keratinocyte Proliferation

Psoriasis is defined by abnormal growth and maturation of keratinocytes, resulting in excessive epidermal lesions [2]. Keratinocytes often experience regulated proliferation and differentiation as a component of the skin's healing mechanism. In psoriasis, the signaling pathways involving Nuclear Factor kappa B [NF-κB], Mitogen-Activated Protein Kinases [MAPKs], and Janus Kinase/Signal Transducer and Activator of Transcription [JAK/STAT] are not functioning properly, as shown in Fig. (**1**). This leads to an excessive growth of keratinocytes and a disruption in their normal development. This leads to the development of distinctive psoriatic plaques, which are characterized by a thicker outer layer of skin, longitudinal folds in the lower layer of skin, and the presence of abnormal keratinization [5, 6].

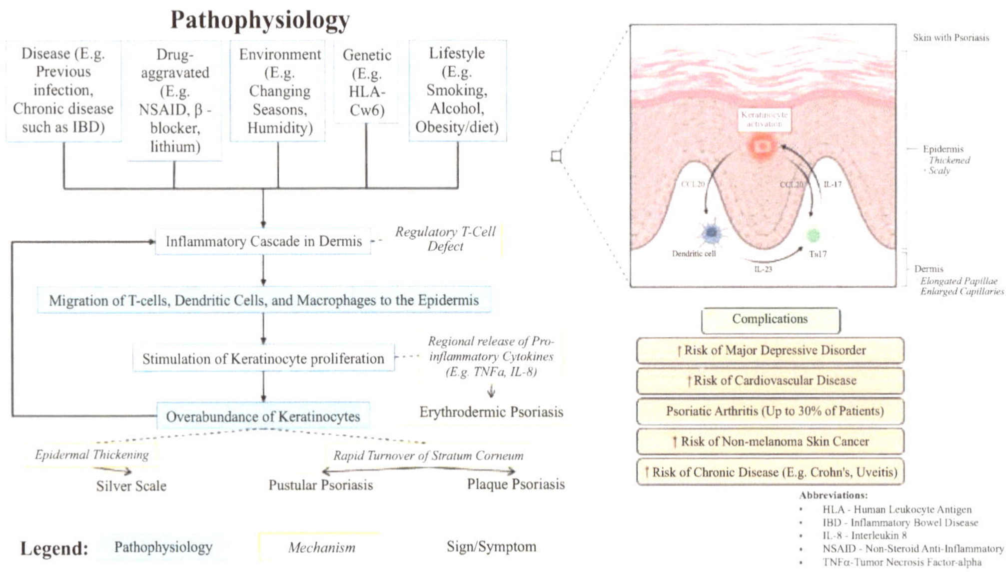

Fig. (1). Pathophysiology of psoriasis.

Role of Genetic and Environmental Factors

The development of psoriasis is significantly influenced by genetic predisposition, including a complex interaction of many susceptibility genes. Genetic variations in genes that code for immune-related components, including Human Leukocyte Antigens [HLA], cytokines, and cytokine receptors, have a role in the abnormal immunological responses seen in psoriasis, as shown in Fig. (**1**). Genetic factors alone are not sufficient to cause the onset of psoriasis, and environmental triggers are crucial in triggering disease flare-ups. Psoriasis may be worsened or triggered in those who are genetically prone to environmental factors such as stress, infections, trauma, smoking, obesity, and certain drugs. In addition, an imbalance in the skin's microbial community and changes in the control of gene activity may also affect the likelihood and intensity of psoriasis [7, 8].

To fully comprehend the pathophysiology of psoriasis and effectively develop targeted therapeutic interventions for this chronic inflammatory disorder, it is crucial to understand the intricate relationship between immune dysregulation, abnormal keratinocyte proliferation, and genetic and environmental factors.

CURRENT TREATMENT OPTIONS

The management of psoriasis involves a wide variety of therapeutic methods aimed at relieving symptoms, decreasing inflammation, and preventing abnormal growth of skin cells called keratinocytes. Treatment choices may be customized based on the severity and scope of the ailment, as well as the specific preferences and concurrent medical conditions of the patient [8].

Topical Therapies

Topical treatments are often used as the first therapy for mild to severe psoriasis. These therapies are topically applied to the afflicted regions of the skin. Typical examples of topical agents include:

- **Corticosteroids:** Potent anti-inflammatory agents that reduce redness, swelling, and itching [9].
- **Vitamin D analogs (*e.g.*, calcipotriene):** Inhibit keratinocyte proliferation and promote normal skin cell growth [10].
- **Retinoids (*e.g.*, tazarotene):** Normalize skin cell turnover and reduce inflammation [11].
- **Coal tar preparations:** Slow skin cell growth and alleviate itching and inflammation [12].
- **Emollients and moisturizers:** Hydrate the skin and relieve dryness and scaling [13].

Phototherapy [Light Therapy]

Phototherapy, often known as light therapy, is a treatment method that includes exposing the skin to Ultraviolet (UV) radiation. This exposure helps decrease inflammation and slow down the excessive proliferation of skin cells that are typical of psoriasis. Typical forms of phototherapy include:

- **UVB phototherapy:** Exposure to UVB light suppresses immune responses and reduces inflammation [13, 14].
- **PUVA therapy:** Psoralen, a light-sensitizing medication, is combined with UVA light to slow down the growth of skin cells [13].

Systemic Medications

Systemic treatments are indicated for cases of moderate to severe psoriasis that do not respond well to topical or phototherapy. These drugs aim to address inflammation and immunological dysregulation throughout the body. Systemic pharmaceuticals include a variety of drugs that are administered throughout the body to achieve a desired effect [14].

- **Methotrexate:** Suppresses the immune system and inhibits cell proliferation [15].

- **Cyclosporine:** Modulates immune responses by inhibiting T-cell activation [16].
- **Acitretin:** Derived from retinoids, it reduces inflammation and abnormal skin cell growth [16].
- **Apremilast:** Phosphodiesterase-4 inhibitor that reduces inflammation and modulates immune responses [15].

Biologic Agents

Biologic agents, or biologics, are immunomodulatory medicines that specifically target and disrupt components of the immune system that contribute to the development of psoriasis. Biologics are often prescribed for patients with moderate to severe psoriasis and include the following:

- **TNF-alpha inhibitors (*e.g.*, etanercept, adalimumab):** Block the action of TNF-alpha, a pro-inflammatory cytokine.
- **IL-17 inhibitors (*e.g.*, secukinumab, ixekizumab):** Target IL-17A, a key cytokine involved in psoriasis inflammation [1, 4, 6].
- **IL-23 inhibitors (*e.g.*, ustekinumab, guselkumab):** Block IL-23, a cytokine implicated in immune dysregulation in psoriasis [1].

LIMITATIONS OF MONOTHERAPY

Although monotherapy with topical medications, phototherapy, systemic drugs, or biologic agents may provide substantial benefits to many psoriasis patients, some restrictions might affect the effectiveness of treatment and long-term results.

Efficacy Challenges

Variability in Response

Psoriasis is a diverse condition, and the way patients respond to therapy might differ greatly. The effectiveness of a therapy may vary across patients, making it difficult to accurately predict the outcomes [17].

Limited Disease Control

Monotherapy may be insufficient in achieving adequate disease control for individuals with moderate to severe psoriasis, resulting in chronic symptoms, flare-ups, and functional impairment [18].

Partial Response

Certain individuals may only achieve partial relief with the use of a single medication, resulting in persistent regions of involvement or continued symptoms despite treatment [19].

Side Effects and Safety Concerns

Topical Agents

Prolonged use of topical corticosteroids, vitamin D analogs, and other topical therapies might lead to skin irritation, thinning, or discoloration. Additional possible adverse effects include hypersensitivity responses, follicular inflammation, and increased susceptibility to light [20].

Systemic Medications

Systemic drugs such as methotrexate and cyclosporine, and biological treatments may lead to several harmful consequences, including liver damage, kidney damage, digestive problems, suppression of bone marrow function, high blood pressure, and increased susceptibility to infections. Prolonged use of systemic drugs might also give rise to worries over the accumulation of harmful substances and problems associated with therapy [21].

Biologic Agents

Although biologic treatments are typically well-tolerated, they can pose risks such as immunosuppression, injection site responses, infusion reactions, and increased vulnerability to infections. Biologic treatment has been associated with infrequent but severe side effects, including demyelinating diseases, cancers, and congestive heart failure [22].

Development of Treatment Resistance

Primary Resistance

Certain individuals may not show a response to the first use of a single medication or may have a natural resistance to certain medicines due to unique variables, such as genetic variations or the intrinsic severity of their ailment [23].

Secondary Resistance

Even individuals who initially show a positive response to therapy may eventually develop secondary resistance, which may result in treatment failure or a decrease in effectiveness. This issue is especially significant for systemic drugs and biological agents, as the presence of antidrug antibodies or changes in drug metabolism might undermine the efficacy of therapy [22, 23].

To overcome the drawbacks of using a single psoriasis treatment, a comprehensive strategy is needed. This strategy should take into account several elements, such as the patient's specific characteristics, the severity of the illness, the desired treatment outcomes, and the balance between potential benefits and risks. To achieve optimal treatment results and enhance patient satisfaction in the management of psoriasis, a combination of medication, lifestyle adjustments, and diligent monitoring may be required.

RATIONALE FOR COMBINATION APPROACH

Psoriasis is a condition caused by a combination of hereditary factors, problems with the immune system, and exposure to certain environmental triggers. It is an autoimmune illness with several causes. Due to the varied and ever-changing nature of how psoriasis develops, using a combination strategy that addresses many ways the disease progresses at the same time has significant benefits compared to using just one treatment [24].

Multifactorial Nature of Psoriasis

Psoriasis is not exclusively caused by a single pathogenic process, but instead, it is influenced by an intricate combination of genetic, immunologic, and environmental variables. Psoriatic lesions are caused by a combination of genetic susceptibility variations, abnormal immune responses, disrupted cytokine signaling, and environmental stimuli. Therefore, no one therapy drug can adequately target the diverse and complex nature of psoriasis pathogenesis [25].

Targeting Multiple Pathogenic Pathways

A combined strategy enables the concurrent targeting of multiple pathogenic pathways involved in the development of psoriasis. Combining several treatments may have a more profound impact on disease activity, symptoms, and long-term results by targeting the main causes of inflammation, immunological dysfunction, and aberrant growth of skin cells. By combining medicines that hinder various pro-inflammatory cytokines or signaling pathways, it is possible to interrupt the inflammatory cascade at numerous stages. This may lead to synergistic therapeutic benefits and improved management of the illness [26].

Potential Synergistic Effects

Combining several therapies has the potential to produce synergistic benefits that are greater than the individual effectiveness of each treatment alone. Combining several therapy methods that work together and have similar goals may improve treatment results, speed up the elimination of symptoms, and extend the periods of remission. Synergistic interactions may happen at several levels, such as the regulation of cytokine production, inhibition of immunological responses, stabilization of keratinocyte proliferation, and restoration of skin barrier function. In addition, the use of combination therapy may help prevent the development of treatment resistance by concurrently targeting numerous pathways. This reduces the chances of illness recurrence or flare-ups in the long term [27].

CLINICAL EVIDENCE FOR COMBINATION THERAPY

Combining several treatment methods, known as combination therapy, is an effective approach for attaining the best results in treating psoriasis. Empirical research has conclusively shown that combination treatment plans are preferable to single-drug therapy in terms of effectiveness, safety, and the capacity to be tolerated by patients [28].

Clinical Studies

Multiple clinical studies have examined the effectiveness and safety of combining different treatments for managing psoriasis. These studies have explored combinations of topical medicines, phototherapy, systemic drugs, and biologic agents. The studies have examined various treatment plans, dosage methods, and groups of patients to see how combination therapy affects the activity of the illness, control of symptoms, and overall quality of life [29].

Comparative Efficacy of Combination vs. Monotherapy

Multiple Randomized Controlled Trials (RCTs) and observational studies have examined the effectiveness of combination treatment compared to monotherapy in treating psoriasis. These studies repeatedly show that combining several treatments yields greater improvements in the severity of the condition, earlier commencement of action, and better rates of treatment response compared to using a single medication alone. Furthermore, combination therapy has been shown to prolong the period of remission, decrease the occurrence of illness flares, and improve patient satisfaction with treatment results [30].

Safety and Tolerability Profiles

Combination therapy in psoriasis management involves using numerous treatment methods at the same time. Research studies have consistently shown that combination regimens are typically safe and well-tolerated. The adverse effects linked to combination treatment are generally mild to moderate in intensity and temporary in duration, with only a few cases of significant adverse events documented. Furthermore, healthcare practitioners may reduce treatment-related risks and enhance patient outcomes by customizing treatment regimens to suit specific patient requirements and continuously monitoring for any negative effects [31].

In general, clinical data confirms that combination therapy is a successful and well-tolerated method for treating psoriasis, providing better results than using a single treatment and leading to improved outcomes for patients. Combination regimens may effectively manage psoriasis by using the combined benefits of numerous therapy modalities. This approach not only reduces the occurrence of treatment-related side effects but also improves the overall quality of life for patients [31, 32].

ADVANTAGES OF COMBINATION THERAPY

Enhanced Therapeutic Efficacy

Synergistic Effects

Combination therapy utilizes the combined effects of many treatment methods, leading to improved therapeutic effectiveness as compared to using a single treatment method. Combination regimens may have a more significant and comprehensive impact on disease activity by concurrently addressing numerous pathogenic pathways [32].

Complementary Mechanisms of Action

Every part of a combination treatment may have distinct effects on the underlying causes of psoriasis, such as reducing inflammation, regulating immune responses, or preventing excessive growth of skin cells. Combining medicines with complementary modes of action in combination therapy may enhance treatment results and expedite the elimination of symptoms [33].

Improved Disease Control

Concurrently addressing numerous harmful pathways in psoriasis results in improved disease management, decreasing the intensity and size of skin lesions, minimizing symptoms, and extending remission times. Improved disease control leads to better overall treatment of psoriasis and more favorable long-term results for patients [34].

Reduced Risk of Treatment Resistance

Mitigation of Resistance Development

Combination therapy reduces the likelihood of treatment resistance by targeting numerous factors involved in the development of psoriasis. Combination regimens reduce the chances of selective pressure and the development of resistance mutations by interfering with the inflammatory cascade at various stages [35].

Diverse Mechanisms of Action

Utilizing a variety of therapeutic methods that have different ways of functioning decreases the chances of developing resistance to several drugs. Combination therapy utilizes several therapeutic targets that complement each other and do not overlap in their effects. This approach helps reduce the development of treatment resistance and maintains the efficacy of the treatment over a longer period [36].

Prevention of Flare-Ups

Combination therapy reduces the occurrence and intensity of illness flares, hence decreasing the need for increasing the dosage or making changes to the treatment. This contributes to the preservation of therapeutic effectiveness and hinders the development of disease phenotypes that are resistant to therapy [37].

Improved Patient Outcomes and Quality of Life

Enhanced Symptom Relief

Combining several therapies provides greater relief from symptoms compared to using a single treatment alone, leading to enhanced patient comfort, decreased itching, scaling, and redness, and improved overall management of symptoms [38].

Longer Remission Periods

Combination regimens that target many parts of psoriasis pathophysiology have the effect of extending periods of remission and decreasing the frequency of disease flares. As a result, there is enhanced disease management, reduced hospital admissions, and enhanced overall patient well-being [39].

Greater Treatment Satisfaction

Combining several treatments leads to improved effectiveness and lowers the chances of developing resistance to treatment. This, in turn, increases patient satisfaction, adherence to therapy, and trust in the results of the treatment. Patients encounter fewer treatment failures and have enhanced illness management, resulting in increased emotional well-being and overall quality of life [40].

CHALLENGES AND CONSIDERATIONS

Treatment Complexity

Multimodal Approach

The management of psoriasis often requires a multimodal strategy that involves several therapeutic methods, including topical medicines, phototherapy, systemic drugs, and biologic agents. Managing and improving the effectiveness of various treatment methods may be difficult, especially in individuals with moderate to severe illness or other health conditions [40].

Individualized Treatment Plans

Given the diverse nature of psoriasis, it is necessary to customize treatment programs based on the individual patient's specific requirements, preferences, and features of the illness. When creating personalized treatment plans, healthcare practitioners need to take into account several criteria, including the severity of the condition, the degree of its impact, the patient's prior reactions to therapy, and the patient's preferences [41].

Treatment Adherence

Patient adherence may be affected by the complexity of treatment regimens, which may include the use of various drugs, distinct formulations, and diverse dose schedules. Adherence rates may be affected by factors such as pharmaceutical side effects, inconvenience, and expense, which might undermine the efficacy of therapy [42].

Cost Considerations

Financial Burden

Psoriasis therapy, especially biological medicines and systemic drugs, may place a substantial economic strain on patients. Expensive medicine, restrictions on insurance coverage, copayments, and personal fees may restrict access to the best therapy and influence treatment choices [43].

Cost-Effectiveness

Healthcare practitioners must take into account the cost-efficiency of treatment alternatives in relation to their effectiveness, safety, and long-term results. It is crucial to optimize value for patients and healthcare systems by carefully considering the cost of therapy in relation to its potential benefits [42, 43].

Drug Interactions and Toxicities

Polypharmacy Risks

Psoriasis patients often get many drugs simultaneously, which heightens the likelihood of drug interactions and negative responses. Healthcare practitioners must thoroughly evaluate possible drug-drug interactions, closely observe for negative effects, and modify treatment plans as needed to reduce risks and enhance patient safety [44, 45].

Toxicity Monitoring

Certain therapies for psoriasis, such as systemic medicines and biologic drugs, might have unique toxicities or side effects. It is crucial to regularly monitor laboratory measures, such as liver function tests, renal function tests, lipid profiles, and complete blood counts, to rapidly diagnose and manage any toxicities linked to the medication [44, 45].

Patient Monitoring and Management

Regular Follow-Up

Psoriasis is a persistent condition that needs continuous monitoring and management to evaluate the effectiveness of therapy, track the activity of the disease, and make necessary adjustments to treatment plans. Regular follow-up appointments with healthcare practitioners are crucial for assessing the efficacy of therapy, addressing patient concerns, and maximizing treatment results [8].

Patient Education

Providing patients with information and knowledge about their situation is very important in managing psoriasis. This helps patients to understand their condition better, follow their treatment plans, and identify any worsening of the illness or negative consequences caused by the medication. Providing a thorough education on treatment alternatives, lifestyle adjustments, and self-management techniques may enhance treatment adherence and improve patient outcomes [8].

FUTURE DIRECTIONS

Emerging Therapeutic Targets

Precision Medicine

Progress in molecular biology and genetics has resulted in the discovery of new therapeutic targets involved in the development of psoriasis. Targeted medicines that specifically target cytokines, signaling pathways, immune cells, and inflammatory mediators show potential for more accurate and efficient therapy of psoriasis [30, 31].

Biologic Innovations

Further investigation into the pathophysiology of psoriasis has the potential to reveal novel biological medicines that possess distinctive modes of action and enhanced treatment profiles. Novel biotechnological advancements aimed at developing cytokines, interleukins, or cellular targets can potentially broaden the range of available therapeutic choices for psoriasis [20].

Personalized Treatment Approaches

Genomic Profiling

Genomic profiling and biomarker analysis provide prospects for individualized treatment strategies in psoriasis. Healthcare practitioners may optimize therapy effectiveness and minimize unwanted effects by tailoring treatment regimens to meet specific patient features, such as genetic predispositions, immunological profiles, and disease subtypes [19, 28, 45].

Precision Medicine Algorithms

The incorporation of genomic data, biomarker analysis, and clinical phenotyping into precision medicine algorithms has the potential to allow healthcare providers to anticipate treatment responses, categorize patients based on risk profiles, and tailor treatment plans to meet individualized patient needs and preferences [30, 32, 38].

Innovation in Combination Therapy

Optimized Combination Regimens

Innovation in combination therapy involves the creation of improved treatment regimens that use synergistic interactions between several treatment methods. Combining medicines with different modes of action, targeted delivery methods, or new formulations may increase the effectiveness of treatment, reduce resistance to treatment, and improve patient results [37, 43].

Integrated Treatment Platforms

Incorporating existing systemic drugs, biologic agents, topical treatments, and new therapy methods into integrated treatment platforms may provide comprehensive ways to manage psoriasis. These platforms may integrate patient education, lifestyle adjustments, telemedicine, and multidisciplinary care to provide thorough and well-coordinated treatment for individuals with psoriasis [41, 44].

CONCLUSION AND TAKEAWAYS

Psoriasis is a multifaceted autoimmune condition affected by genetic, immunological, and environmental factors. Using only one treatment method, such as topical medicines, phototherapy, systemic pharmaceuticals, or biologics, has limitations in terms of how effective it is, how safe it is, and the likelihood of the treatment becoming ineffective over time [2, 17]. Simultaneously employing numerous therapies in a combination strategy can offer substantial benefits. The combination technique exploits the combinatorial impact of addressing multiple pathogenic pathways implicated in the development of psoriasis. By considering the multiple factors contributing to the condition and implementing a comprehensive treatment plan, healthcare providers can increase the effectiveness of therapy, reduce the chances of treatment resistance, and enhance the overall results and quality of life for patients. This holistic strategy is especially advantageous for individuals with moderate to severe psoriasis or those who have not had a satisfactory response to a single medication [7]. When incorporating combination therapy into clinical practice, healthcare professionals must take into account the intricacy of managing numerous treatment modalities, potential drug interactions, and the monitoring of toxicity. Prudent selection of patients, personalized planning of therapy, and vigilant monitoring are crucial to guarantee the secure and efficient utilization of combination medicines. Providing patients with information about the reasoning and anticipated results of the combined strategy can enhance their adherence to therapy and improve overall outcomes [15, 27]. Promising areas for future advancements in psoriasis management involve investigating novel therapeutic targets, devising precision medicine approaches, and incorporating diverse treatment modalities into integrated care platforms. Further research in these fields has the potential to enhance the optimization of combination therapy and offer more individualized and effective care for this persistent and complex skin condition [44, 45].

REFERENCES

[1] Ghoreschi K, Balato A, Enerbäck C, Sabat R. Therapeutics targeting the IL-23 and IL-17 pathway in psoriasis. Lancet 2021; 397(10275): 754-66.
[http://dx.doi.org/10.1016/S0140-6736(21)00184-7] [PMID: 33515492]

[2] Boehncke WH, Schön MP. Psoriasis. Lancet 2015; 386(9997): 983-94.
[http://dx.doi.org/10.1016/S0140-6736(14)61909-7] [PMID: 26025581]

[3] Tait Wojno ED, Hunter CA, Stumhofer JS. The immunobiology of the interleukin-12 family: room for discovery. Immunity 2019; 50(4): 851-70.
[http://dx.doi.org/10.1016/j.immuni.2019.03.011] [PMID: 30995503]

[4] McGeachy MJ, Cua DJ, Gaffen SL. The IL-17 family of cytokines in health and disease. Immunity 2019; 50(4): 892-906.
[http://dx.doi.org/10.1016/j.immuni.2019.03.021] [PMID: 30995505]

[5] Bugaut H, Aractingi S. Major role of the IL17/23 axis in psoriasis supports the development of new targeted therapies. Front Immunol 2021; 12: 621956.
[http://dx.doi.org/10.3389/fimmu.2021.621956] [PMID: 33717124]

[6] Gallais Sérézal I, Classon C, Cheuk S, *et al.* Resident T cells in resolved psoriasis steer tissue responses that stratify clinical outcome. J Invest Dermatol 2018; 138(8): 1754-63.
[http://dx.doi.org/10.1016/j.jid.2018.02.030] [PMID: 29510191]

[7] Wang CY, Wang CW, Chen CB, *et al.* Pharmacogenomics on the treatment response in patients with psoriasis: an updated review. Int J Mol Sci 2023; 24(8): 7329.
[http://dx.doi.org/10.3390/ijms24087329] [PMID: 37108492]

[8] Guidelines for the diagnosis and treatment of psoriasis in China: 2019 concise edition#. International Journal of Dermatology and Venereology 2020; 3(1): 14-26.
[http://dx.doi.org/10.1097/JD9.0000000000000074]

[9] Gossec L, Smolen JS, Ramiro S, *et al.* European league against rheumatism (EULAR) recommendations for the management of psoriatic arthritis with pharmacological therapies: 2015 update. Ann Rheum Dis 2016; 75(3): 499-510.
[http://dx.doi.org/10.1136/annrheumdis-2015-208337] [PMID: 26644232]

[10] Smith CH, Jabbar-Lopez ZK, Yiu ZZ, *et al.* British association of dermatologists guidelines for biologic therapy for psoriasis 2017. Br J Dermatol 2017; 177(3): 628-36.
[http://dx.doi.org/10.1111/bjd.15665] [PMID: 28513835]

[11] Puig L. PASI 90 response: the new standard in therapeutic efficacy for psoriasis. J Eur Acad Dermatol Venereol 2015; 29(4): 645-8.
[http://dx.doi.org/10.1111/jdv.12817] [PMID: 25370811]

[12] Torres T, Puig L. Treatment goals for psoriasis: Should PASI 90 become the standard of care? Actas Dermo-Sifiliográficas (English Edition) 2015; 106(3): 155-7.
[http://dx.doi.org/10.1016/j.adengl.2014.10.005] [PMID: 25455503]

[13] Coates LC, Kavanaugh A, Mease PJ, *et al.* Group for research and assessment of psoriasis and psoriatic arthritis 2015 treatment recommendations for psoriatic arthritis. Arthritis Rheumatol 2016; 68(5): 1060-71.
[http://dx.doi.org/10.1002/art.39573] [PMID: 26749174]

[14] Armstrong AW, Bagel J, Van Voorhees AS, Robertson AD, Yamauchi PS. Combining biologic therapies with other systemic treatments in psoriasis: evidence-based, best-practice recommendations from the medical board of the national psoriasis foundation. JAMA Dermatol 2015; 151(4): 432-8. [http://dx.doi.org/10.1001/jamadermatol.2014.3456] [PMID: 25517130]

[15] Ramiro S, Smolen JS, Landewé R, *et al.* Pharmacological treatment of psoriatic arthritis: a systematic literature review for the 2015 update of the EULAR recommendations for the management of psoriatic arthritis. Ann Rheum Dis 2016; 75(3): 490-8. [http://dx.doi.org/10.1136/annrheumdis-2015-208466] [PMID: 26660203]

[16] Gossec L, Coates LC, de Wit M, *et al.* Management of psoriatic arthritis in 2016: a comparison of EULAR and GRAPPA recommendations. Nat Rev Rheumatol 2016; 12(12): 743-50. [http://dx.doi.org/10.1038/nrrheum.2016.183] [PMID: 27829672]

[17] Kaushik SB, Lebwohl MG. Psoriasis: Which therapy for which patient. J Am Acad Dermatol 2019; 80(1): 27-40. [http://dx.doi.org/10.1016/j.jaad.2018.06.057] [PMID: 30017705]

[18] Jiang Y, Chen Y, Yu Q, Shi Y. Biologic and small-molecule therapies for moderate-to-severe psoriasis: focus on psoriasis comorbidities. BioDrugs 2023; 37(1): 35-55. [http://dx.doi.org/10.1007/s40259-022-00569-z] [PMID: 36592323]

[19] Strober B, Ryan C, van de Kerkhof P, *et al.* Recategorization of psoriasis severity: Delphi consensus from the international psoriasis council. J Am Acad Dermatol 2020; 82(1): 117-22. [http://dx.doi.org/10.1016/j.jaad.2019.08.026] [PMID: 31425723]

[20] Mahil SK, Wilson N, Dand N, *et al.* Psoriasis treat to target: defining outcomes in psoriasis using data from a real-world, population-based cohort study (the British Association of Dermatologists Biologics and Immunomodulators Register, BADBIR). Br J Dermatol 2020; 182(5): 1158-66. [http://dx.doi.org/10.1111/bjd.18333] [PMID: 31286471]

[21] Brownstone ND, Hong J, Mosca M, *et al.* Biologic treatments of psoriasis: an update for the clinician. Biologics 2021; 15: 39-51. [PMID: 33623366]

[22] Marotte H, Cimaz R. Etanercept – TNF receptor and IgG1 Fc fusion protein: is it different from other TNF blockers? Expert Opin Biol Ther 2014; 14(5): 569-72. [http://dx.doi.org/10.1517/14712598.2014.896334] [PMID: 24611432]

[23] Singh R, Koppu S, Perche PO, Feldman SR. The cytokine mediated molecular pathophysiology of psoriasis and its clinical implications. Int J Mol Sci 2021; 22(23): 12793. [http://dx.doi.org/10.3390/ijms222312793] [PMID: 34884596]

[24] Goel N, Stephens S. Certolizumab pegol. MAbs 2010; 2(2): 137-47. [http://dx.doi.org/10.4161/mabs.2.2.11271] [PMID: 20190560]

[25] Veronese FM, Mero A. The impact of PEGylation on biological therapies. BioDrugs 2008; 22(5): 315-29. [http://dx.doi.org/10.2165/00063030-200822050-00004] [PMID: 18778113]

[26] Mariette X, Förger F, Abraham B, *et al.* Lack of placental transfer of certolizumab pegol during pregnancy: results from CRIB, a prospective, postmarketing, pharmacokinetic study. Ann Rheum Dis 2018; 77(2): 228-33. [http://dx.doi.org/10.1136/annrheumdis-2017-212196] [PMID: 29030361]

[27] Yang K, Oak ASW, Elewski BE. Use of IL-23 inhibitors for the treatment of plaque psoriasis and psoriatic arthritis: a comprehensive review. Am J Clin Dermatol 2021; 22(2): 173-92. [http://dx.doi.org/10.1007/s40257-020-00578-0] [PMID: 33301128]

[28] Kulig P, Musiol S, Freiberger SN, *et al.* IL-12 protects from psoriasiform skin inflammation. Nat Commun 2016; 7(1): 13466. [http://dx.doi.org/10.1038/ncomms13466] [PMID: 27892456]

[29] Blauvelt A, Kimball AB, Augustin M, *et al.* Efficacy and safety of mirikizumab in psoriasis: results from a 52-week, double-blind, placebo-controlled, randomized withdrawal, phase III trial (OASIS-1). Br J Dermatol 2022; 187(6): 866-77.
[http://dx.doi.org/10.1111/bjd.21743] [PMID: 35791755]

[30] Zhou L, Wang Y, Wan Q, *et al.* A non-clinical comparative study of IL-23 antibodies in psoriasis. MAbs 2021; 13(1): 1964420.
[http://dx.doi.org/10.1080/19420862.2021.1964420] [PMID: 34460338]

[31] Ghazawi FM, Mahmood F, Kircik L, *et al.* A review of the efficacy and safety for biologic agents targeting IL-23 in treating psoriasis with the focus on tildrakizumab. Front Med (Lausanne) 2021; 8: 702776.
[http://dx.doi.org/10.3389/fmed.2021.702776] [PMID: 34447766]

[32] ten Bergen LL, Petrovic A, Krogh Aarebrot A, Appel S. The TNF/IL-23/IL-17 axis—Head-to-head trials comparing different biologics in psoriasis treatment. Scand J Immunol 2020; 92(4): e12946.
[http://dx.doi.org/10.1111/sji.12946] [PMID: 32697374]

[33] Facheris P, Valenti M, Pavia G, Guanziroli E, Narcisi A, Borroni RG, *et al.* Brodalumab: A new way to inhibit <scp>IL</scp> -17 in psoriasis. Dermatol Ther (Heidelb) 2020; 33. [3].

[34] Ruggiero A, Potestio L, Camela E Snr, Fabbrocini G, Megna M. Bimekizumab for the treatment of psoriasis: a review of the current knowledge. Psoriasis (Auckl) 2022; 12: 127-37.
[http://dx.doi.org/10.2147/PTT.S367744] [PMID: 35707807]

[35] Torres T, Filipe P. Small molecules in the treatment of psoriasis. Drug Dev Res 2015; 76(5): 215-27.
[http://dx.doi.org/10.1002/ddr.21263] [PMID: 26255795]

[36] Gao JC, Wu AG, Contento MN, Maher JM, Cline A. Apremilast in the treatment of plaque psoriasis: differential use in psoriasis. Clin Cosmet Investig Dermatol 2022; 15: 395-402.
[http://dx.doi.org/10.2147/CCID.S266036] [PMID: 35300435]

[37] Warren RB, Strober B, Silverberg JI, *et al.* Oral orismilast: Efficacy and safety in moderate-to-severe psoriasis and development of modified release tablets. J Eur Acad Dermatol Venereol 2023; 37(4): 711-20.
[http://dx.doi.org/10.1111/jdv.18812] [PMID: 36478476]

[38] Dodson J, Lio PA. Biologics and small molecule inhibitors: an update in therapies for allergic and immunologic skin diseases. Curr Allergy Asthma Rep 2022; 22(12): 183-93.
[http://dx.doi.org/10.1007/s11882-022-01047-w] [PMID: 36348149]

[39] Hoy SM. Deucravacitinib: First approval. Drugs 2022; 82(17): 1671-9.
[http://dx.doi.org/10.1007/s40265-022-01796-y] [PMID: 36401743]

[40] Zhang J, Qi F, Dong J, Tan Y, Gao L, Liu F. Application of baricitinib in dermatology. J Inflamm Res 2022; 15: 1935-41.
[http://dx.doi.org/10.2147/JIR.S356316] [PMID: 35330989]

[41] Thakur V, Mahajan R. Novel therapeutic target(s) for psoriatic disease. Front Med (Lausanne) 2022; 9: 712313.
[http://dx.doi.org/10.3389/fmed.2022.712313] [PMID: 35265634]

[42] Mascarenhas-Melo F, Carvalho A, Gonçalves MBS, Paiva-Santos AC, Veiga F. Nanocarriers for the topical treatment of psoriasis - pathophysiology, conventional treatments, nanotechnology, regulatory and toxicology. Eur J Pharm Biopharm 2022; 176: 95-107.
[http://dx.doi.org/10.1016/j.ejpb.2022.05.012] [PMID: 35605927]

[43] Wang X, Kaiser H, Kvist-Hansen A, *et al.* IL-17 pathway members as potential biomarkers of effective systemic treatment and cardiovascular disease in patients with moderate-to-severe psoriasis. Int J Mol Sci 2022; 23(1): 555.
[http://dx.doi.org/10.3390/ijms23010555] [PMID: 35008981]

[44] Bai F, Zheng W, Dong Y, *et al.* Serum levels of adipokines and cytokines in psoriasis patients: a systematic review and meta-analysis. Oncotarget 2018; 9(1): 1266-78. [http://dx.doi.org/10.18632/oncotarget.22260] [PMID: 29416693]

[45] Dickerson T, Lee BI, Montgomery P, *et al.* Mind.Px – personalized medicine for psoriasis biologic treatment. SKIN The Journal of Cutaneous Medicine 2021; 5(6): s46. [http://dx.doi.org/10.25251/skin.5.supp.46]

CHAPTER 4

Gene Therapies in the Management of Psoriasis

Nidhi Gairola[1,*], **Shalu Verma**[1] and **Bhawna**[1]

[1] *Uttaranchal Institute of Pharmaceutical Sciences, Uttaranchal University, Dehradun 248001, Uttarakhand, India*

Abstract: Psoriasis is a long-lasting autoimmune dermatological disorder affecting millions of individuals globally, causing substantial physical and psychological distress. While various treatment options, including topical creams, phototherapy, and systemic medications, resulted in relief for several sufferers, a significant portion of those affected by psoriasis remains inadequately treated. In recent years, gene therapy has emerged as a promising frontier in the field of dermatology, offering the potential for more effective and targeted treatments. This chapter reviews the current landscape of gene therapies for the management of psoriasis. It explores the underlying genetic factors contributing to psoriasis susceptibility, emphasizing the role of the immune system and the dysregulation of keratinocyte proliferation. The chapter also explores the various gene therapy approaches being developed to target these specific mechanisms. Recent advancements in gene editing technologies, such as CRISPR-Cas9, have paved the way for precise and targeted modification of genes associated with psoriasis. Researchers are developing strategies to either suppress overactive immune responses or correct genetic mutations that contribute to the pathogenesis of psoriasis. Promising preclinical and clinical results suggest that gene therapies hold the potential to provide long-lasting relief and even a cure for some patients. While gene therapy for psoriasis is still in its experimental stages, early trials have shown encouraging results with minimal side effects. It is essential to acknowledge the challenges and ethical considerations associated with gene therapy, including the need for rigorous safety and efficacy assessments. In conclusion, gene therapies offer a promising avenue for treating psoriasis, with the potential to revolutionize the management of this chronic condition. Ongoing research and clinical trials will determine the safety and effectiveness of these innovative approaches, ultimately providing hope for those suffering from psoriasis and paving the way for personalized, precision medicine in dermatology.

Keywords: Autoimmune, CRISPR-Cas9, Gene Therapy, Keratinocyte Proliferation, Psoriasis Management.

* **Corresponding author Nidhi Gairola:** Uttaranchal Institute of Pharmaceutical Sciences, Uttaranchal University, Dehradun 248001, Uttarakhand, India; E-mail: nidhigairola@uumail.in

Anjali Sharma, Prerna Sharma, Roy Rillera Marzo & Ahmed A. Al Karmalawy (Eds.)

INTRODUCTION

Psoriasis is a prevalent, persistent papulosquamous dermatological disorder that can develop at any age and varies in prevalence depending on the nation, indicating that environmental variables, genetic background, and ethnicity all influence its emergence [1]. It is related to a multitude of significant medical dysfunctions, such as psoriatic arthritis, depression, and cardiometabolic syndrome. Psoriasis is an inflammatory dermatological condition that affects approximately 60 million people and children worldwide [2]. One of the WHO's primary research priorities is determining the worldwide burden of psoriasis. It is characterized by erythematous plaques that are well-defined and covered with silvery-white scales, usually affecting the elbows, knees, trunk, and scalp in a symmetrical pattern. This is at least three times more than the number of DALYs caused by inflammatory bowel disease [3]. When genetic and/or environmental factors activate plasmacytoid dendritic cells, proinflammatory cytokines such as tumor necrosis factor [TNF]-α, interferon [IFN]-γ, interleukin [IL]-17, IL-22, IL-23, and IL-1β are produced; this refers to the initial stage of psoriasis [4]. Among the acknowledged environmental causes and correlations are streptococcal infections, physical trauma, specific medications (including antidepressants, antihypertensive meds, and anti-cytokine therapy), smoking, and alcohol addiction. It wasn't until 1841 that von Hebra recognized psoriasis as a distinct medical condition, dispelling the earlier belief that it was a variant of leprosy [5]. Hereditary factors primarily influence the pathophysiology of psoriasis. Situated on chromosome 6p21, inside a roughly 220 kb length of the major histocompatibility complex, is a substantial susceptibility locus for psoriasis known as PSORS1. An early onset of severe and unstable sickness is associated with the susceptibility allele within PSORS1, HLA-Cw6 [6]. The three primary histologic features of psoriasis are epidermal hyperplasia, dilated and prominent blood vessels in the dermis, and an inflammatory leukocyte infiltrate, primarily in the dermis. In addition to the skin, psoriasis also affects the joints and nails. The three main clinical manifestations of psoriasis are Generalised Pustular Psoriasis [GPP], psoriasis vulgaris, and psoriatic arthritis. Obesity, diabetes, metabolic syndrome, hypertension, hyperlipidaemia, psoriatic march, inflammatory march, and chronic kidney disease are other systemic disorders that may occur with psoriasis. Psoriasis patients frequently experience psychological difficulties and psychiatric conditions, including depression [7]. Fig. (**1**) illustrates the key symptoms of psoriasis, providing an overview of its clinical presentation, and Fig. (**2**) highlights the risk factors associated with the onset and worsening of psoriasis.

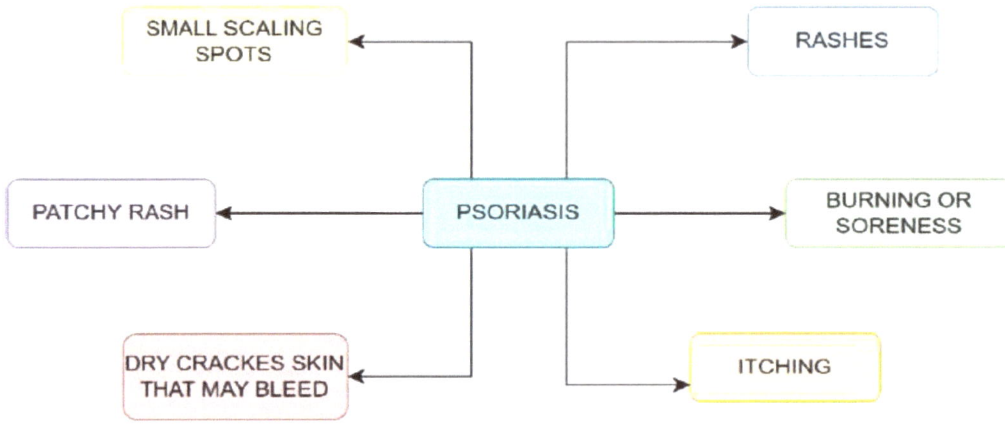

Fig. (1). Symptoms of psoriasis.

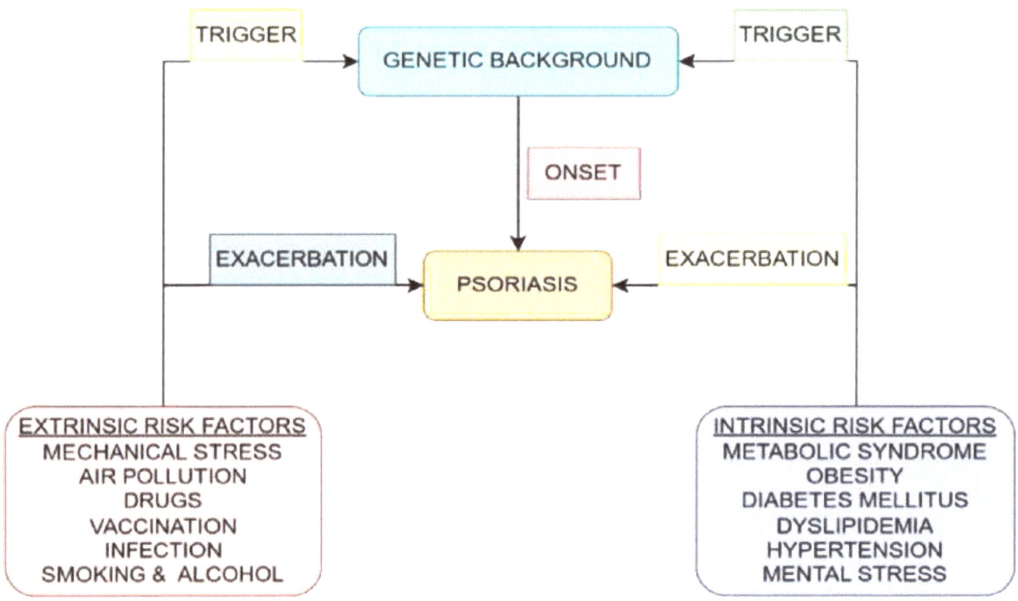

Fig. (2). Risk factors for onset and worsening of psoriasis [8].

PREVALENCE

Studies conducted recently indicate that around 8 million Americans suffer from psoriasis [9]. The World Psoriasis Day consortium estimates that approximately 125 million individuals worldwide, or 2-3% of the global population, suffer from psoriasis. Approximately thirty percent of individuals with psoriasis are likely to develop psoriatic arthritis [10]. 3.6 percent of Caucasians and 1.5 percent of African Americans suffer from psoriasis [11]. Due to variations in clinical presentation, psoriasis is probably underdiagnosed in African Americans and other people with skin of color [12]. Although psoriasis can develop in both genders, women and those with a familial history are at risk of developing it earlier. Its age of beginning, peaking 10 years earlier in women and 30–39 and 60–69 years older in men [13]. Psoriasis is estimated to affect approximately 60 million individuals globally; prevalence rates vary by country, ranging from 0.05% in Taiwan to 1.88% in Australia [14]. It is more prevalent in affluent and older demographic areas.

CLINICAL MANIFESTATIONS OF PSORIASIS

Table **1** summarizes the clinical manifestations of psoriasis, distinguishing its various forms and presentations.

Table 1. Clinical manifestations of psoriasis.

Manifestations	Types	Key Findings
Plaque psoriasis	-	> 0.5 cm in diameter, well-circumscribed, erythematous, scaly plaques that can occur as a single lesion or as a widespread illness
-	Flexural	Also called inverted psoriasis or intertriginous psoriasis. Localised to the skin folds (inframammary, axillary, groin, genital, and natal cleft regions), well-defined, thin plaques with minimal scaling.
-	Nail	Can appear separately from concurrent skin plaques. Leukonychia, cracking, red lunular, oil drop sign, splinter haemorrhage, distal onycholysis, and subungual hyperkeratosis. Psoriatic arthritis is predicted by nail involvement.
-	Scalp	Extremely prevalent, challenging to treat.
-	Palmoplantar	Restricted to the hands and foot soles. Confluent redness and scaling ranging from huge plaques covering the palm or sole to ill-defined scaly or fissured areas without evident plaques.
Other variants	Guttate	Sudden outburst of tiny, finely scaled, salmon-pink papules on the trunk or limbs known as "dew drop." Able to track the group's history, specifically for infections such as perianal streptococcal infections, pharyngitis caused by *streptococci*, and dermatitis caused by *Streptococcus*.
-	Pustular	Monomorphic pustule sheets on painful, irritated skin, usually confined to the soles or palms.
-	Erythroderma	Generalised erythema that covers 90% or more of the patient's body and exhibits minimal scaling at the time of acute or subacute onset. May be linked to high-output heart failure, hypoalbuminemia, hypothermia, and electrolyte abnormalities. An emergency that could be fatal.
-	Annular	Erythematous, scaly plaques that are well-defined and have a centre clearing.

PATHOPHYSIOLOGY

The pathogenesis of psoriasis is explained by a variety of causes. The amphipathic structure, positively charged nature, and 12- to 50-amino acid composition of AMPs make them vital for shielding hosts against viruses, bacteria, fungi, and protozoa [15]. Moreover, AMPs influence host inflammatory responses as chemotactic agents, angiogenic factors, and regulators of cell proliferation in vertebrates. In response to cytokine stimulation and damage in psoriasis, keratinocytes, neutrophils, and macrophages significantly generate and release certain AMPs, such as cathelicidin, S100 proteins, and β-defensins [16]. One such autoantigen is the protein A Disintegrin and Metalloprotease Domain Containing Thrombospondin Type 1 Motif-Like 5 [ADAMTSL5], which is generated from melanocytes. Melanocytes expressing ADAMTSL5 are recognized by intra-epidermal CD8 T cells in correlation with HLA-C*06:02. With IL17 stimulation, keratinocytes create ADAMTSL5, and CXCL1, a melanocyte growth factor and neutrophil chemoattractant, induces ADAMTSL5 expression [17]. Increased melanocyte counts and T lymphocytes, particularly cytotoxic T cells, co-localize with melanocytes in psoriasis [18]. Fig. (**3**) explains the pathophysiology of psoriasis, outlining the immune system's role in disease progression.

Dermal conventional DCs (cDCs), derived from bone marrow, inflammatory DCs (iDCs), pDCs, and epidermal Langerhans Cells (LCs) comprise the majority of the complex network of DCs present in the skin. Psoriasis develops because DCs are an important source of TNF-α, IL-12, IL-23, and IFN-α within the cell. pDCs, which come from the bone marrow, migrate to the skin due to pathologic conditions [19]. When pDCs attach themselves to endosomal Toll-Like Receptors (TLRs), such as TLR7 and 9, they are able to recognise viral nucleic acids and produce large amounts of type I IFNs [20, 21]. Psoriatic inflammation starts when pDCs produce IFNα after misidentifying self-nucleic acids. TLR7, 8, and 9 in psoriasis can be activated by AMPs such as LL37, human β-defensin (hBD) 2, hBD3, and lysozyme when self-DNA or RNA is condensed into particles that are endocytosed by pDCs [22, 23].

Skin cells have high levels of expression for the transcription factor and cytosolic ligand-activated receptor AhR. AhR ligands include dioxins and other endogenous and exogenous substances. AhR controls the homeostasis of the Th17/22 system, which is critical for the onset of psoriasis. Moreover, AhR in cutaneous Vascular Endothelial Cells (VECs) plays a critical role in the development of psoriasis [24]. Zhu *et al.* found that AhR in cutaneous VECs downregulates neutrophil recruitment through adhesion molecule ICAM-1 in psoriasis using particular AhR knockout mice [25]. IL17 is produced by innate lymphoid cells, Th17, Tc17, and δT cells in the skin. The production of IL17 is stimulated by dermal DC expression of IL23. TNF, IL-26, IL-29 (IFN-λ1), and IL-17 are produced under certain conditions, such as psoriasis autoantigens and/or specific environmental stimuli (*e.g.*, trauma or infection) [26]. These cytokine signals trigger a feed-forward inflammatory response in keratinocytes by activating STAT1, nuclear factor kB, and CCAAT enhancer-binding protein [C/EBP] β or δ. This feed-forward effect speeds up the progression of psoriasis [27]. Together, TNF and IL-17 promote the transcription of several proinflammatory genes activated by IL-17, including TNF, IL-1β, IL-6, and IL-8. In draining lymph nodes and the skin, they promote the growth of Th17 cells and activate mDCs [28].

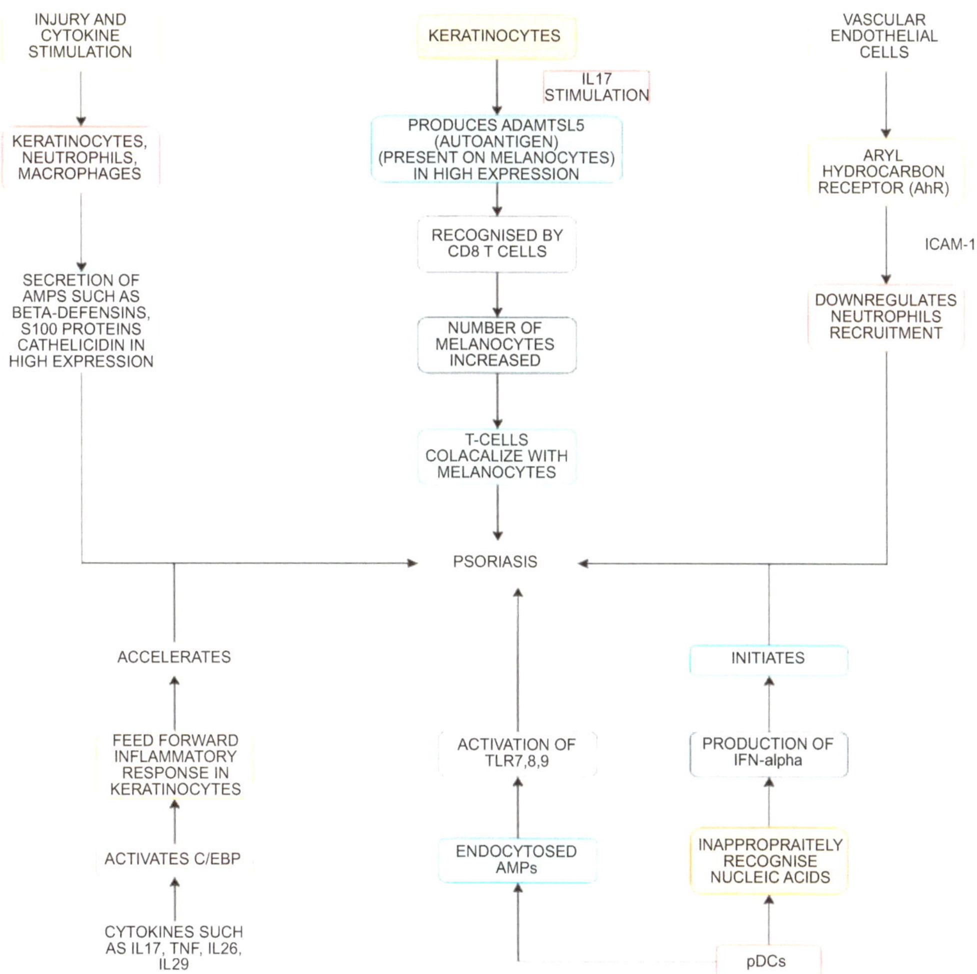

Fig. (3). Pathophysiology of psoriasis.

DIAGNOSIS

Table **2** presents the differential diagnosis of psoriasis, comparing the distinguishable clinical features with those of other dermatological conditions.

Table 2. Differential diagnosis of psoriasis with distinguishable clinical features [29].

Differential Diagnosis	Distinguishing Clinical Features
Atopic dermatitis	The predominant pruritus symptom, with typical form and location (vesicles in infancy, face and extensor papules and lichenification in adults and older children).
Contact dermatitis	Patches or plaques having sharp edges, geometric shapes, and angular corners, depending on how long they were exposed to an allergy or irritation.
Lichen planus	Violaceous lesions and recurrent involvement of the mucosa.
Secondary syphilis	Lesions with a copper hue and a tendency to affect the palms and soles of the feet.
Mycosis fungoides	Lesions of irregular shape, asymmetric distribution, unusual hue, and wrinkles from epidermal atrophy.
Tinea corporis	Fewer lesions in the form of an annulus.
Pityriasis rosea	Oval, tan-pink papules and patches on the trunk like a "Christmas tree," sparing the face and distal extremities.

CURRENT ARMAMENTARIUM

Drugs available for oral systemic therapy. Table 3 lists drugs available for oral systemic therapy, categorizing them based on their mechanism of action.

Table 3. Drugs available for oral systemic therapy [30, 31].

Drug	MOA	Application
Methotrexate	Inhibition of dihydrofolate reductase prevents the synthesis of purines and causes lymphocyte death.	Oral/S.C
Cyclosporin	Inhibition of calcineurin resulting in decreased IL-2.	Oral
Acitretin	Normalisation of keratinocyte differentiation and proliferation through interaction with retinoid receptors.	Oral
Fumarate	Intracellular glutathione, NF-κB, Nrf2, and HIF-1α regulation. Facilitating the transition from pro-inflammatory Th1/Th17 to anti-inflammatory/regulatory Th2 responses.	Oral
Apremilast	Immune and non-immune cell types' intracellular cAMP levels are raised by PDE4 inhibitors, which modulate inflammation.	Oral

Biologics Available

Different biologics are available for treating psoriasis, each with a distinct mechanism. A few examples are provided in the table. Table 4 provides an overview of biologics available for psoriasis treatment, detailing their therapeutic targets.

Table 4. Biologics available for treatment [32 - 34].

Biologics	Category	Mechanism	Route
Adalimumab	TNF-antagonist	Anti-TNF-α human monoclonal antibody	S.C
Certolizumab	TNF-antagonist	Polyethylene glycol-conjugated humanised monoclonal antibody fragment against TNF-α	S.C
Etanercept	TNF-antagonist	Man-made dimeric fusion protein that resembles TNF-αR	S.C
Infliximab	TNF-antagonist	Monoclonal antibody chimeric IgG1κ that binds to both soluble and transmembrane versions of TNF-α	I.V
Brodalumab	IL17-antagonist	IgG2 monoclonal antibody from humans that targets the IL-17RA	S.C
Ixekizumab	IL17-antagonist	Immunoglobulin G4κ monoclonal antibody that has been humanised binds and neutralises IL-17A alone.	S.C
Secukinumab	IL17-antagonist	Monoclonal antibody against IL-17A, human IgG1κ	S.C
Risankizumab	IL23-antagonist	Humanised IgG1 monoclonal antibody that selectively targets the p19 subunit to suppress interleukin-23	S.C
Tildrakizumab	IL23-antagonist	Humanized IgG1κ binds to the p19 component of IL-23, selectively inhibiting it.	S.C
Ustekinumab	IL12 & IL23-antagonist	Monoclonal antibody IgG1k from humans that binds specifically to the p40 protein component required by the cytokines IL-12/IL-23 and interleukin [IL]-12.	S.C

Phototherapy

On a local level, ultraviolet light suppresses immunity. It selectively reduces cutaneous T cells through apoptosis, suppresses angiogenesis and epidermal hyperproliferation, and directly impacts Langerhans' cells. Several phototherapy modalities include targeted phototherapy, broadband [280–320 nm] and narrowband [311–313 nm] UVB radiation, as well as oral psoralen UVA [photo chemotherapy], which is currently less common in some regions of the world due to the cumulative risk of skin cancer. The most popular of these is narrowband UVB radiation, which is typically administered twice or three times a week. In certain nations, the use of home devices is also on the rise. For treating plaque psoriasis, narrowband UVB radiation is effective; however, it is time-consuming, has a burning side effect, and carries a very low risk of photo carcinogenesis compared to photochemotherapy. It is still mixed with dithranol or crude coal tar [Goeckerman regimen] in some places [35].

Topical Therapy

Table **5** showcases examples of topical therapy, summarizing formulations commonly used in clinical practice.

Table 5. Examples of topical therapy available [36].

Drugs	Characteristics
Corticosteroids	Corticosteroids are frequently useful and well tolerated for those with moderate psoriasis. Topical steroids are an effective first treatment for quick symptom relief, available in a variety of formulations, dosages, and combinations.
Vitamin D3 analogues	The first-line topical treatment for moderately severe scalp psoriasis and plaque psoriasis is calcitriol, a vitamin D3 analogue. By limiting T lymphocyte activity and regulating keratinocyte proliferation and differentiation, it lessens symptoms.
Combination products	It has been demonstrated that the combination of betamethasone propionate and calcipotriol is more beneficial than either medication alone for psoriasis.

Advanced Drug Delivery System for Psoriasis

Table **6** examines advanced drug delivery systems for psoriasis, highlighting novel approaches that aim to enhance treatment outcomes.

Table 6. Advanced drug delivery systems for psoriasis.

Formulation	Drug	Entrapment Efficiency	Results	References
Liposomes	Methotrexate	85%	Liposomes coated with methotrexate may provide a less harmful topical formulation.	37
-	Psoralen	75.12%	Psoralen-loaded liposomes exhibit enhanced topical safety and efficacy.	38
Nanostructured lipid carriers	Pentoxifylline	10–90%	Nanostructured lipid carriers loaded with pentoxifylline show promise for topical delivery to psoriatic skin and can be generated quickly without the need for complicated equipment or specialized conditions.	39
-	Methotrexate	62.72%	NLCs demonstrate enhanced skin penetration, longer drug release, and promise as a drug delivery vehicle.	40

(Table 6) cont.....

Formulation	Drug	Entrapment Efficiency	Results	References
Niosomes	Celastrol	-	Celastrol-loaded nanoparticles enhance the anti-psoriatic action by increasing celastrol penetration into the skin.	41
-	Tazarotene	49.50%	The formulation is effective for topical distribution and demonstrates enhanced drug accumulation in the skin layer.	42
Solid lipid nanoparticles	Clobetasol	78.1%	The formulation demonstrates longer medication release and improved skin penetration.	43
Ethosomes	Terbinafine hydrochloride	69.11%	Enhanced retention at the target site.	44
Transfersomes	Betamethasone dipropionate	77.4%	In comparison to its marketed forms, the formulation demonstrates greater safety and efficacy, as well as an efficient carrier for delivering the medication deep into the epidermal layer.	45
Dendrimers	Dithranol	71.33%	By eliminating the restrictions associated with traditional drug delivery, formulation enables the avoidance of auto-oxidation in antipsoriatic medications.	46
-	SiRNA	98.72%	The findings demonstrate improved histological and phenotypic characteristics, as well as a reduction in levels of TNF-α, IL-17, IL-22, and IL-6.	47
Microspheres	Apremilast	90%	Formulation demonstrates that psoriasis can be effectively treated with gel-loaded microspheres.	48
Microemulsion	Anthralin	97.03%	In comparison to its commercialised forms, the formulation has strong anti-psoriatic action.	49
Micelles	Terconazole	92.98%	Terconazole-loaded micelles have been demonstrated, *via* formulation, to be an effective drug delivery system for the skin.	50

Gene Therapy

Gene therapy is the process of treating a disease by integrating genetic material, either DNA or RNA, into the patient's cells. One of the three ways that the transferred genetic material functions is either [i] it allows the transferred gene to be expressed, [ii] it prevents the target gene from being expressed, or [iii] it modifies the target gene [51]. Gene therapy was first proposed for the treatment of inherited monogenic disease approximately fifty years ago. Its potential use was soon expanded to include acquired illnesses, such as cancer. Gene therapy is a particularly appealing concept since it offers the promise of a long-lasting cure with just one application of gene delivery or modification. Gene therapy has shown significant progress over the past 50 years, with more than two dozen gene therapies officially approved for use as therapeutic medications [52, 53]. They have made it possible to cure some diseases that would otherwise be incurable or that would not respond to conventional therapies. For instance, just 8% of patients with Spinal Muscular Atrophy [SMA], a severe infantile monogenic motor neuron disease brought on by an SMN1 mutation, would make it past 20 months without continuous ventilator support. On the other hand, in a clinical experiment, every patient who underwent gene therapy with Zolgensma lived to be 20 months old and showed improved motor ability [54]. Meanwhile, from the inception of gene therapy, concerns have been raised regarding its ethical and safety implications. Many experiments, particularly in the early stages of gene therapy, resulted in unanticipated side effects or even patient deaths, or failed to show any clinical benefits. Fortunately, most safety issues have been resolved or will be resolved in the near future due to the field's rapid advancement in research [55, 56].

GENE THERAPY IN THE TREATMENT OF PSORIASIS

Since gene delivery or alteration can potentially result in a permanent cure with just one application, gene therapy is an especially alluring prospect. One promising method of treating psoriasis is gene therapy. Given that psoriasis is believed to have a strong genetic origin, gene therapy appears to be a plausible treatment option. The gene therapy approach involves identifying a specific functional gene or gene fragment and replacing a defective gene in order to treat diseases caused by genetic abnormalities. Adenosine deaminase gene mutations are the source of normal gene sequence problems [57]. Once the replacement gene has been identified, the next step is to insert it into the corresponding location within the genome. In this exercise, choosing the activity is a crucial step. A study by Al-Raawi *et al.* revealed that N-JARID2, a JARID2 fragment, contributes to maintaining the skin's native architecture. Finding that N-JARID2 protein maintains skin cells in their normal differentiation stage could have therapeutic implications for psoriasis [58].

Small interfering [si]RNA, miRNA, and antisense oligonucleotides are examples of nucleic acids that can impede the transcription and translation of genes that are overexpressed in psoriasis. Antisense oligonucleotides specifically target proteins linked to inflammation (IL-2 and IL-8), proliferation (epidermal growth factor), and neovascularization (VEGF). Their low cellular absorption results in restricted bioavailability upon injection, and the absorbed protein is susceptible to enzymatic degradation. However, research is being conducted to transfer nucleic acids using liposomes and polymeric micelles, two different types of nanocarriers [59, 60].

RNA interference is a technique used to induce post-transcriptional gene silencing by degrading specific messenger RNA in the cytoplasm of the cell. This approach is very promising for silencing disease-promoting genes, as seen by the decrease in protein expression that results, which is relevant to several biological goals. For inflammatory skin conditions such as psoriasis, vitiligo, and atopic dermatitis, as well as abnormal cell behavior, including squamous cell carcinoma and melanoma, and damage, including burns and wounds, small interfering RNA therapy has been deemed appropriate for monogenic skin disorders, such as pachyonychia congenita. This is because there are specific molecular targets for these illnesses that can be suppressed to produce beneficial treatment effects. Small interfering RNA has the potential to be given topically to the skin due to its accessibility, ease of administration, and ability to bypass first-pass metabolism. However, the skin's outermost layer, the stratum corneum, acts as a strong barrier to stop substances from entering the skin. The limitations associated with the size of small interfering RNA molecules, their rapid enzymatic breakdown, and the strong anionic charge of their phosphate backbone, which results in electrostatic repulsion from the anionic cell membrane surface, are overcome by novel delivery techniques. Using nonviral vectors, nanocarriers, small interfering RNA complexes with positively charged compounds (*e.g.*, cationic polymers, lipids, dendrimers, peptides, or proteins), conjugates with small molecules (*e.g.*, cholesterol), antibodies, polymers, and lipids, there have been encouraging results in small interfering RNA delivery to knock down specific targets in various cell lines and tissues [61].

Another way to reduce psoriasis is to use cytokines that block the ability of T cells to trigger an immune response. Interleukin-4, or IL-4, is the only cytokine that has the ability to selectively neutralise the effects of Th1 cells, or T cells that cause psoriasis, and produce a Th2 phenotype. A clinical trial involving patients with severe psoriasis demonstrated the efficacy of this pleiotropic cytokine in suppressing human psoriasis. Li *et al.* investigated the antipsoriatic effect of transdermal distribution of IL-4 plasmid using ultra-deformable cationic liposomes using a K14-VEGF transgenic mouse model [a psoriasis model]. A daily application of 15 μg of plasmid DNA may be an effective treatment for psoriasis. A novel transdermal delivery technique for psoriasis treatment was studied. Using dimethyl sulfoxide as a penetration enhancer, the IL-4 expression plasmid (pIL-4) is used in this procedure. Significant amounts of IL-4 were found in the dermis and epidermis. When the antipsoriatic efficacy of this treatment was evaluated in mice, the symptoms of psoriasis were alleviated.173 Only in psoriatic lesions is the intermediate filament protein Keratin 17 (K17) abundantly expressed, and it has been suggested that K17 plays a role in the disease's aetiology. Chang *et al.* used RNA interference [siRNA] and Antisense Oligo-Deoxy Nucleotides (ASODN) to downregulate K17, a novel and promising psoriasis therapeutic method. They looked at the effects of liposome-encapsulated siRNA and topically administered K-17-specific ASODN in murine models of psoriasis. This medication was found to downregulate K-17 expression, which prevented keratinocyte proliferation and caused apoptosis. It was discovered that this drug downregulated the expression of K-17, which stopped keratinocyte growth and triggered apoptosis. Nonviral somatic [antiangiogenic] gene therapy targeting angiogenesis has been shown to be a highly successful treatment for psoriasis, as it is thought to block the progression of psoriatic illness [62].

Gene Therapy for Psoriasis in the K14-VEGF Transgenic Mouse Model by Topical Transdermal Delivery of Interleukin-4 Using Ultra-Deformable Cationic Liposome

Topical transdermal gene delivery to the skin holds promise for the painless, non-invasive administration of vaccinations and medications. Clinical studies have demonstrated that interleukin-4 (IL-4) treatments have a significant antipsoriatic effect. To transfer plasmid DNA transdermally to mouse skin, a suitable formula was developed at UCL. Next, to evaluate the antipsoriatic efficacy, UCL was utilised to deliver mIL-4 transdermally to the K14-VEGF transgenic mouse model. Plasmid DNA was applied transdermally to the proximal regions of the epidermis and hair follicles using this optimised solution. Expression of plasmid DNA was detected in the skin of the ears. The likelihood of plasmid promoter integration into genomic DNA may be reduced if plasmid DNA is not found in the liver or blood serum 24 hours following topical treatment. Mice treated with UCL/mIL-4 displayed a modest psoriasis phenotype. Histological analysis of the abnormal score using the Baker grading method demonstrated an antipsoriatic effect. Immunohistochemical analysis revealed that inflammatory and hyperplastic arteries were suppressed. These results demonstrate that topical transdermal mIL-4 therapy is an effective treatment for psoriasis. Transdermal topical gene transfer is therefore intriguing and may be applied in the future to treat other dermatological conditions in individuals [63].

Halting Engiogenesis by Non-Viral Somatic Gene Therapy Alleviates Psoriasis and Murine Psoriasiform Skin Lesions

Dysregulated angiogenesis characterizes chronic inflammatory disorders, such as psoriasis, a common skin condition that affects approximately 2% of the population. It has been demonstrated that antiangiogenic non-viral somatic gene therapy reduces cutaneous microvasculature and relieves chronic inflammatory skin conditions. Studies on human psoriasis in two complementary xenotransplantation models and psoriasis-like skin lesions in transgenic mice expressing human TGF-β1 in the epidermis have demonstrated this. Using *in vivo* electroporation, metargidin's Recombinant Disintegrin Domain (RDD), also known as ADAM-15, was transiently expressed in the muscles, which reduced cutaneous angiogenesis and vascularization in all three models. Red fluorescent protein-coupled RDD demonstrated that the therapy induced the gene product to be produced in the muscles and deposited in the cutaneous hyperangiogenic connective tissue. High-resolution ultrasound revealed decreased cutaneous blood flow *in vivo* after electroporation with RDD, but not with control plasmids. Moreover, keratinocyte proliferation, clinical disease scores, epidermal thickness, and molecular markers associated with inflammation and angiogenesis were all downregulated in all models. Thus, non-viral antiangiogenic gene therapy is effective in treating psoriasis and may also help treat other inflammatory skin disorders associated with angiogenesis.

Pharmacogenomics

It is now feasible to understand the reasons behind the different therapy reactions due to pharmacogenomics research. This healthcare approach includes the exploration of the human genome to identify different genetic variants (single-nucleotide variants, or SNVs; copy number variations, or CNVs; small insertions and deletions, or INDELs) that are related to disease susceptibility, drug response degree, and Adverse Drug Reactions (ADRs). In particular, the collection of these data might be used to develop personalised treatments based on the genetic makeup of the patient. Its clinical importance is demonstrated by the increase in pharmacological efficacy and the decrease in the incidence of adverse drug responses. One useful tool that can enhance the pharmacological treatment of various disorders is pharmacogenomics. Further research is needed to identify a set of biomarkers that can be used in clinical practice, as research on genes related to the metabolism of biological drugs (tumor necrosis factor inhibitors and cytokine inhibitors) and small molecules (apremilast, dimethyl fumarate, and tofacitinib) has produced inconsistent results. We can target the specific gene for therapeutic accuracy in psoriasis by studying pharmacogenomics. Currently, the approaches of genomic and epigenetic research are useful in identifying novel targets for Psoriasis treatment. In terms of therapeutic techniques for psoriasis, numerous medications are available today to help control comorbidities, reduce symptoms, and address clinical presentations. In reality, the presence of comorbidities related to the illness must be taken into account when selecting a treatment plan [64].

Anti-Tumour Necrosis Factor Drugs

The TNF or TNF-α gene, located on the short arm of chromosome 6 [6p21.33], codes for a multifunctional pro-inflammatory cytokine that is a member of the TNF superfamily. Primarily released by macrophages, this cytokine regulates a range of unique biological processes, including cell differentiation, proliferation, and lipid metabolism. Furthermore, TNF plays a key role in the etiopathogenesis of psoriatic lesions by promoting the production of T-cells, which in turn drive localised proliferation of epidermal keratinocytes. Psoriasis therapy utilizes TNF-α inhibitors, including etanercept (ETN), certolizumab (CTL), adalimumab (ADA), and infliximab (INF). INF, ADA, and CTL are monoclonal antibodies against TNF-α, and there is a recombinant fusion protein named ETN [65]. The effectiveness of these monoclonal antibodies is influenced by several genetic variants on the TNF-α gene [66, 67]. As pharmacogenetics or risk biomarkers, the polymorphisms TNF-857 [C/T, rs1799724], TNF-238 [G/A, rs361525], and TNF-308 [A/G, rs1800629] have all been extensively investigated. It was discovered that in European individuals, a favourable response to anti-TNF drugs was significantly linked [$p = 0.000086$ and $p = 0.016$, respectively] with the G alleles of rs1800629 and rs361525. Another genotyping study has linked TNF-1031 [T/C, rs1799964] in the promoter region of the TNF gene to a favorable response to anti-TNF treatments. Furthermore, the bioinformatics study demonstrated that rs361525 and rs1800629 alter the regulatory regions associated with specific biological processes, such as the Epithelial–Mesenchymal Transition (EMT). EMT results in morphological changes in cells. This method enhances the capacity of polarized epithelial cells to move, become invasive, and exhibit strong resistance to apoptosis by enabling them to mimic mesenchymal cells. This finding suggests that epithelial changes may be associated with EMT in patients affected by Psoriasis [68]. Two polymorphisms in TNFAIP3 [rs610604, G/A/C/T and rs6920220, G/A] have been found through pharmacogenomics research in particular, and they may be the cause of the different reactions to different drugs. The SNP rs2546890 [A/G] on the IL-12B gene [5q33.3] may affect an individual's response to ETN, ADA, and INF treatment. Moreover, variations in IL-1B [2q14.1] [rs1143623, C/A/G; rs1143627, G/A] could affect the way the body responds to anti-TNF drugs.

The genotype CT of rs763780 [C/T], located in the IL-17A gene [6p12.2], indicated a favourable outcome in patients undergoing INF treatment. The rs4819554 [G/A/C] locus, located in the IL-17-RA gene [22q11.1], may influence the body's response to anti-TNF drugs. Anti-TNF treatment was more effective for psoriatic patients carrying the A allele. Another IL that could have a role in Ps pharmacogenomics is IL-23R, which is encoded by the IL-23R gene located on the 1p31.3 locus. The Human Leukocyte Antigen (HLA) system is a transplantation antigen with clinical significance and is crucial for modulating the immune response. It is located on the short arm of chromosome 6 [6p21]. HLA polymorphisms have been described as risk and pharmacogenetic biomarkers. More specifically, rs1048554 [G/A/C, HLA-C] showed a positive response to anti-TNF medicines, while rs13437088 [C/T, HLA-B] was associated with the reaction to ETN. There is evidence that the HLA-Cw*06 alleles are associated with a lower risk of responding to ADA, ETN, or INF. The Genome-Wide Association Study (GWAS) identified new putative candidate genes (AKAP13, HNRNPKP3, SUPT3H, NPFFR2, and CDH12) that may be involved in the metabolism of anti-TNF drugs. Table **7** identifies genes and genetic variants that may be involved in the response to anti-TNF therapy, highlighting pharmacogenomics considerations.

Table 7. Genes and genetic variants potentially involved in the response to anti-tnf therapy.

GENE	LOCUS	GENETIC VARIANTS
TNF-α	6p21.33	rs1800629 A/G rs361525 G/A rs1799724 C/T rs1799964 T/C
TNFAIP3	6q23.3	rs610604 G/A/C/T rs6920220 G/A
IL-12B	5q33.3	rs2546890 A/G
IL-1B	2q14.1	rs1143623 C/A/G rs1143627 G/A
IL-6	7p15.3	rs1800795 C/G/T
IL-17A	6p12.2	rs763780 C/T
IL-17-RA	22q11.1	rs4819554 G/A/C
IL-23R	1p31.3	rs11209026 A/G
HLA-B	6p21	rs13437088 C/T
HLA-C	6p21	rs1048554 G/A/C HLA-Cw*06
AKAP13	15q25.3	rs28461892 C/A
HNRNPKP3	11p12	rs11037360 G/A rs7481533 T/A/C/G rs11037342 A/C/T rs145304743 G/A/T/C rs1845821 A/G/T
SUPT3H	6p21.1	rs9472377 A/G
NPFFR2	4q13.3	rs13139992 G/A rs77656238 C/A/T

(Table 7) cont.....

GENE	LOCUS	GENETIC VARIANTS
CDH12	5p14.3	rs1487419 G/A rs77497886 G/T rs80063785 A/G

Cytokine Inhibitors

Cytokine-targeted therapy for psoriasis patients involves administering IL-17 inhibitors that target the IL-17RA receptor, such as brodalumab (BDL), ixekizumab (IXE), and secukinumab (SCK). Other cytokine inhibitors used in psoriasis therapy include ustekinumab (USTK), guselkumab (GUS), tildrakizumab (TDK), and risankizumab (RSK). In particular, GSL, TDK, and RSK block IL-23 or its receptor, IL-23R. Estimates state that 50–70% of psoriatic individuals respond differently to anti-IL therapy [69]. The IL-17A gene, a member of the IL-17 receptor family, codes for a pro-inflammatory cytokine. The creation of remodelling proteins, chemokines, antimicrobial peptides, and inflammatory compounds is aided by IL-17A. High levels of IL-17 have been linked to a number of chronic inflammatory diseases, such as multiple sclerosis, Psoriasis, and rheumatoid arthritis [70]. The SNP rs4819958 [G/A] may have an impact on IL-17RA's [22q11.1] ability to interact with PAX1 and NR2F1 in the process of keratinocyte hyper-proliferation. SCK and IXE are fully human monoclonal antibodies that target IL-17A. IXE interacts with IL-17A/F, a protein in its heterodimer form. These drugs have a potent safety record and a long-lasting, prompt first reaction [71]. The majority of pharmacogenetics research focuses on single-nucleotide polymorphisms (SNPs). Preliminary data suggest that the HLA-C*06:02 allele might affect SCK's security and effectiveness [72]. The genes and polymorphisms summarized in Table 8 may potentially affect how cytokine inhibitors work. Table **8** presents genes and genetic variants influencing response to cytokine inhibitors, shedding light on personalized psoriasis therapy.

Table 8. Genes and genetic variants potentially involved in the response to cytokine inhibitors [73]

GENE	LOCUS	GENETIC VARIANTS
IL-17	6p12.2	rs763780 C/T rs3748067 C/T rs2275913 C/G/T rs3819025 A/G rs7747909 A/G rs8193037 A/C/T
IL-17RA	22q11.1	rs4819958 G/A
HLA-C	6p21	HLA-C*06:02
MICB-DT	6p21.33	rs9267325 G/C

(Table 8) cont.....

GENE	LOCUS	GENETIC VARIANTS
DDX58	9p21.1	rs34085293 T/G
TYK2	19p13.2	rs2304255 C/T
IL-12B	5q33.3	rs2546890 A/G rs3213094 C/G/T
IL-1B	2q14.1	rs1143623 C/G/T rs1143627 A/G
TNFAIP3	6q23.3	rs610604 G/A/C/T
TLR2	4q31.	rs4696480 A/T rs11938228 A/G/T
TLR5	1q41	rs5744174 A/G
TLR9	3p21.2	rs352139 G/A/T/C
PGLYRP4	1q21.3	rs2916205 C/T
FBXL19	16p11.2	rs10782001 G/A/C
CARD14	17q25.3	rs11652075 C/T

CHALLENGES TO GENE THERAPY

Safety is one of the most significant concerns with gene therapy. After Jesse Gelsinger passed away in 1999 from a severe immunological response to the AdV vector that had been employed to cure his ornithine transcarbamylase deficiency, gene therapy research took a turn for the worse. Even though AAVs are widely acknowledged to have a low immunogenicity and high safety profile, they have been demonstrated to elicit an immune response in a range of animal models examined, covering several diseases. Apart from initiating an immunological reaction, AAVs have been linked to renal failure, hepatotoxicity, and human thrombocytopenia. Modified by CRISPR-Cas9, genome editing presents distinct safety issues, chief among them being the worry about off-target consequences. These off-target occurrences may cause genomic instability and hazardous alterations in vital genes, such as tumor suppressors. Single-gene mutations are the cause of certain disorders, like sickle cell anemia and cystic fibrosis. Nevertheless, a large number of hereditary illnesses that make excellent candidates for gene therapy are very genetically diverse, which adds extra complexity to the development process of these therapies. Finding the causing gene is the first difficulty in treating genetically diverse disorders. Besides the difficulties involved in identifying genes, gene treatments also face an extremely expensive and challenging procedure before being commercialized. The current range of estimates for the price of clinical studies needed to introduce a new medication into the market is $161 million to $2 billion [74].

CONCLUSION

To cure diseases originating from hereditary conditions, the gene therapy procedure involves identifying a particular functioning gene or specific portion and replacing it with a defective one. Adenosine deaminase is an enzyme, and its mutation causes disturbance in normal gene structure. Placing the newly discovered gene in the appropriate location throughout the genome is the next necessary step. Identifying the activity is a crucial stage in this endeavor. Medical knowledge has advanced, yet a comprehensive remedy for this illness remains pending. As a result, the quality of life when a disease is discovered is undoubtedly greatly influenced and requires deliberate efforts and routines since disease management is a crucial tool for keeping the illness under control. Psoriasis management is made more promising by gene therapy, which holds forth the possibility of more targeted and potent therapies. Gene therapy seeks to mitigate the hereditary causes of this debilitating and chronic illness in order to provide long-term support and maybe even a cure. In contrast to conventional therapies, which mostly target symptom management, gene therapy may address the underlying biological causes of psoriasis. Cutting-edge gene editing tools, including CRISPR-Cas9, have shown tremendous promise in early research, paving the way for innovative therapeutic approaches. Although there are still challenges to overcome, such as ensuring safety and efficacy in humans, the achievements so far demonstrate the potential of gene therapy to transform the field of psoriasis treatment. With further research, gene therapy has the potential to be a key component of a comprehensive psoriasis treatment plan, offering hope to millions of people worldwide. To develop more effective medications for treatment plans, further research on psoriasis is needed to identify the precise causes of the condition. Ongoing research is exploring innovative methods for delivering medication more effectively using novel carriers, aiming to reduce costs, enhance efficacy, and minimize adverse effects. Novel dermal delivery systems are being researched extensively to help overcome these obstacles and improve the bioavailability and potential of drugs. Recent biotechnology advancements, in conjunction with pharmaceutical carriers and delivery systems, have a promising potential role in the diagnosis, mitigation, management, and treatment of psoriasis and diseases that resemble it.

REFERENCES

[1] Michalek IM, Loring B, John SM. A systematic review of worldwide epidemiology of psoriasis. J Eur Acad Dermatol Venereol 2017; 31(2): 205-12. [http://dx.doi.org/10.1111/jdv.13854] [PMID: 27573025]

[2] WHO. Global report on psoriasis. Geneva: World Health Organization 2016.

[3] Hay SI, Abajobir AA, Abate KH, *et al.* Global, regional, and national disability-adjusted life-years (DALYs) for 333 diseases and injuries and healthy life expectancy (HALE) for 195 countries and territories, 1990–2016: a systematic analysis for the Global Burden of Disease Study 2016. Lancet

2017; 390(10100): 1260-344.
[http://dx.doi.org/10.1016/S0140-6736(17)32130-X] [PMID: 28919118]

[4] Mahil SK, Capon F, Barker JN. Update on psoriasis immunopathogenesis and targeted immunotherapy. Semin Immunopathol 2016; 38(1): 11-27.
[http://dx.doi.org/10.1007/s00281-015-0539-8] [PMID: 26573299]

[5] Grän F, Kerstan A, Serfling E, Goebeler M, Muhammad K. Current developments in the immunology of psoriasis. Yale J Biol Med 2020; 93(1): 97-110.
[PMID: 32226340]

[6] Chen L, Tsai TF. *HLA-Cw6* and psoriasis. Br J Dermatol 2018; 178(4): 854-62.
[http://dx.doi.org/10.1111/bjd.16083] [PMID: 29072309]

[7] Tang L, Yang X, Liang Y, Xie H, Dai Z, Zheng G. Transcription factor retinoid-related orphan receptor γt: A promising target for the treatment of psoriasis. Front Immunol 2018; 9: 1210.
[http://dx.doi.org/10.3389/fimmu.2018.01210] [PMID: 29899748]

[8] Kamiya K, Kishimoto M, Sugai J, Komine M, Ohtsuki M. Risk factors for the development of psoriasis. Int J Mol Sci 2019; 20(18): 4347.
[http://dx.doi.org/10.3390/ijms20184347] [PMID: 31491865]

[9] National psoriasis foundation. Psoriasis Statistics 2022.

[10] Mease PJ, Gladman DD, Papp KA, *et al.* Prevalence of rheumatologist-diagnosed psoriatic arthritis in patients with psoriasis in European/North American dermatology clinics. J Am Acad Dermatol 2013; 69(5): 729-35.
[http://dx.doi.org/10.1016/j.jaad.2013.07.023] [PMID: 23981683]

[11] Armstrong AW, Mehta MD, Schupp CW, Gondo GC, Bell SJ, Griffiths CEM. Psoriasis prevalence in adults in the united states. JAMA Dermatol 2021; 157(8): 940-6.
[http://dx.doi.org/10.1001/jamadermatol.2021.2007] [PMID: 34190957]

[12] Alexis AF, Blackcloud P. Psoriasis in skin of color: epidemiology, genetics, clinical presentation, and treatment nuances. J Clin Aesthet Dermatol 2014; 7(11): 16-24.
[PMID: 25489378]

[13] Parisi R, Iskandar IYK, Kontopantelis E, Augustin M, Griffiths CEM, Ashcroft DM. National, regional, and worldwide epidemiology of psoriasis: systematic analysis and modelling study. BMJ 2020; 369: m1590.
[http://dx.doi.org/10.1136/bmj.m1590] [PMID: 32467098]

[14] Global psoriasis atlas. Statistics. GPA 15 March 2021].

[15] Ogawa E, Sato Y, Minagawa A, Okuyama R. Pathogenesis of psoriasis and development of treatment. J Dermatol 2018; 45(3): 264-72.
[http://dx.doi.org/10.1111/1346-8138.14139] [PMID: 29226422]

[16] Rendon A, Schäkel K. Psoriasis pathogenesis and treatment. Int J Mol Sci 2019; 20(6): 1475.
[http://dx.doi.org/10.3390/ijms20061475] [PMID: 30909615]

[17] Arakawa A, Siewert K, Stöhr J, *et al.* Melanocyte antigen triggers autoimmunity in human psoriasis. J Exp Med 2015; 212(13): 2203-12.
[http://dx.doi.org/10.1084/jem.20151093] [PMID: 26621454]

[18] Krueger JG. An autoimmune "attack" on melanocytes triggers psoriasis and cellular hyperplasia. J Exp Med 2015; 212(13): 2186.
[http://dx.doi.org/10.1084/jem.21213insight3] [PMID: 26666753]

[19] Wang A, Bai Y. Dendritic cells: The driver of psoriasis. J Dermatol 2020; 47(2): 104-13.
[http://dx.doi.org/10.1111/1346-8138.15184] [PMID: 31833093]

[20] Macri C, Pang ES, Patton T, O'Keeffe M. Dendritic cell subsets. Semin Cell Dev Biol 2018; 84: 11-21.

[http://dx.doi.org/10.1016/j.semcdb.2017.12.009] [PMID: 29246859]

[21] Panda SK, Kolbeck R, Sanjuan MA. Plasmacytoid dendritic cells in autoimmunity. Curr Opin Immunol 2017; 44: 20-5.
[http://dx.doi.org/10.1016/j.coi.2016.10.006] [PMID: 27855321]

[22] Takagi H, Arimura K, Uto T, *et al.* Plasmacytoid dendritic cells orchestrate TLR7-mediated innate and adaptive immunity for the initiation of autoimmune inflammation. Sci Rep 2016; 6(1): 24477.
[http://dx.doi.org/10.1038/srep24477] [PMID: 27075414]

[23] Kopfnagel V, Wagenknecht S, Harder J, *et al.* RNase 7 strongly promotes TLR9-mediated DNA sensing by human plasmacytoid dendritic cells. J Invest Dermatol 2018; 138(4): 872-81.
[http://dx.doi.org/10.1016/j.jid.2017.09.052] [PMID: 29157732]

[24] Furue M, Hashimoto-Hachiya A, Tsuji G. Aryl hydrocarbon receptor in atopic dermatitis and psoriasis. Int J Mol Sci 2019; 20(21): 5424.
[http://dx.doi.org/10.3390/ijms20215424] [PMID: 31683543]

[25] Zhu Z, Chen J, Lin Y, *et al.* Aryl hydrocarbon receptor in cutaneous vascular endothelial cells restricts psoriasis development by negatively regulating neutrophil recruitment. J Invest Dermatol 2020; 140(6): 1233-1243.e9.
[http://dx.doi.org/10.1016/j.jid.2019.11.022] [PMID: 31899186]

[26] Hawkes JE, Chan TC, Krueger JG. Psoriasis pathogenesis and the development of novel targeted immune therapies. J Allergy Clin Immunol 2017; 140(3): 645-53.
[http://dx.doi.org/10.1016/j.jaci.2017.07.004] [PMID: 28887948]

[27] Kim J, Krueger JG. Highly effective new treatments for psoriasis target the IL-23/Type 17 T cell autoimmune axis. Annu Rev Med 2017; 68(1): 255-69.
[http://dx.doi.org/10.1146/annurev-med-042915-103905] [PMID: 27686018]

[28] Tokuyama M, Mabuchi T. New treatment addressing the pathogenesis of psoriasis. Int J Mol Sci 2020; 21(20): 7488.
[http://dx.doi.org/10.3390/ijms21207488] [PMID: 33050592]

[29] Kim WB, Jerome D, Yeung J. Diagnosis and management of psoriasis. Can Fam Physician 2017; 63(4): 278-85.
[PMID: 28404701]

[30] West J, Ogston S, Foerster J. Safety and efficacy of methotrexate in psoriasis: A meta-analysis of published trials. PLoS One 2016; 11(5): e0153740.
[http://dx.doi.org/10.1371/journal.pone.0153740] [PMID: 27168193]

[31] Raaby L, Zachariae C, Østensen M, *et al.* Methotrexate use and monitoring in patients with psoriasis: A consensus report based on a danish expert meeting. Acta Derm Venereol 2017; 97(4): 426-32.
[http://dx.doi.org/10.2340/00015555-2599] [PMID: 27958611]

[32] Griffiths CEM, Armstrong AW, Gudjonsson JE, Barker JNWN. Psoriasis. Lancet 2021; 397(10281): 1301-15.
[http://dx.doi.org/10.1016/S0140-6736(20)32549-6] [PMID: 33812489]

[33] Menter A, Strober BE, Kaplan DH, Kivelevitch D, Prater EF, Stoff B, *et al.* Joint AAD-NPF guidelines of care for the management and treatment of psoriasis with biologics. J Am Acad Dermatol. 2019. April; 80(4): 1029–72.
[http://dx.doi.org/10.1016/j.jaad.2018.11.057]

[34] Papp KA, Blauvelt A, Bukhalo M, Gooderham M, Krueger JG, Lacour JP, *et al.* Risankizumab versus ustekinumab for moderate-to-severe plaque psoriasis. N Engl J Med. 2017. April; 376(16): 1551–60.
[http://dx.doi.org/10.1056/NEJMoa1607017]

[35] Morita A. Current developments in phototherapy for psoriasis. J Dermatol 2018; 45(3): 287-92.
[http://dx.doi.org/10.1111/1346-8138.14213] [PMID: 29369396]

[36] Elmets CA, Lim HW, Stoff B, *et al.* Joint american academy of dermatology–national psoriasis foundation guidelines of care for the management and treatment of psoriasis with phototherapy. J Am Acad Dermatol 2019; 81(3): 775-804. [http://dx.doi.org/10.1016/j.jaad.2019.04.042] [PMID: 31351884]

[37] Bahramizadeh M, Bahramizadeh M, Kiafar B, *et al.* Development, characterization and evaluation of topical methotrexate-entrapped deformable liposome on imiquimod-induced psoriasis in a mouse model. Int J Pharm 2019; 569: 118623. [http://dx.doi.org/10.1016/j.ijpharm.2019.118623] [PMID: 31419462]

[38] Doppalapudi S, Jain A, Chopra DK, Khan W. Psoralen loaded liposomal nanocarriers for improved skin penetration and efficacy of topical PUVA in psoriasis. Eur J Pharm Sci 2017; 96: 515-29. [http://dx.doi.org/10.1016/j.ejps.2016.10.025] [PMID: 27777066]

[39] Ghate VM, Kodoth AK, Shah A, Vishalakshi B, Lewis SA. Colloidal nanostructured lipid carriers of pentoxifylline produced by microwave irradiation ameliorates imiquimod-induced psoriasis in mice. Colloids Surf B Biointerfaces 2019; 181: 389-99. [http://dx.doi.org/10.1016/j.colsurfb.2019.05.074] [PMID: 31170645]

[40] Tripathi P, Kumar A, Jain PK, Patel JR. Carbomer gel bearing methotrexate loaded lipid nanocontainers shows improved topical delivery intended for effective management of psoriasis. Int J Biol Macromol 2018; 120(Pt A): 1322-34. [http://dx.doi.org/10.1016/j.ijbiomac.2018.08.136] [PMID: 30171962]

[41] Meng S, Sun L, Wang L, *et al.* Loading of water-insoluble celastrol into niosome hydrogels for improved topical permeation and anti-psoriasis activity. Colloids Surf B Biointerfaces 2019; 182: 110352. [http://dx.doi.org/10.1016/j.colsurfb.2019.110352] [PMID: 31306831]

[42] Prasad V, Chaurasia S. Performance evaluation of non-ionic surfactant based tazarotene encapsulated proniosomal gel for the treatment of psoriasis. Mater Sci Eng C 2017; 79: 168-76. [http://dx.doi.org/10.1016/j.msec.2017.05.036] [PMID: 28629004]

[43] K.R. Redddy, S.V. Satyanarayana, V.J. Reddy, Development and evaluation of clobetasol–loaded solid lipid nanoparticles for topical treatment of psoriasis, Int. J. Appl. Pharm. (2019) 143–150. [http://dx.doi.org/10.22159/ijap.2019v11i5.33592]

[44] Of E, Gel H. Formulation and evaluation of niosomal gel containing ketoprofen 2012; 2: 54-9.

[45] Gizaway SE, Fadel M, Mourad B, Elnaby FEA. Betamethasone dipropionate gel for treatment of localized plaque psoriasis. Int J Pharm Pharm Sci 2017; 9(8): 173. [http://dx.doi.org/10.22159/ijpps.2017v9i8.18571]

[46] Tripathi PK, Gorain B, Choudhury H, Srivastava A, Kesharwani P. Dendrimer entrapped microsponge gel of dithranol for effective topical treatment. Heliyon 2019; 5(3): e01343. [http://dx.doi.org/10.1016/j.heliyon.2019.e01343] [PMID: 30957038]

[47] Pandi P, Jain A, Kommineni N, Ionov M, Bryszewska M, Khan W. Dendrimer as a new potential carrier for topical delivery of siRNA: A comparative study of dendriplex vs. lipoplex for delivery of TNF-α siRNA. Int J Pharm 2018; 550(1-2): 240-50. [http://dx.doi.org/10.1016/j.ijpharm.2018.08.024] [PMID: 30165098]

[48] Priyanka NVSAI, Neeraja P, Mangilal T, Kumar MR. Formulation and evaluation of gel loaded with microspheres of apremilast for transdermal delivery system. 2019; p. 12.

[49] Dixit GR, Shende AB. Formulation and evaluation of anthralin microemulsion gel using karanj oil. Int J Pharm Sci Res 2014; 5: 2041-50. [http://dx.doi.org/10.13040/IJPSR.0975-8232.5(5).2041-50]

[50] Abd-Elsalam WH, El-Zahaby SA, Al-Mahallawi AM. Formulation and *in vivo* assessment of terconazole-loaded polymeric mixed micelles enriched with Cremophor EL as dual functioning mediator for augmenting physical stability and skin delivery. Drug Deliv 2018; 25(1): 484-92.

[http://dx.doi.org/10.1080/10717544.2018.1436098] [PMID: 29411650]

[51] Tang R, Xu Z. Gene therapy: a double-edged sword with great powers. Mol Cell Biochem 2020; 474(1-2): 73-81.
[http://dx.doi.org/10.1007/s11010-020-03834-3] [PMID: 32696132]

[52] Shahryari A, Saghaeian Jazi M, Mohammadi S, *et al.* Development and clinical translation of approved gene therapy products for genetic disorders. Front Genet 2019; 10: 868.
[http://dx.doi.org/10.3389/fgene.2019.00868] [PMID: 31608113]

[53] Ma CC, Wang ZL, Xu T, He ZY, Wei YQ. The approved gene therapy drugs worldwide: from 1998 to 2019. Biotechnol Adv 2020; 40: 107502.
[http://dx.doi.org/10.1016/j.biotechadv.2019.107502] [PMID: 31887345]

[54] Mendell JR, Al-Zaidy S, Shell R, *et al.* Single-dose gene-replacement therapy for spinal muscular atrophy. N Engl J Med 2017; 377(18): 1713-22.
[http://dx.doi.org/10.1056/NEJMoa1706198] [PMID: 29091557]

[55] Dunbar CE, High KA, Joung JK, Kohn DB, Ozawa K, Sadelain M. Gene therapy comes of age. Science 2018; 359(6372): eaan4672.
[http://dx.doi.org/10.1126/science.aan4672] [PMID: 29326244]

[56] High KA, Roncarolo MG. Gene Therapy. N Engl J Med 2019; 381(5): 455-64.
[http://dx.doi.org/10.1056/NEJMra1706910] [PMID: 31365802]

[57] What is Gene Therapy? Genetics Home Reference NIH.

[58] Al-Raawi D, Jones R, Wijesinghe S, *et al.* A novel form of JARID2 is required for differentiation in lineage-committed cells. EMBO J 2019; 38(3): e98449.
[http://dx.doi.org/10.15252/embj.201798449] [PMID: 30573669]

[59] Martins AM, Ascenso A, Ribeiro HM, Marto J. Current and future therapies for psoriasis with a focus on serotonergic drugs. Mol Neurobiol 2020; 57(5): 2391-419.
[http://dx.doi.org/10.1007/s12035-020-01889-3] [PMID: 32062841]

[60] Rapali V.K., Dubet S.K., *et al.* Psoriasis: pathological mechanisms, current pharmacological therapies, and emerging drug delivery systems. Dug discovery Today. 2020. Vol 25, Issue 12, pages- 2212-2226.
[http://dx.doi.org/10.1016/j.drudis.2020.09.023] [PMID: 33011340]

[61] Sawarkar SP, Yadav V. Novel drug delivery strategies and gene therapy regimen as a promising perspective for management of psoriasis. Indian J Dermatol Venereol Leprol 2021; 87(3): 333-40.
[http://dx.doi.org/10.25259/IJDVL_470_19] [PMID: 33943062]

[62] Raut AS, Prabhu RH, Patravale VB. Psoriasis clinical implications and treatment: a review. Crit Rev Ther Drug Carrier Syst 2013; 30(3): 183-216.
[http://dx.doi.org/10.1615/CritRevTherDrugCarrierSyst.2013005268] [PMID: 23614646]

[63] Li J, Li X, Zhang Y, *et al.* Gene therapy for psoriasis in the K14-VEGF transgenic mouse model by topical transdermal delivery of interleukin-4 using ultradeformable cationic liposome. J Gene Med 2010; 12(6): 481-90.
[http://dx.doi.org/10.1002/jgm.1459] [PMID: 20527041]

[64] Coates LC, Corp N, van der Windt DA, Soriano ER, Kavanaugh A. GRAPPA treatment recommendations: An update from the 2020 GRAPPA annual meeting. J Rheumatol Suppl 2021; 97: 65-6.
[PMID: 34074672]

[65] Muñoz-Aceituno E, Martos-Cabrera L, Ovejero-Benito MC, Reolid A, Abad-Santos F, Daudén E. Pharmacogenetics update on biologic therapy in psoriasis. Medicina (Kaunas) 2020; 56(12): 719.
[http://dx.doi.org/10.3390/medicina56120719] [PMID: 33419370]

[66] Wang L, Zhou H. A meta-analysis of the relationship between tumor necrosis factor-α polymorphisms and psoriasis. Dermatology 2021; 237(1): 39-45.

[http://dx.doi.org/10.1159/000502255] [PMID: 31775137]

[67] Membrive Jiménez C, Pérez Ramírez C, Sánchez Martín A, *et al.* Influence of genetic polymorphisms on response to biologics in moderate-to-severe psoriasis. J Pers Med 2021; 11(4): 293. [http://dx.doi.org/10.3390/jpm11040293] [PMID: 33921427]

[68] Ruiz Ramírez AV, Flores-Saiffe Farías A, Chávez Álvarez RC, Prado Montes de Oca E. Predicted regulatory SNPs reveal potential drug targets and novel companion diagnostics in psoriasis. J Transl Autoimmun 2021; 4: 100096. [http://dx.doi.org/10.1016/j.jtauto.2021.100096] [PMID: 33898962]

[69] Brownstone ND, Hong J, Mosca M, *et al.* Biologic treatments of psoriasis: An update for the clinician. Biologics 2021; 15: 39-51. [PMID: 33623366]

[70] Bernardini N, Skroza N, Tolino E, *et al.* *IL-17* and its role in inflammatory, autoimmune, and oncological skin diseases: state of art. Int J Dermatol 2020; 59(4): 406-11. [http://dx.doi.org/10.1111/ijd.14695] [PMID: 31663126]

[71] Costanzo A, Bianchi L, Flori ML, *et al.* Secukinumab shows high efficacy irrespective of *HLA-Cw6* status in patients with moderate-to-severe plaque-type psoriasis: SUPREME study. Br J Dermatol 2018; 179(5): 1072-80. [http://dx.doi.org/10.1111/bjd.16705] [PMID: 29704432]

[72] Sabry D, Aboraia N, Samir M. A potential association between psoriasin to rs4819554 of IL-17RA gene polymorphism in psoriasis Egyptian patients. Arch Dermatol Res 2020; 312(4): 273-81. [http://dx.doi.org/10.1007/s00403-019-02011-x] [PMID: 31745628]

[73] Caputo V, Strafella C, Cosio T, *et al.* Pharmacogenomics: An update on biologics and small-molecule drugs in the treatment of psoriasis. Genes (Basel) 2021; 12(9): 1398. [http://dx.doi.org/10.3390/genes12091398] [PMID: 34573380]

[74] Cring MR, Sheffield VC. Gene therapy and gene correction: targets, progress, and challenges for treating human diseases. Gene Ther 2022; 29(1-2): 3-12. [http://dx.doi.org/10.1038/s41434-020-00197-8] [PMID: 33037407]

CHAPTER 5

Conventional Therapies and Challenges in the Treatment of Psoriasis

Himani Bajaj[1,*], **Seema B. Chauhan**[1], **Mayank Yadav**[1] and **Anjali Sharma**[2]

[1] *Adarsh Vijendra Institute of Pharmaceutical Sciences, Shobhit University, Gangoh, Saharanpur, India*

[2] *Department of Pharmaceutics, Guru Gobind Singh College of Pharmacy, Yamunanagar, Haryana, India*

Abstract: Psoriasis is an autoimmune disease that re-emerges through the proliferation of keratinocytes. It occurs at any age, but is usually observed in temperate regions. It has a global population of 2 to 5 percent on average. The treatment of psoriasis remains a daunting task, with various challenges affecting treatment, including patient compliance and adherence, delicate patient profiles, psychological aspects, and skin as an obstacle to current delivery. Psoriasis is characterized by an excessive proliferation of cells, resulting in painful skin spots due to the absence of normal skin cell replacement, which occurs every 3 to 4 weeks. Treatment strategies for psoriasis depend on the severity and location of the injuries. The current chapter reviews the therapies and challenges associated with current treatments, including topical therapy, oral therapy, biological therapy, parenteral therapy, and phototherapy.

Keywords: Challenges, Psoriasis, Therapies, Treatment.

INTRODUCTION

Psoriasis is a frequently occurring, autoimmune, and inflammatory disease characterized by red, inflamed plaques and macules resulting from increased keratin-producing epidermal cell proliferation and poor differentiation. These plaques are often accompanied by silvery scales [1]. The highly inflamed lesions appear as a result of defective signals produced by the immune system to increase the mitosis rate of keratin-producing cells by tenfold [2]. This, in turn, leads to nuclear retention and incomplete cornification of stratum corneum cells. This disease develops at an early stage of life and progresses slowly throughout life. Psoriasis varies according to the affected tissues [3 - 6]. The prevalence of psoriasis has been reported to range between 0.09% and 11.43% [7]. Psoriasis, on

* **Corresponding author Himani Bajaj:** Adarsh Vijendra Institute of Pharmaceutical Sciences, Shobhit University, Gangoh, Saharanpur, India; E-mail: himanibajaj@gmail.com

average, affects 2% to 5% of the population worldwide [8]. Even if it spreadsglobally, its prevalence differs depending on the location and ethnicity. In general, the higher the latitude, the greater the prevalence [9].

As a result, compared to countries farther from the equator like Europe and Australia, Asia and Africa had lower rates of psoriasis [10].

Men and women are equally affected by psoriasis; however, women experience the disease's beginning substantially sooner [11]. The prevalence of the condition has multiplied during the past few years, according to recent studies [12]. A full cure remains elusive despite the plethora of therapeutic choices available today to lessen the disease's signs and symptoms. Some of the drawbacks of traditional medication delivery methods, such as topical treatments, include excessive dose frequency, poor drug penetration, and low patient compliance [13]. Conventional remedies are also limited by the toxicity of phototherapy and systemic therapy. Thus, it is crucial to investigate and create new safe and effective delivery methods for the treatment of psoriasis [14].

Current choices for Treatment

Conventional methods of treating psoriasis include topical, oral, biological, and parenteral treatments (Fig. **1**). Another treatment option for symptoms is phototherapy.

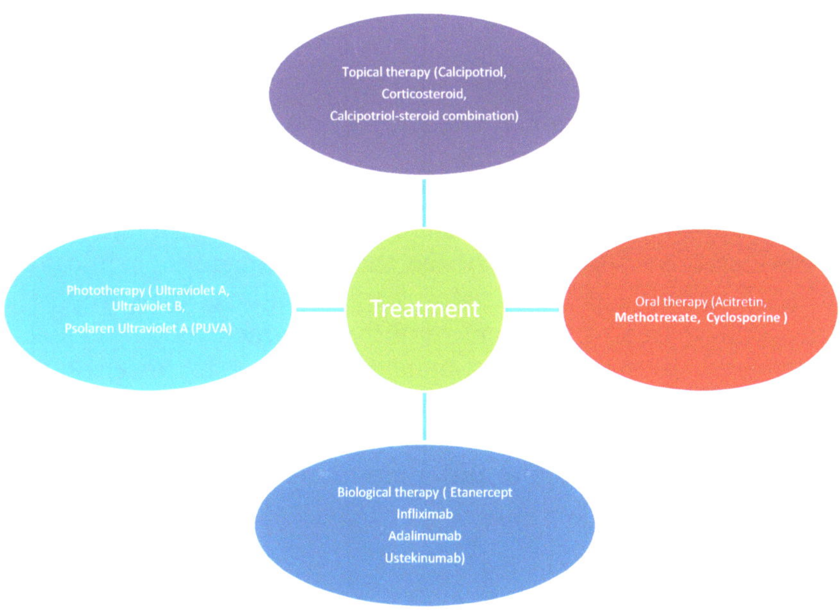

Fig. (1). Current Treatment choices for psoriasis.

Topical Therapy

Topical therapy for psoriasis typically yields moderately to unsatisfactory results and is often accompanied by irritation [15]. For mild to moderate psoriasis, topical therapy is considered the primary form of treatment. On the other hand, systemic administration combined with topical therapy may be helpful in extreme situations. Topical treatments may cause unwanted skin interactions, such as burning and irritation, which could lead to patient non-compliance [16].

Oral therapy

The majority of medications used in oral therapy for psoriasis are those that may be taken orally and administered successfully. When it comes to side effects, oral medications have more than topical treatments. As a result, it is not often acknowledged. To reduce adverse effects and increase efficacy, it is used as monotherapy, in combination with biologics, and phototherapy. When topical therapy is unable to alleviate symptoms, oral therapy is typically employed. Drugs frequently used in oral treatment include the following:

Acitretin

Since the 1970s, this acid metabolite of etretinate has been employed as a therapeutic agent. It is a retinoid that works by preventing keratinocytes from proliferating [17]. It is not immunosuppressive and is derived from vitamin A.

Methotrexate

It functions as an inhibitor of dihydrofolate reductase, an enzyme that is required for the synthesis of purines and pyrimidines during the synthesis of DNA. It is the most established and least expensive systemic medication for treating mild to moderate psoriasis. It reduces inflammation by breaking down into polyglutamate analogues, which raise the amount of the anti-inflammatory chemical adenosine [18]. It raises T-cell apoptosis and reduces epithelial layer hypertrophy [19]. It is also an immunosuppressive and anti-proliferative medication. Typically, folic acid supplements are advised in conjunction with it to lessen any potential negative effects. When used repeatedly, it might be harmful to the liver. There are many interactions between methotrexate and other medications, including salicylates and antibiotics. As a result, precautions should be taken while taking these medications.

Cyclosporine

For decades, this putative calcineurin inhibitor has been used to treat moderate to severe cases of psoriasis. It reduces the synthesis of IL2 as a result of this inhibition. Moreover, it prevents the synthesis of gamma interferon. Hypertension, nausea, headaches, and heightened sensitivity are typical adverse effects. It starts working fairly quickly. It is said that the medication is safe to take when pregnant [20].

Apremilast

It functions by inhibiting phosphodiesterase-4 (PDE-4), which lowers the thickness of epidermal layers and decreases the manufacture of pro-inflammatory cytokines. It has a reputation for having a favourable safety profile. The typical adverse effects that may occur are headache, nausea, and vomiting. Weight loss is another side effect of long-term apremilast therapy; the underlying mechanism is unknown. This medicine is known to be effective in treating psoriasis of the nails and scalp [21, 22].

Fumaric Acid Esters

In 1959, these were originally mentioned as a psoriasis therapy. This substance is a blend of monoethyl and dimethyl fumarate. These have anti-proliferative, anti-inflammatory, and antioxidative properties. It has demonstrated a strong safety and effectiveness record. Fumaric acid esters are known to cause several adverse gastrointestinal effects [23]. Its treatment has been found to cause a drop in the leukocyte count. Some of the less frequent adverse effects that are reported during treatment include pruritis, headaches, weariness, and lower extremity edoema. Therefore, a combinition of topical psoriasis treatment with fumaric acid ester therapy is advised.

Mycophenolate Mofetil

This prodrug is metabolised to mycophenolic acid, an inhibitor of purine synthesis that is important for B and T cell development. Research indicates that mycophenolate mofetil is more effective in treating psoriasis than both methotrexate and cyclosporine [24]. Treatment-related side effects include nausea, diarrhoea, and reversible hematologic abnormalities, which are frequent, therefore, it is not advised in pregnancy. Antibiotics, thymidine kinase inhibitors, non-steroidal anti-inflammatory medicines (NSAIDs), and opioids are among the medications that interact with mycophenolate mofetil.

Biological Therapy and Parenteral Therapy

Parenterally administered small biologics can also have a systemic effect. Glycoproteins derived from living things are known as biologics. These have the capacity to engage with specific immune system targets. Monoclonal antibodies, cytokines, antisense oligonucleotides, fusion proteins, and RNA are examples of biologics.

Phototherapy

Phototherapy involves the application of UV radiation to the skin in order to reduce the appearance of skin plaques and associated itching. These radiations have a wavelength range of 100–400 nm, and their therapeutically active wavelength range is 290–400 nm. Light therapy aids in the management of the disease's symptoms but does not treat the illness itself. It works by suppressing the immune system, reducing uncontrollably growing cells, and changing the expression of cytokines [25]. Every human body responds to phototherapy differently. Usually, three to five therapy sessions per week are required, and the entire treatment period lasts between two and three months. This means that the therapy takes a significant time duration. Patients receiving phototherapy have a chance of getting skin cancer. UV-A, UV-B, and UVA1 phototherapy are the possible forms of administration. Longer wavelengths make up UV-A, which has the ability to reach deep skin layers. Psoralen, which increases the skin's receptivity to UVA treatment, is typically administered in addition to UVA treatment. Because UV-B has short wavelengths, it cannot penetrate deeper skin tissues. Fig. (**2**). demonstrates the preference ranking for different psoriasis treatment methods.

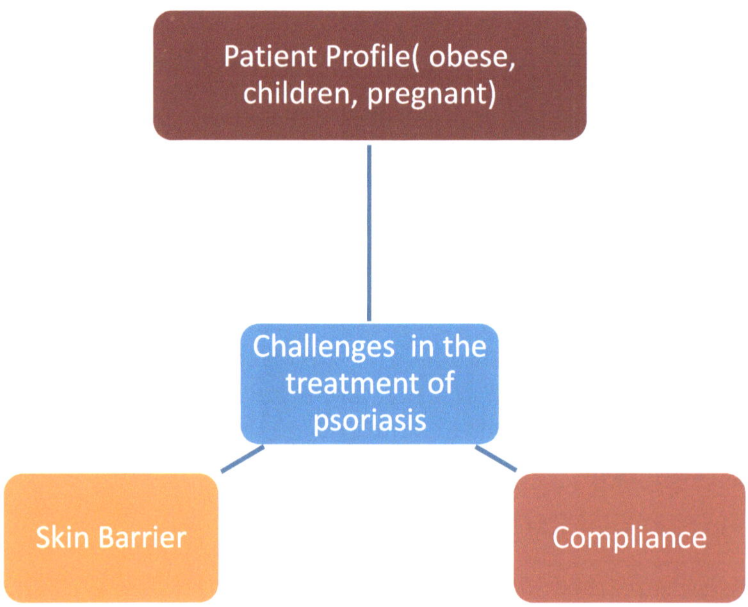

Fig. (2). Treatment challenges.

Marketed Formulations

Psoriasis has been treated using a variety of commercial medications, the details of which are compiled in Table **1**, along with the active medication and associated risk.

Table 1. Anti-psoriatic drugs under conventional treatment [24 - 50].

Class/type	Therapeutic Agents	Adverse Effects
Topical medicaments	Calcipotriol, Corticosteroid, Calcipotriol-steroid combination	Irritation, burning, and itching. Hypercalcemia may occur if excessive amounts are absorbed.
Phototherapy and Photochemotherapy	Ultraviolet A, Ultraviolet B, Psoralen Ultraviolet A (PUVA)	May lead to skin irritation, burning, erythema, photosensitivity, and potential long-term risks such as hyperpigmentation and an increased risk of skin cancer.
Systemic treatment	Acitretin	Mucocutaneous effects such as dryness of the skin and mucous membranes, cheilitis (inflammation of the lips), and scaling. Additionally, potential side effects may involve elevated levels of blood lipids (hyperlipidemia), hepatotoxicity, teratogenicity (a risk for congenital disabilities if used during pregnancy), and musculoskeletal symptoms.
	Cyclosporine	Renal dysfunction, hypertension.
	Methotrexate	Methotrexate, a systemic treatment for psoriasis, may lead to adverse effects such as gastrointestinal symptoms, hepatotoxicity, hematological abnormalities, and an increased risk of infection, necessitating close monitoring during therapy.
Biologics treatments	Etanercept	Injection site reactions, increased risk of infections, and, rarely, development of anti-drug antibodies.
	Infliximab	Adverse effects on psoriasis management may encompass infusion reactions, heightened susceptibility to infections, and the potential development of anti-infliximab antibodies.
	Adalimumab	Injection site reactions, Upper respiratory tract infections, Nasopharyngitis, Increased risk of opportunistic infections, Reactivation of latent tuberculosis, Lymphoma, and solid tumors.
	Ustekinumab	Upper respiratory tract infections, headache, and rare instances of serious infections or allergic reactions.

Role of Traditional Medicine in Psoriasis:

Psoriasis has long been treated with plant resources in the form of extracts, fractions, isolated chemicals, or formulations. Numerous benefits come with using natural medications derived from plants, including their accessibility, non-toxicity, improved patient tolerance, fewer side effects, cost, multiple biochemical action modes, and acceptability. A list of certain medicinal herbs and their mode of action for psoriasis was compiled [26 - 37]. (Table **2**).

Table. 2: Anti-psoriatic plants and their mechanism of action.

Plant (Family)	Mechanism of Action	Challenges
Aloe vera (Liliaceae)	Anthrones are responsible for their activity; mechanism of action involves inhibition of oxygen utilization by cells, inhibition of enzymes associated with cell proliferation and inflammation	Aloe vera for psoriasis may not be effective for everyone, and it could lead to skin irritation or allergies in some individuals. Scientific evidence supporting its effectiveness is limited, and the quality of Aloe vera products may differ.
Alpinia galanga (Zingiberaceae)	Increased expression of Tumour necrosis factor alpha induced protein 3 (TNFAIP3). Reduced expression of Colony stimulating factor 1(CSF-1), Nuclear factor kappa B Subunit 2 (NF-κB2). The ethanolic rhizome extract of the plant is the major constituent.	With a scarcity of research on its effectiveness and potential safety concerns, including unknown interactions and individual variability, relying on Alpinia galanga as a primary or alternative treatment for psoriasis may present risks.
Annona squamosa (Annonaceae)	Lower the expression of cluster of differentiation 40 (CD40) and Nuclear factor kappa B Subunit 1 (NF-κB1), Epidermal growth factor receptor (EGFR), and Inhibitor of Differentiation protein (ID1)	The mechanisms by which sugar-apple could potentially alleviate psoriasis symptoms are not well-understood, and the safety of its use specifically for psoriasis is unknown.
Curcuma longa (Zingiberaceae)	Decrease the expression of Colony stimulating Factor 1 (CSF-1), Interleukin-8 (IL-8), NF-κB2, NF-κB1, REL-associated protein A (RelA)	Limited clinical evidence supports its effectiveness, and the specific mechanisms by which curcumin, the active compound in turmeric, may alleviate psoriasis symptoms are not fully understood. Challenges include issues related to bioavailability, as curcumin absorption can be limited. Moreover, individual responses may vary, and its use as a sole or primary treatment may not provide comprehensive relief for all individuals with psoriasis.

(Table 2) cont.....

Plant (Family)	Mechanism of Action	Challenges
Matricaria chamomilla (Asteraceae)	Inhibition of leukotriene B4 (LTB4)	Chamomile has been traditionally praised for its anti-inflammatory and soothing properties; its specific impact on psoriasis remains unclear. Challenges include the lack of standardized formulations, potential variations in chamomile products, and the risk of skin irritation or allergic reactions in some individuals.
Inula viscosa (Asteraceae)	Inhibition of Nuclear factor kappa B (NF-κB), Cyclooxygenase -1 (COX-1) and Lipoxygenase (LOX) activity	While Inula viscosa has been utilized in traditional medicine for various purposes, comprehensive clinical studies validating its effectiveness in treating psoriasis are limited. The plant's complex chemical composition, influenced by factors such as geographic location and cultivation conditions, makes standardization of herbal preparations challenging, leading to variability in therapeutic outcomes.
Artemisia arborescens (Asteraceae)	Inhibition of NF-κB activation, (COX-1), (LOX) activity	Limited understanding of its varied bioactive compounds, potential side effects, interactions with medications, and individual responses complicate its integration into psoriasis management.
Achillea ligustica (Asteraceae)	Enhance the biosynthesis of 15-Hydroxyeicosatetraenoic acid (15(S)-HETE), Inhibition of NF-κB, COX-1 and LOX activity	Individual variability in responses, potential herb-drug interactions, and concerns about product quality and standardization are noteworthy issues. Safety concerns, such as allergic reactions or skin irritation, may also arise, emphasizing the importance of individualized care.
Acanthus mollis (Acanthaceae)	Enhance the biosynthesis of HETE, Inhibition of COX-1 and LOX activity	The incorporation of Acanthus mollis, a member of the Acanthaceae family, into psoriasis management encounters challenges rooted in the scarcity of scientific evidence substantiating its efficacy for this skin condition. Insufficient clinical trials hinder the establishment of specific benefits and risks associated with its use.

(Table 2) cont.....

Plant (Family)	Mechanism of Action	Challenges
Smilax china (Smilacaceae)	Inhibits the development of pleural exudates and leukocyte migration	Smilax china has been traditionally used in certain traditional medicine systems for its potential anti-inflammatory properties. There is a lack of well-established clinical studies to validate its effectiveness in treating psoriasis. Additionally, variations in the plant's chemical composition, inadequate standardization of herbal preparations, and potential side effects or interactions with conventional psoriasis treatments raise concerns about its safety and reliability.

Treatment Challenges

Even though psoriasis treatment has advanced greatly, some patients still do not respond well to the medication. The main obstacles to treating psoriasis are the patient profile, since various patient populations react to treatment in different ways, skin barriers, difficulties with topical therapy, and patient satisfaction or adherence to the regimen, as depicted in Fig. (**2**).

Profile of Patients

The management of elderly patients presents a number of challenges, including the co-occurrence of secondary disorders in addition to the main illness, a higher risk of medication interactions, and the requirement for dosage modifications. It thus results in ineffective illness treatment. According to study data, compared to conventional medications, biotechnology products were used less frequently for therapy. Inverse psoriasis, pustular psoriasis, and psoriatic arthritis are the three types of psoriasis that affect the older population most commonly. The quality of life is negatively impacted by the disease's comorbidities. The possible side effects, medication, patient history, current state, and patient preferences should all be taken into consideration while framing the therapy objectives. For senior patients, topical medications such as salicylic acid, corticosteroids, dithranol, and vitamin analogues are the preferred course of treatment. UVB phototherapy is also a part of the accepted standard therapy. Only in severe cases, systemic therapy is given . Corticosteroid therapy in the elderly can cause infection, purple patches on the skin, and skin thinning [38].

Pregnant Women

Pregnancy and nursing are typically unaffected by psoriasis. Pregnancy has been associated with a documented variability in illness symptoms. Low birth weight kids are born to psoriasis-affected moms, according to research. Pregnancy should not be the time to administer certain medications, such as acitretin and methotrexate. Cyclosporine can be taken throughout pregnancy; however, since it suppresses an infant's immune system, it is not advised to use it while nursing. Treatment options include topical, phototherapy, biologics, and oral medication. The best times to use topical therapy are during pregnancy and lactation. Typically, these consist of vitamin D analogues and steroids. It is not recommended to use tazarotene as it may cause birth defects. In addition, using sunscreen protection is generally advised in conjunction with UVB phototherapy to prevent the development of melasma. It is advised that the biotechnology-derived goods be discontinued before the infant is born and are linked to half-life monitoring [39].

Obese Patients

An elevated risk of psoriasis can result from obesity. Genetic and metabolic factors influence this relationship between psoriasis and obesity. Visceral organ obesity is mostly linked to atherosclerosis and inflammation. Inappropriate selection of systemic treatment options affects metabolic parameters, including lipid, kidney, and liver enzyme levels. The cell-signaling proteins known as adipokines, or adipocytokines, are secreted by adipose tissue. Through the inhibition of hunger, the adipocytokine leptin aids in the regulation of body weight and energy balance. Leptin levels have been shown to rise during psoriasis, and hyperleptinemia is linked to obesity [40]. Adipose tissue is the source of the cysteine-rich protein known as resistin. It also goes by the name "secretory factor specific to adipose tissue." It has been discovered to establish a connection between type 2 diabetes and obesity. Psoriasis has been linked to elevated serum resistin levels.

Children

According to reports, there is a connection between multifactorial metabolic and cardiovascular illnesses and childhood psoriasis [41]. Children's symptoms are challenging to diagnose since they resemble childhood rashes. The scalp is the primary target area for children with plaque psoriasis. Another prevalent type of psoriasis that affects children is guttate. It frequently manifests as small, patchy drops due to a streptococcal throat infection. Flexural psoriasis, a type of psoriasis characterised by big red areas, is commonly seen in children. Stress, upper respiratory tract infections, and drug reactions are the main causes of psoriasis in children. The epidermal absorption process, drug kinetics, and the physical integration of the body and metabolism present difficulties for safe and successful treatment of children. Consideration must be given to increased skin penetration during topical treatment, especially with steroids, as this can result in toxicity.

Compared to adults, children are more likely to develop guttate psoriasis, which can be treated with antibiotics. Thin skin and a higher surface area to body weight ratio can lead to toxicity and enhanced topical medication absorption. The only conditions for which systemic therapy should be used are severe psoriasis and immature livers that cannot properly metabolise many medications. In addition, the kidneys are not fully formed to eliminate medications. Antimitotic medications are more likely to have an impact on the active hematopoietic system. Adolescents and children do not substantially follow treatment plans [42].

Skin Barrier

Skin serves as a barrier, especially against pathogen invasion. The mechanical, immunity, and permeability barriers are just a few of the obstacles that make up the skin barrier. A large number of cell-signalling molecules, including chemokines and cytokines, are produced as a result of psoriasis. The epidermal cells divide far more quickly than they would under normal skin conditions, and the barrier that shields the skin from infections and pathogens becomes compromised. It is more difficult to elicit an immunological response in psoriatic skin due to a decrease in T cells [43]. Psoriatic skin additionally expresses integrins, granular products, and cornified envelope proteins, which causes the skin to thicken [44]. The majority of solutes travel *via* intracellular lipids to enter the skin. Reduced ceramide levels and elevated cholesterol cause psoriatic skin to stiffen; moreover, psoriatic skin is devoid of moisture. All of them make it difficult to apply topical medications to psoriatic skin. Due to side effects or their failure to adhere to traditional vehicles, none of the topical treatments now available for the treatment of psoriasis is regarded as the perfect alternative. Numerous issues arise, including patient adherence and therapeutic compliance [45].

Patient's point of view

Psoriasis adversely affects one's quality of life. Although psoriasis is not entirely curable, even with a wide range of therapeutic choices, including topical therapy, parenteral therapy, small molecule therapy, and phototherapy, there has been no full symptom relief and skin clearance.

Patients become dissatisfied with the available therapeutic alternatives as a result [46]. Throughout the illness, individuals in numerous situations stick to unsatisfactory and ineffective treatment alternatives, which exacerbate symptoms and cause psoriatic skin inflammation [47].

Compliance with Therapy

It is a significant obstacle to the management of psoriasis. Ineffectiveness and patient dissatisfaction are primary factors that lead to low therapy adherence [48]. It is essential to select treatment alternatives that will best support achieving the intended goals. The World Health Organisation states that the main element in the successful eradication of a chronic disease is adherence to treatment. Evaluating adherence is a difficult undertaking. A study report states that treatment adherence is observed in the following sequence; according to a study on psoriatic patients, therapeutic adherence was assessed to be between 27 and 29%, but for treatment to be effective, adherence should be between 50 and 60% [49]. The method used to administer the medication affects adherence as well. Adherence is also impacted by drug administration convenience and less frequent dosing. Adherence is also negatively impacted by the expense of medication . Some psoriatic patients struggle to afford the costly biological drugs due to their low wages.

Psychological Impact

In addition to cutaneous effects, psoriasis has a significant psychological influence on its patients. It has a significant impact on an individual's quality of life. It negatively affects mood and self-esteem, causing worry and despair. The person with psoriasis frequently experience prejudice and loneliness. Patients frequently experience emotional stress and irritability. Abuse of alcohol is also linked to depression, which exacerbates the illness and lengthens its course. Patients who have facial psoriasis have a distinct type of depression, a conscious depressive state, and a need for social distancing. Patients consequently become irritated and annoyed with the existing course of treatment and react poorly to the care approach [50].

Compliance with Treatment

Treatment decision-making and patient compliance are linked. Compared to other treatment options, the majority of patients comply with systemic medication, according to a study. Additionally, it has been observed that less than 40% of people comply with traditional treatment alternatives. Both the estimation of clinical attendance and the evaluation of the Dermatology Life Quality Index (DLQI) can be used to evaluate patient compliance. A technique that divides the patient population into compliers, and non-compliers based on median compliance level is used to examine compliance. An alternate method of assessing compliance is also employed, in which a compliance cutoff level is initially approximated using data from accessible studies and past investigations. It is also possible to employ a method that aids in the investigation of how specific traits affect compliance. Several objective techniques, including the quality of life evaluation tool, clinical attendance, and median adherence, can be used to assess compliance [51, 52].

CONCLUSION

Patients still have unmet medical demands despite the wide range of traditional therapeutic choices available for illness management because of low patient satisfaction and therapy adherence. Consequently, in order to control psoriasis, it is necessary to investigate new and emerging therapeutic perspectives. Research on widely accepted biological therapies must be taken into consideration in order to create methods that are more satisfying and effective.

Subsequent investigations will focus on the utilisation of combined multi-omics data for patient stratification and therapy guidance. The ideas of early systemic treatment intervention and better access to care are being explored . This is the area where research and service development intersect, necessitating creative ways and research techniques to accomplish this.

REFERENCES

[1] Sala M, Elaissari A, Fessi H. Advances in psoriasis physiopathology and treatments: Up to date of mechanistic insights and perspectives of novel therapies based on innovative skin drug delivery systems (ISDDS). J Control Release 2016; 239: 182-202.
[http://dx.doi.org/10.1016/j.jconrel.2016.07.003] [PMID: 27381248]

[2] Lowes MA, Suárez-Fariñas M, Krueger JG. Immunology of psoriasis. Annu Rev Immunol 2014; 32(1): 227-55.
[http://dx.doi.org/10.1146/annurev-immunol-032713-120225] [PMID: 24655295]

[3] Danielsen K, Olsen AO, Wilsgaard T, Furberg AS. Is the prevalence of psoriasis increasing? A 30-year follow-up of a population-based cohort. Br J Dermatol 2013; 168(6): 1303-10.
[http://dx.doi.org/10.1111/bjd.12230] [PMID: 23374051]

[4] Mehlis SL, Gordon KB. The immunology of psoriasis and biologic immunotherapy. J Am Acad Dermatol 2003; 49(2) (Suppl.): 44-50.
[http://dx.doi.org/10.1016/S0190-9622(03)01134-4] [PMID: 12894125]

[5] Fitch E, Harper E, Skorcheva I, Kurtz SE, Blauvelt A. Pathophysiology of psoriasis: Recent advances on IL-23 and Th17 cytokines. Curr Rheumatol Rep 2007; 9(6): 461-7.
[http://dx.doi.org/10.1007/s11926-007-0075-1] [PMID: 18177599]

[6] Hawkes JE, Chan TC, Krueger JG. Psoriasis pathogenesis and the development of novel targeted immune therapies. J Allergy Clin Immunol 2017; 140(3): 645-53.
[http://dx.doi.org/10.1016/j.jaci.2017.07.004] [PMID: 28887948]

[7] Eberle FC, Brück J, Holstein J, Hirahara K, Ghoreschi K. Recent advances in understanding psoriasis. F1000 Res 2016; 5: 770.
[http://dx.doi.org/10.12688/f1000research.7927.1] [PMID: 27158469]

[8] Pradhan M, Singh D, Singh MR. Influence of selected variables on fabrication of Triamcinolone acetonide loaded solid lipid nanoparticles for topical treatment of dermal disorders. Artif Cells Nanomed Biotechnol 2016; 44(1): 392-400.
[http://dx.doi.org/10.3109/21691401.2014.955105] [PMID: 25229831]

[9] Takeshita J, Gelfand JM, Li P, *et al.* Psoriasis in the US Medicare population: prevalence, treatment, and factors associated with biologic use. J Invest Dermatol 2015; 135(12): 2955-63. [http://dx.doi.org/10.1038/jid.2015.296] [PMID: 26214380]

[10] Gupta R, Debbaneh MG, Liao W. Genetic epidemiology of psoriasis. Curr Dermatol Rep 2014; 3(1): 61-78. [http://dx.doi.org/10.1007/s13671-013-0066-6] [PMID: 25580373]

[11] Griffiths CEM, van der Walt JM, Ashcroft DM, *et al.* The global state of psoriasis disease epidemiology: a workshop report. Br J Dermatol 2017; 177(1): e4-7. [http://dx.doi.org/10.1111/bjd.15610] [PMID: 28555722]

[12] Gudjonsson JE, Elder JT. Psoriasis: epidemiology. Clin Dermatol 2007; 25(6): 535-46. [http://dx.doi.org/10.1016/j.clindermatol.2007.08.007] [PMID: 18021890]

[13] Icen M, Crowson CS, McEvoy MT, Dann FJ, Gabriel SE, Maradit Kremers H. Trends in incidence of adult-onset psoriasis over three decades: A population-based study. J Am Acad Dermatol 2009; 60(3): 394-401. [http://dx.doi.org/10.1016/j.jaad.2008.10.062] [PMID: 19231638]

[14] Bhatia A, Singh B, Wadhwa S, Raza K, Katare OP. Novel phospholipid-based topical formulations of tamoxifen: evaluation for antipsoriatic activity using mouse-tail model. Pharm Dev Technol 2014; 19(2): 160-3. [http://dx.doi.org/10.3109/10837450.2013.763260] [PMID: 23369039]

[15] Finlay AY, Ortonne JP. Patient satisfaction with psoriasis therapies: an update and introduction to biologic therapy. J Cutan Med Surg 2004; 8(5): 310-20. [http://dx.doi.org/10.1177/120347540400800502] [PMID: 15868312]

[16] Fouéré S, Adjadj L, Pawin H. How patients experience psoriasis: results from a European survey. J Eur Acad Dermatol Venereol 2005; 19(s3) (Suppl. 3): 2-6. [http://dx.doi.org/10.1111/j.1468-3083.2005.01329.x] [PMID: 16274404]

[17] Dogra S, Yadav S. Acitretin in psoriasis: an evolving scenario. Int J Dermatol 2014; 53(5): 525-38. [http://dx.doi.org/10.1111/ijd.12365] [PMID: 24601982]

[18] Montesinos MC, Desai A, Delano D, *et al.* Adenosine A_{2A} or A_3 receptors are required for inhibition of inflammation by methotrexate and its analog MX-68. Arthritis Rheum 2003; 48(1): 240-7. [http://dx.doi.org/10.1002/art.10712] [PMID: 12528125]

[19] Elango T, Dayalan H, Gnanaraj P, Malligarjunan H, Subramanian S. Impact of methotrexate on oxidative stress and apoptosis markers in psoriatic patients. Clin Exp Med 2014; 14(4): 431-7. [http://dx.doi.org/10.1007/s10238-013-0252-7] [PMID: 23949337]

[20] Salvarani C, Boiardi L, MacChioni P, Pipitone N, Catanoso M, Pigatto P. Multidisciplinary focus on cyclosporin A. J Rheumatol Suppl 2009; 83(0): 52-5. [http://dx.doi.org/10.3899/jrheum.090225] [PMID: 19661542]

[21] Papp K, Reich K, Leonardi CL, *et al.* Apremilast, an oral phosphodiesterase 4 (PDE4) inhibitor, in patients with moderate to severe plaque psoriasis: Results of a phase III, randomized, controlled trial (Efficacy and Safety Trial Evaluating the Effects of Apremilast in Psoriasis [ESTEEM] 1). J Am Acad Dermatol 2015; 73(1): 37-49. [http://dx.doi.org/10.1016/j.jaad.2015.03.049] [PMID: 26089047]

[22] Schadler ED, Ortel B, Mehlis SL. Biologics for the primary care physician: Review and treatment of psoriasis. Dis Mon 2019; 65(3): 51-90. [http://dx.doi.org/10.1016/j.disamonth.2018.06.001] [PMID: 30037762]

[23] Balak DM. Fumaric acid esters in the management of psoriasis. Psoriasis (Auckl) 2015; 5: 9-23. [http://dx.doi.org/10.2147/PTT.S51490] [PMID: 29387578]

[24] Pedraz J, Daudén E, Delgado-Jiménez Y, García-Río I, García-Díez A. Sequential study on the

treatment of moderate-to-severe chronic plaque psoriasis with mycophenolate mofetil and cyclosporin. J Eur Acad Dermatol Venereol 2006; 20(6): 702-6.
[http://dx.doi.org/10.1111/j.1468-3083.2006.01577.x] [PMID: 16836499]

[25] Wong T, Hsu L, Liao W. Phototherapy in psoriasis: a review of mechanisms of action. J Cutan Med Surg 2013; 17(1): 6-12.
[http://dx.doi.org/10.2310/7750.2012.11124] [PMID: 23364144]

[26] Masood E. 'Medicinal plants threatened by over-use'. Nature 1997; 385(6617): 570.
[http://dx.doi.org/10.1038/385570a0] [PMID: 9024646]

[27] Müller K. Antipsoriatic anthrones: Aspects of oxygen radical formation, challenges and prospects. Gen Pharmacol 1996; 27(8): 1325-35.
[http://dx.doi.org/10.1016/S0306-3623(96)00075-4] [PMID: 9304402]

[28] Saelee C, Thongrakard V, Tencomnao T. Effects of Thai medicinal herb extracts with anti-psoriatic activity on the expression on NF-κB signaling biomarkers in HaCaT keratinocytes. Molecules 2011; 16(5): 3908-32.
[http://dx.doi.org/10.3390/molecules16053908] [PMID: 21555979]

[29] Ronpirin C, Charueksereesakul T, Thongrakard V, Tencomnao T. Effects of ethanolic extract of *Annona squamosa* L. leaves on the expression of EGFR. J Chem Pharm Res 2014; 6(4): 791-7.
[http://dx.doi.org/10.1055/s-0032-1320823]

[30] Kawjit N, Charueksereesakul T, Thongrakard V, Sangsuthum S, Tencomnao T. Suppressive effect of ethanolic extract of *Annona squamosa* L. leaves on the expression of Id1 biomarker: Phytochemical investigation and antioxidant activity study. J Chem Pharm Res 2014; 6(1): 499-506.

[31] Azadeh Izadyari Aghmiuni and Azim Akbarzadeh Khiavi. Medicinal plants to calm and treat psoriasis. Aromatic and Medicinal Plants - Back to Nature InTech publishers. El-Shemy HA, Ed. 2017; pp. 1-28.
[http://dx.doi.org/10.5772/67062]

[32] Safayhi H, Sabieraj J, Sailer ER, Ammon H. Chamazulene: an antioxidant-type inhibitor of leukotriene B4 formation. Planta Med 1994; 60(5): 410-3.
[http://dx.doi.org/10.1055/s-2006-959520] [PMID: 7997466]

[33] Alalaiwe A, Hung CF, Leu YL, *et al.* The active compounds derived from *Psoralea corylifolia* for photochemotherapy against psoriasis-like lesions: The relationship between structure and percutaneous absorption. Eur J Pharm Sci 2018; 124(124): 114-26.
[http://dx.doi.org/10.1016/j.ejps.2018.08.031] [PMID: 30153523]

[34] Bader A, Martini F, Schinella GR, Rios JL, Prieto JM. Modulation of Cox-1, 5-, 12- and 15-Lox by popular herbal remedies used in southern Italy against psoriasis and other skin diseases. Phytother Res 2015; 29(1): 108-13.
[http://dx.doi.org/10.1002/ptr.5234] [PMID: 25278440]

[35] Palaniswamy D, Nithyanantham M, Raghu PS, Dwarampudi LP. Antipsoriatic activity and cytotoxicity of ethanolic extract of *Nigella sativa* seeds. Pharmacogn Mag 2012; 8(32): 268-72.
[http://dx.doi.org/10.4103/0973-1296.103650] [PMID: 24082629]

[36] Okasha EF, Bayomy NA, Abdelaziz EZ. Effect of topical application of black seed oil on imiquimodinduced psoriasislike lesions in the thin skin of adult male albino rats. Anat Rec (Hoboken) 2018; 301(1): 166-74.
[http://dx.doi.org/10.1002/ar.23690] [PMID: 28926201]

[37] Vijayalakshmi A, Ravichandiran V, Velraj M, Nirmala S, Jayakumari S. Screening of flavonoid "quercetin" from the rhizome of *Smilax china* Linn. for anti–psoriatic activity. Asian Pac J Trop Biomed 2012; 2(4): 269-75.
[http://dx.doi.org/10.1016/S2221-1691(12)60021-5] [PMID: 23569912]

[38] Vide J, Magina S. Moderate to severe psoriasis treatment challenges through the era of biological drugs. An Bras Dermatol 2017; 92(5): 668-74.

[http://dx.doi.org/10.1590/abd1806-4841.20175603] [PMID: 29166504]

[39] Mervic L. Management of moderate to severe plaque psoriasis in pregnancy and lactation in the era of biologics. Acta Dermatovenerol Alp Panonica Adriat 2014; 23(2): 27-31. [http://dx.doi.org/10.15570/actaapa.2014.7] [PMID: 24964946]

[40] Chen YJ, Wu CY, Shen JL, *et al.* Psoriasis independently associated with hyperleptinemia contributing to metabolic syndrome. Arch Dermatol 2008; 144(12): 1571-5. [http://dx.doi.org/10.1001/archderm.144.12.1571] [PMID: 19075139]

[41] Badaoui A, Tounian P, Mahé E. Psoriasis and metabolic and cardiovascular comorbidities in children: A systematic review. Arch Pediatr 2019; 26(2): 86-94. [http://dx.doi.org/10.1016/j.arcped.2018.12.005] [PMID: 30638928]

[42] Thomas J, Parimalam K. Treating pediatric plaque psoriasis: challenges and solutions. Pediatric Health Med Ther 2016; 7: 25-38. [http://dx.doi.org/10.2147/PHMT.S75834] [PMID: 29388608]

[43] Sugiyama H, Gyulai R, Toichi E, *et al.* Dysfunctional blood and target tissue CD4+CD25high regulatory T cells in psoriasis: mechanism underlying unrestrained pathogenic effector T cell proliferation. J Immunol 2005; 174(1): 164-73. [http://dx.doi.org/10.4049/jimmunol.174.1.164] [PMID: 15611238]

[44] Roberson EDO, Bowcock AM. Psoriasis genetics: breaking the barrier. Trends Genet 2010; 26(9): 415-23. [http://dx.doi.org/10.1016/j.tig.2010.06.006] [PMID: 20692714]

[45] Armstrong AW, Robertson AD, Wu J, Schupp C, Lebwohl MG. Undertreatment, treatment trends, and treatment dissatisfaction among patients with psoriasis and psoriatic arthritis in the United States: findings from the National Psoriasis Foundation surveys, 2003-2011. JAMA Dermatol 2013; 149(10): 1180-5. [http://dx.doi.org/10.1001/jamadermatol.2013.5264] [PMID: 23945732]

[46] Nast A, Boehncke WH, Mrowietz U, *et al.* S3 – Guidelines on the treatment of psoriasis vulgaris (English version). Update. J Dtsch Dermatol Ges 2012; 10(s2) (Suppl. 2): S1-S95. [http://dx.doi.org/10.1111/j.1610-0387.2012.07919.x] [PMID: 22386073]

[47] Thorneloe RJ, Bundy C, Griffiths CEM, Ashcroft DM, Cordingley L. Adherence to medication in patients with psoriasis: a systematic literature review. Br J Dermatol 2013; 168(1): 20-31. [http://dx.doi.org/10.1111/bjd.12039] [PMID: 22963128]

[48] Augustin M, Holland B, Dartsch D, Langenbruch A, Radtke MA. Adherence in the treatment of psoriasis: a systematic review. Dermatology 2011; 222(4): 363-74. [http://dx.doi.org/10.1159/000329026] [PMID: 21757881]

[49] Kerdel F, Zaiac M. An evolution in switching therapy for psoriasis patients who fail to meet treatment goals. Dermatol Ther 2015; 28(6): 390-403. [http://dx.doi.org/10.1111/dth.12267] [PMID: 26258910]

[50] Griffiths CEM, Richards HL. Psychological influences in psoriasis. Clin Exp Dermatol 2001; 26(4): 338-42. [http://dx.doi.org/10.1046/j.1365-2230.2001.00834.x] [PMID: 11422186]

[51] Nijsten T, Margolis DJ, Feldman SR, Rolstad T, Stern RS. Traditional systemic treatments have not fully met the needs of psoriasis patients: Results from a national survey. J Am Acad Dermatol 2005; 52(3): 434-44. [http://dx.doi.org/10.1016/j.jaad.2004.10.862] [PMID: 15761421]

[52] Zaghloul SS, Goodfield MJD. Objective assessment of compliance with psoriasis treatment. Arch Dermatol 2004; 140(4): 408-14. [http://dx.doi.org/10.1001/archderm.140.4.408] [PMID: 15096368]

CHAPTER 6

Phytopharmaceuticals in the Management of Psoriasis

Bhawna Chopra[1,*], **Ashwani Kumar Dhingra**[2] and **Priyanka Kriplani**[3]

[1] *Department of Pharmaceutical Chemistry, Guru Gobind Singh College of Pharmacy, Yamuna Nagar 135001, Haryana, India*

[2] *Department of Pharmaceutical Sciences, Global Research Institute of Pharmacy, Yamuna Nagar 135001, Haryana, India*

[3] *Department of Pharmaceutics, Guru Gobind Singh College of Pharmacy, Yamuna Nagar 135001, Haryana, India*

Abstract: Psoriasis is a globally prevalent chronic inflammatory condition. Traditional treatment methods often rely on immunosuppressive agents, which can have adverse effects on the human body. As a result, alternative therapies, particularly those utilizing phytoconstituents with immunomodulatory, antioxidant, and anti-inflammatory properties, have gained attention. This chapter explores the potential of medicinal plants and phytoconstituents in managing psoriasis symptoms and supporting long-term disease control. However, to fully harness the therapeutic benefits of these plant-derived compounds and integrate them into standard dermatological care for psoriasis patients, further research and rigorous clinical validation are essential.

Keywords: Bioactive components, Medicinal plants, Psoriasis, Pathology, *Psoralea corylifola.*

INTRODUCTION

Psoriasis, a longstanding autoimmune disease, has been recognized since ancient times [1]. It is one of the most common hereditary skin diseases, characterized by the abnormal proliferation and shedding of skin cells, leading to the formation of psoriatic plaques, pustules, and scaly patches [2]. The papillary dermis, the topmost layer of the dermis, is where the first lesions show up. At this point, blood vessels dilate and become more curved, allowing granulocytes and neutrophil-absorbing lymphocytes to migrate towards the epidermis, which remains visible as normal. This marks the beginning of abnormal keratinocyte proliferation and migration. As psoriasis progresses, the epidermis thickens and

* **Corresponding author Bhawna Chopra:** Department of Pharmaceutical Chemistry, Guru Gobind Singh College of Pharmacy, Yamuna Nagar 135001, Haryana, India; E-mail: bhawna8486@gmail.com

Anjali Sharma, Prerna Sharma, Roy Rillera Marzo & Ahmed A. Al Karmalawy (Eds.)

keratinocytes fail to fully differentiate. This leads to the loss of the granular layer and the development of parakeratosis, a condition in which keratinocytes rctaintheir nuclei. In the later stages, certain skin cell populations proliferate excessively, resulting in the expansion of the spinous layer—a condition known as acanthosis. Removal of psoriatic plaques may lead to pinpoint bleeding due to the presence of dilated blood vessels extending into the upper dermis [3].

Psoriasis is categorized as an autoimmune disease, resulting from the dysfunction of key pathways and elements in the immune system [4]. Individuals who have severe psoriasis also have an elevated risk for metabolic syndrome, such as obesity, hypertension [5 - 7]. Although conventional therapies alleviate psoriasis symptoms, the literature suggests that a complete cure remains unattainable. This results in an urgent need to develop safe and effective, yet affordable, treatments for psoriasis. Recent research suggests targeting or regulating the activity of progressive cells involved in psoriasis using herbal drugs. Literature reviews have documented the effectiveness of herbal remedies in managing psoriasis, highlighting the supportive role of phytochemicals in treating psoriasis [8, 9]. Highlighting the impact of phytochemicals on oxidative stress and immune pathways, the review consolidates evidence on the anti-inflammatory and immunomodulatory effects of natural compounds, as well as their molecular interactions, which alleviate psoriatic inflammation and progression.

SUBSTANCES OF NATURAL ORIGIN—PLANTS AND PHYTOCHEMICALS WITH POTENTIAL THERAPEUTIC SIGNIFICANCE

In the ongoing exploration of innovative therapies, natural compounds have become a focal point, drawing attention due to their extensive diversity, favorable safety profile, and widespread availability [10]. Various clinical studies have demonstrated that specific natural substances of diverse origins exhibit the ability to alleviate psoriasis. These substances work by promoting apoptosis, inhibiting angiogenesis, suppressing inflammation triggered by reactive oxygen species, and overexpressing inducible nitric oxide synthase, among other molecular pathways [11, 12]. Some of the medicinal plants and their bioactive components are explained below:

Vegetal Medicinal Plants

Aloe vera

Aloe vera has earned global recognition as a traditional remedy for various ailments, including antiseptic, anti-inflammatory, wound-healing, and antidiabetic properties, particularly for skin disorders. Its gel, widely utilized in cosmetics and pharmaceuticals, contains a plethora of potentially active components. Research suggests that these components play a role in mitigating the progression of psoriasis by alleviating skin itching and reducing inflammation. Research on a psoriatic model using TNF-α-stimulated HaCaT cells demonstrated promising outcomes, with various doses of Aloe vera extract administered over 24 hours supporting cell viability in these stimulated cells [13, 14]. Notably, an ethanolic extract derived from *Aloe vera* gel showed results comparable to tazarotene, indicating its potential as an effective treatment option for psoriasis. In essence, *Aloe Vera's* multifaceted therapeutic properties, supported by both traditional wisdom and scientific research, underscore its significance as a promising natural remedy for various health conditions, including psoriasis [15 - 17].

Artemisia capillaris

Artemisia capillaris has historically been employed in East Asia to address pyrexia and liver disorders as an herbal remedy [18]. Regarding psoriasis, the extract derived from *Artemisia capillaris* holds promise to inhibit excessive keratinocyte proliferation. Additionally, it reduces leukocyte influx by suppressing the expression of ICAM-1 and lowering nitric oxide levels through the inhibition of iNOS production [19, 20].

Hypericum perforatum

St. John's Wort (*Hypericum perforatum*) has a long history of traditional use [21]. In clinical trials, the topical application of St. John's Wort ointment demonstrated significant reductions in redness scores and the thickness of skin flakes compared to the placebo group [22]. Another study assessed the clinical effects of *Hypericum perforatum* as a topical treatment for plaque-type psoriasis. The results indicate a substantial reduction in erythema, scaling, and thickness [23].

Rehmannia glutinosa

Research indicates that *Rehmannia glutinosa* extract exhibits strong antioxidative effects, including scavenging free radicals, inhibiting iNOS, and reducing pro-inflammatory cytokines. It also lowers prostaglandin production by blocking the COX enzyme and thus suppresses chemotaxis through JAK-STAT inhibition, with efficacy demonstrated in both *in vivo* and *in vitro* studies [24 - 26].

Salvia miltiorrhiza

Salvia miltiorrhiza and its active compounds, known for anti-inflammatory, antioxidant, and antiproliferative effects, show potential antipsoriatic properties. *In vitro* studies on HaCaT cells and *in vivo* studies in IMQ-induced mice reveal that *Salvia miltiorrhiza* reduces inflammation, inhibits Akt and ERK1/2 phosphorylation, thins lesions, and reduces scaling while promoting keratinocyte apoptosis. Although the precise mode of action remains unclear, it may be connected to STAT3 activation and/or yes-associated protein (YAP) inhibition [27, 28].

Psoralea corylifolia

Psoralea corylifolia, an esteemed medicinal plant, holds a significant place in various traditional medicines due to its efficacy in treating skin ailments such as psoriasis, leukoderma, and leprosy [29]. The plant extract exhibits a spectrum of medicinal properties, including antimicrobial and anti-inflammatory effects [30 - 33]. The chemical compounds isopsoralen, psoralen, and bakuchiol, primarily derived from Babchi oil, are recognized for their diverse properties. Recent advancements involve formulating Babchi oil into various formulations, such as emulgel [34] and nanoemulsion-based hydrogel, to enhance its application. Microemulsion gel represents a promising vehicle for enhancing the topical delivery of psoralen, thereby serving as a potential means to improve the topical delivery of Babchi oil [35].

Curcuma longa

Turmeric is renowned for its numerous medicinal properties. With a history deeply rooted in traditional Chinese medicine, turmeric has been utilized for centuries to address various health issues, including respiratory and cardiovascular diseases, liver and gastrointestinal ailments, and arthritis [36].

Polyherbal formulations

PSORI-CM01 has demonstrated antipsoriatic properties in animal studies, primarily by inducing autophagy and inhibiting cytokines and chemokines associated with psoriasis. In BALB/c mice, PSORI-CM02, a combination of five widely used plants in China—*Curcuma longa*, Peonies radix, *Smilax glabra*, and *Sarcandrae herb*—did not cause any adverse effects. Furthermore, it increased the mice's body mass, which is a crucial sign of general health, especially in cases of imiquimod-induced inflammation. By lowering T cell infiltration, interferon-γ, and IL-17A levels while raising IL-4, an anti-inflammatory agent, this formula demonstrates immunomodulatory effects, identifying the GATA3 pathway as a key therapeutic target [36]. Other studies have explored extracts from various herbs with pharmacological properties, as well as other natural substances that can be used in complementary and alternative treatments for psoriasis [36 - 42].

Additionally, the methanol extract-based ointment of *Kigelia africana* demonstrated a dose-dependent increase in orthokeratosis and a reduction in epidermal thickness [43].

Phytoconstituents

Capsaicin

Capsaicin exhibits a strong affinity for vanilloid receptors and modulates inflammation by inhibiting NF-κB and AP-1 signaling pathways [44]. However, its practical application as a topical treatment is limited due to the pain and discomfort associated with its use [45].

Resveratrol

Resveratrol, a stilbenoid polyphenol found in grapes, berries, and *Polygonum cuspidatum*, is renowned for its potent pharmacological actions [46, 47]. In an imiquimod-induced psoriasis model, resveratrol reduced proinflammatory cytokines, promoted keratinocyte death, and inhibited AQP3 expression [48, 49].

Curcumin

Curcumin is known for its antioxidant, anti-inflammatory, antimicrobial, and anticancer effects [50]. Notably, curcumin has been demonstrated to be safe and non-toxic to humans, even with a daily intake of up to 8 g [51]. Evidence suggests that curcumin can be taken daily up to 8 g. It may have potential in combating psoriasis. In a molecular docking study, curcumin interacts with the receptor-binding sites of TNF [52]. Clinical trials with oral curcumin have shown tolerability among patients with psoriasis, with some positive responses observed. While Kurd *et al.* acknowledged the possibility of a placebo effect or natural disease reversal, massive, placebo-controlled trials are deemed necessary to definitively establish the potential of oral curcumin as a psoriasis remedy [53].

Sun *et al.* found curcumin inhibits TNF-induced NF-κB activation and IL-6/8 in HaCaT cells. Curcumin also reduces phosphorylase kinase activity, suggesting its suitability for treating psoriasis and other hyperproliferative diseases [54]. Curcumin reduces TNF-induced IL-1ß, IL-6, and TNF production in TNF-treated HaCaT cells, according to *in vitro* research. The inhibition of MAPKs and NF-κB is probably the cause of this action, indicating curcumin's potential as an immunomodulatory drug to reverse TNF's anti-apoptotic effects in psoriasis.

Turmeric, containing over a hundred active components, mainly relies on curcumin for its therapeutic effects. It works by suppressing certain pathways, such as NF-κB, and reducing the activity of inflammatory molecules [55, 56]. Studies often used BALB/c mice and applied imiquimod to induce psoriasis-like symptoms on their skin. They then treated the mice with curcumin ointments or gels. They assessed the severity of the lesions using the Psoriasis Area and Severity Index (PASI), which evaluates redness, scaling, and thickness of the affected skin [56 - 60]. Curcumin effectively combats psoriasis by reducing hyperkeratosis and skin thickening, as observed under the microscope and reflected in the PASI scores. It also decreases the presence of inflammatory cells, such as CD8+ T cells, and inhibits signaling pathways, including JNK [55, 56, 36]. In one study, curcumin was delivered using ethosomes, resulting in reduced levels of inflammatory mediators and improved PASI scores. Another study combined curcumin with *Aloe vera* extract, resulting in reduced skin thickness and inflammation, attributed to decreased cytokine levels and inhibition of the STAT-3 pathway. Further research is needed to understand its effects on the skin microbiome [36].

Rottlerin

Rottlerin is extracted from *Mallotus phillippinensis* [61]. Rottlerin is a potent inhibitor of keratinocyte proliferation, preventing both basal and H_2O_2-stimulated elevation of NF-κB [62]. Doses of 0, 1, 5, and 10 μM demonstrate that rottlerin not only inhibits keratinocyte proliferation but also induces apoptosis. It also impairs the secretion of key psoriasis-driving cytokines [63].

Quercetin

Quercetin can be isolated from the plants *Ginkgo biloba* [64 - 67] or *Hypericum perforatum* [68] and is known to possess a wide range of pharmacological potential [69]. The study carried out by Kiekow *et al.* [70] revealed that quercetin exhibits anti-inflammatory activity, impacting the modulation of MAPK signaling and the NF-κB pathway. Chen *et al.* conducted studies on psoriatic models and IMQ-stimulated mice to investigate the effect of quercetin on cytokine levels. Their results showed a significant reduction in TNF-α, IL-6, and IL-17 levels following quercetin administration [71].

Apigenin

Apigenin has antibacterial, anti-inflammatory, and antioxidant properties. This plant flavonoid effectively inhibits NF-κB activation in autoimmune cells. In *in vivo* studies by Miroeva *et al.*, 5 μmol of apigenin reduced IL-6 and IL-12 levels in mice, cytokines typically elevated in psoriasis [72 - 74].

Kaempferol

Kaempferol, a flavonoid found in foods like tea, broccoli, apples, and strawberries, plays a crucial role in managing inflammation-related diseases such as psoriasis. In Liu *et al.*'s study, kaempferol reduced psoriatic skin lesions and inflammation, while also decreasing the expression of proinflammatory cytokines. *In vivo*, mice with IMQ-induced psoriasis were treated with kaempferol (50 and 100 mg/kg) for seven days. The results indicated that kaempferol inhibits Th17 levels and suppresses the phosphorylation of NF-κB, a typical proinflammatory signal in psoriasis [75, 76].

Genistein

Genistein, found in soybeans and fava beans, exhibits pharmacological potential against numerous ailments. In *in vivo* studies by Wang *et al.*, genistein (50-100 μM) reduced cytokine levels and inhibited STAT3 phosphorylation and NF-κB activation in psoriasis models. *In vitro*, Smolińska *et al.* found that genistein (1 μg/mL) suppressed ROS generation in TNF-α or LPS-stimulated HaCaT cells [77 - 79].

Rutin

Rutin is found in various foods, such as citrus fruits. It is known for its antioxidant and anti-inflammatory properties [80]. In studies on *Memecylon malabaricum*, rutin (100 mg/mL) exhibited strong antipsoriatic effects in a mouse tail test. While it showed limited activity in three *in vitro* tests on HaCaT cells, the plant demonstrated the highest potential in the LOX inhibition assay. These findings confirm that the entire M. malabaricum leaf exhibits antipsoriatic properties [81].

Naringenin

Naringenin, a flavanone, is known for its pharmacological activities, including anticancer, antioxidant, anti-inflammatory, antibacterial, and cardioprotective properties [82]. The compound naringenin significantly reduces the cytokine level and thus produces an anti-inflammatory effect in a psoriasis model [83].

Naringin

The bioactive constituent naringin, commonly found in citrus fruits, beans, and oregano, has been reported in the literature to offer several therapeutic benefits relevant to psoriasis pathogenesis, particularly its anti-inflammatory effects. It also inhibits the chemokine production [84]. Deenonpoe and his co-workers discovered that naringin exhibits an inhibitory effect on the production of TNF-alpha and IL-6, and thus possesses a significant role in immunological effects associated with psoriasis [85].

Epigallocatechin-3-gallate (EGCG)

EGCG, a flavonoid, is known for its pharmacological potential against inflammation and cancer. In *in vivo* studies, Zhang and his coworkers observed that EGCG reduces PCNA expression and thus inhibits abnormal cell proliferation. The study suggests that EGCG may improve psoriasis symptoms by regulating antioxidant factors [86, 87].

Anthocyanidins

Anthocyanidins, green water-soluble flavonoids, are abundant in berries, such as strawberries, and in red cabbage. In *in vivo* research, Chamcheu *et al.* [88] discovered that delphinidin, a type of anthocyanin, suppresses the proliferation and inflammation. The study also found that delphinidin inhibited the elevated release of inflammatory cytokines associated with psoriasis.

Lycopene

Lycopene is found in red fruits. The literature indicates that lycopene inhibits IMQ-induced psoriasis-like inflammation in keratinocytes, both through topical and oral treatment (0.12 mg/kg for 42 days). Moreover, it not only provides local symptomatic relief but also reduces the monocytic cell adhesion in an IMQ-induced psoriasis [89].

Emodin

Emodin, an anthraquinone derivative, exhibits a diverse range of pharmacological activities. The study concludes that the topical application of a natural compound combination at a dose of 10 μM, including emodin, reduces the proliferation rate of IL-22-stimulated keratinocytes and alleviates IMQ-induced psoriasis [90].

EPIDEMIOLOGY AND PATHOPHYSIOLOGY OF PSORIASIS

Psoriasis affects approximately 2% of the global population, with the lowest prevalence observed among Black populations. It is more common in colder regions than in tropical areas, with incidence rates in Europe ranging from 0.6% to 6.5%, and higher prevalence observed in northern countries. While psoriasis can develop at any age, it most commonly begins between the ages of 15 and 20. However, diagnosis is sometimes delayed due to postponed clinical consultation. Psoriasis affects various aspects of the skin, nails, joints, and the immune system, making its pathophysiology complex. Various newer technologies and therapies target immune cells and cytokines. It also explores the role of skin microbiota, as abnormal immune cell activation is triggered by bacteria present in the skin,

which contributes to psoriasis. In addition to this, genetic factors, gene mutations also influence the cytokine expression and keratinocyte proliferation.

CONCLUSION

The chapter concludes that psoriasis remains a challenging condition for individuals seeking a definitive cure, as current treatments primarily focus on immune suppression or symptom management. However, these treatments often come with undesirable side effects, including mood swings, digestive issues, and other related complications. In recent years, natural compounds have gained considerable attention as potential therapeutic options for psoriasis. Post-treatment observations suggest improvements in immune system responses and reductions in oxidative stress; however, further studies are necessary to comprehensively explore these effects. While additional research is required for confirmation, growing evidence indicates that natural substances may enhance clinical outcomes for individuals undergoing systemic treatments, whether conventional or immunobiological. The increasing interest in phytotherapeutic research highlights the demand for safer and more effective psoriasis treatments, offering hope for improved management of this complex condition.

REFERENCES

[1] Krueger JG. The immunologic basis for the treatment of psoriasis with new biologic agents. J Am Acad Dermatol 2002; 46(1): 1-26.
[http://dx.doi.org/10.1067/mjd.2002.120568] [PMID: 11756941]

[2] Griffiths CEM, Christophers E, Barker JNWN, *et al.* A classification of psoriasis vulgaris according to phenotype. Br J Dermatol 2007; 156(2): 258-62.
[http://dx.doi.org/10.1111/j.1365-2133.2006.07675.x] [PMID: 17223864]

[3] Di Meglio P, Villanova F, Nestle FO. Psoriasis. Cold Spring Harb Perspect Med 2014; 4(8): a015354.
[http://dx.doi.org/10.1101/cshperspect.a015354] [PMID: 25085957]

[4] Benhadou F, Mintoff D, Schnebert B, Thio HB. Psoriasis and microbiota: A systematic review. Diseases 2018; 6(2): 47.
[http://dx.doi.org/10.3390/diseases6020047] [PMID: 29865237]

[5] Bowcock AM, Krueger JG. Getting under the skin: the immunogenetics of psoriasis. Nat Rev Immunol 2005; 5(9): 699-711.
[http://dx.doi.org/10.1038/nri1689] [PMID: 16138103]

[6] Barak A, Sharma A, Arora D, Mittal V, Gupta A, Grover R. From pathophysiology to personalized treatment strategies for psoriasis. Curr Drug Ther 2025; 20(1): 57-75.
[http://dx.doi.org/10.2174/0115748855279099240119110656]

[7] Carvalho AVE, Romiti R, Souza CS, Paschoal RS, Milman LM, Meneghello LP. Psoriasis comorbidities: complications and benefits of immunobiological treatment. An Bras Dermatol 2016; 91(6): 781-9.

[http://dx.doi.org/10.1590/abd1806-4841.20165080] [PMID: 28099601]

[8] Aghmiuni AI, Khiavi AA. Medicinal plants to calm and treat psoriasis disease. Aromat Med Plants Back Nat 2016; 1: 1-28.
[http://dx.doi.org/10.5772/67062]

[9] Kaur A, Kumar S. Plants and plant products with potential antipsoriatic activity – a review. Pharm Biol 2012; 50(12): 1573-91.
[http://dx.doi.org/10.3109/13880209.2012.690430] [PMID: 22971237]

[10] Svendsen MT, Jeyabalan J, Andersen KE, Andersen F, Johannessen H. Worldwide utilization of topical remedies in treatment of psoriasis: a systematic review. J Dermatolog Treat 2017; 28(5): 374-83.
[http://dx.doi.org/10.1080/09546634.2016.1254331] [PMID: 27786594]

[11] Farahnik B, Sharma D, Alban J, Sivamani RK. Topical botanical agents for the treatment of psoriasis: A systematic review. Am J Clin Dermatol 2017; 18(4): 451-68.
[http://dx.doi.org/10.1007/s40257-017-0266-0] [PMID: 28289986]

[12] May BH, Deng S, Zhang AL, Lu C, Xue CCL. *In silico* database screening of potential targets and pathways of compounds contained in plants used for psoriasis vulgaris. Arch Dermatol Res 2015; 307(7): 645-57.
[http://dx.doi.org/10.1007/s00403-015-1577-8] [PMID: 26142738]

[13] Radha MH, Laxmipriya NP. Evaluation of biological properties and clinical effectiveness of Aloe vera: A systematic review. J Tradit Complement Med 2015; 5(1): 21-6.
[http://dx.doi.org/10.1016/j.jtcme.2014.10.006] [PMID: 26151005]

[14] Leng H, Pu L, Xu L, Shi X, Ji J, Chen K. Effects of aloe polysaccharide, a polysaccharide extracted from Aloe-vera, on TNF-α-induced HaCaT cell proliferation and the underlying mechanism in psoriasis. Mol Med Rep 2018; 18(3): 3537-43.
[http://dx.doi.org/10.3892/mmr.2018.9319] [PMID: 30066937]

[15] Zhou Q, Mrowietz U, Rostami-Yazdi M. Oxidative stress in the pathogenesis of psoriasis. Free Radic Biol Med 2009; 47(7): 891-905.
[http://dx.doi.org/10.1016/j.freeradbiomed.2009.06.033] [PMID: 19577640]

[16] Kröncke KD, Fehsel K, Kolb-Bachofen V. Inducible nitric oxide synthase and its product nitric oxide, a small molecule with complex biological activities. Biol Chem Hoppe Seyler 1995; 376(6): 327-43.
[PMID: 7576227]

[17] Förstermann U, Sessa WC. Nitric oxide synthases: regulation and function. Eur Heart J 2012; 33(7): 829-837, 837a-837d.
[http://dx.doi.org/10.1093/eurheartj/ehr304] [PMID: 21890489]

[18] Ha H, Lee H, Seo CS, *et al.* *Artemisia capillaris* inhibits atopic dermatitis-like skin lesions in Dermatophagoides farinae-sensitized Nc/Nga mice. BMC Complement Altern Med 2014; 14(1): 100.
[http://dx.doi.org/10.1186/1472-6882-14-100] [PMID: 24624888]

[19] Lee SY, Nam S, Hong IK, Kim H, Yang H, Cho HJ. Antiproliferation of keratinocytes and alleviation of psoriasis by the ethanol extract of *Artemisia capillaris*. Phytother Res 2018; 32(5): 923-32.
[http://dx.doi.org/10.1002/ptr.6032] [PMID: 29377339]

[20] Lee SY, Nam S, Kim S, *et al.* Therapeutic efficacies of *Artemisia capillaris* extract cream formulation in imiquimod-induced psoriasis models. Evid Based Complement Alternat Med 2018; 2018(1): 3610494.
[http://dx.doi.org/10.1155/2018/3610494] [PMID: 30210571]

[21] Najafizadeh P, Hashemian F, Mansouri P, Farshi S, Surmaghi MS, Chalangari R. The evaluation of the clinical effect of topical St Johns wort (*Hypericum perforatum L.*) in plaque type psoriasis vulgaris: A pilot study. Australas J Dermatol 2012; 53(2): 131-5.
[http://dx.doi.org/10.1111/j.1440-0960.2012.00877.x] [PMID: 22571563]

[22] Wölfle U, Seelinger G, Schempp CM. Topical application of St. John's wort (*Hypericum perforatum*). Planta Med 2014; 80(2-3): 109-20.
[PMID: 24214835]

[23] Mansouri P, Mirafzal S, Najafizadeh P, Safaei-Naraghi Z, Salehi-Surmaghi MH, Hashemian F. The impact of topical Saint John's Wort (*Hypericum perforatum*) treatment on tissue tumor necrosis factor-alpha levels in plaque-type psoriasis. J Postgrad Med 2017; 63(4): 215-20.
[http://dx.doi.org/10.4103/0022-3859.201423] [PMID: 28272075]

[24] Yan X, Zhang H, Dang M, Chen X. *Rehmannia radix* extract ameliorates imiquimod-induced psoriasis-like skin inflammation in a mouse model *via* the janus-kinase signal transducer and activator of transcription pathway. Pharmacogn Mag 2020; 16(71): 613.
[http://dx.doi.org/10.4103/pm.pm_218_19]

[25] Liu CL, Cheng L, Ko CH, *et al.* Bioassay-guided isolation of anti-inflammatory components from the root of *Rehmannia glutinosa* and its underlying mechanism *via* inhibition of iNOS pathway. J Ethnopharmacol 2012; 143(3): 867-75.
[http://dx.doi.org/10.1016/j.jep.2012.08.012] [PMID: 23034094]

[26] Baek GH, Jang YS, Jeong SI, *et al. Rehmannia glutinosa* suppresses inflammatory responses elicited by advanced glycation end products. Inflammation 2012; 35(4): 1232-41.
[http://dx.doi.org/10.1007/s10753-012-9433-x] [PMID: 22327862]

[27] Jia J, Mo X, Liu J, *et al.* Mechanism of danshensu-induced inhibition of abnormal epidermal proliferation in psoriasis. Eur J Pharmacol 2020; 868: 172881.
[http://dx.doi.org/10.1016/j.ejphar.2019.172881] [PMID: 31866405]

[28] Tang L, He S, Wang X, *et al. Cryptotanshinone* reduces psoriatic epidermal hyperplasia *via* inhibiting the activation of STAT 3. Exp Dermatol 2018; 27(3): 268-75.
[http://dx.doi.org/10.1111/exd.13511] [PMID: 29427477]

[29] Alam A, Alqarni MH, Foudah AI, Raish M, Salkini MA. Babchi oil-based nanoemulsion hydrogel for the management of psoriasis: A novel energy economic approach employing biosurfactants. Gels 2022; 8(12): 761.
[http://dx.doi.org/10.3390/gels8120761] [PMID: 36547285]

[30] Chopra B, Dhingra AK, Dhar KL. *Psoralea corylifolia* L. (Buguchi) — Folklore to modern evidence: Review. Fitoterapia 2013; 90: 44-56.
[http://dx.doi.org/10.1016/j.fitote.2013.06.016] [PMID: 23831482]

[31] Chopra B, Dhingra AK. Therapeutic and health promoting potential of bakuchiol from *Psoralea corylifolia*: A comprehensive review. Endocr Metab Immune Disord Drug Targets 2023; 23(9): 1125-36.
[http://dx.doi.org/10.2174/1871530323666230207123613] [PMID: 36748816]

[32] Chopra B, Dhingra AK, Grewal AS, Jain A, Chaudhary J, Grover P. Bakuchiol: A potential anticancer compound from *Psoralea corylifolia* Linn. Anticancer Agents Med Chem 2023; 23(9): 989-98.
[http://dx.doi.org/10.2174/1871520623666230130102910] [PMID: 36717993]

[33] Chopra B, Dhingra AK, Dhar KL. Antimicrobial activity of *Psoralea corylifolia* Linn. (Baguchi) seeds extracts by organic solvents and supercritical fluids. Int J Pharm Clin Res 2013; 5(1): 13-6.

[34] Marwaha TK. Formulation design and evaluation of herbal anti-psoriatic emulgel. Journal of Pharmaceutical and Scientific Innovation 2013; 2(3): 30-42.
[http://dx.doi.org/10.7897/2277-4572.02334]

[35] Ali J, Akhtar N, Sultana Y, Baboota S, Ahuja A. Antipsoriatic microemulsion gel formulations for topical drug delivery of babchi oil (*Psoralea corylifolia*). Methods Find Exp Clin Pharmacol 2008; 30(4): 277-85.
[http://dx.doi.org/10.1358/mf.2008.30.4.1185802] [PMID: 18773122]

[36] Niculet E, Radaschin D, Nastase F, *et al.* Influence of phytochemicals in induced psoriasis (Review).

Exp Ther Med 2020; 20(4): 3421-4.
[http://dx.doi.org/10.3892/etm.2020.9013] [PMID: 32905089]

[37] Mihăilă B, Dinică RM, Tatu AL, Buzia OD. New insights in vitiligo treatments using bioactive compounds from *Piper nigrum*. Exp Ther Med 2019; 17(2): 1039-44.
[PMID: 30679971]

[38] Dumitriu Buzia O, Fasie V, Mardare N, Diaconu C, Gurau G, Tatu AL. Formulation, preparation, physico-chemical analysis, microbiological peculiarities and therapeutic challenges of extractive solution of Kombucha. Revista de Chimie 2018; 69(3): 720-4.
[http://dx.doi.org/10.37358/RC.18.3.6184]

[39] Tatu A, Ionescu MA. Multiple autoimmune syndrome type III: Thyroiditis, vitiligo and alopecia areata. Acta Endocrinol (Bucur) 2017; 13(1): 124-5.
[http://dx.doi.org/10.4183/aeb.2017.124] [PMID: 31149160]

[40] Chopra B, Dhingra AK, Kapoor RP, Prasad DN. Piperine and its various physicochemical and biological aspects: A review. Open Chem J 2016; 3(1): 75-96.
[http://dx.doi.org/10.2174/1874842201603010075]

[41] Chopra B, Saini N, Dhingra AK. Synergistic effect of piperine and its derivatives: a comprehensive review. Curr Drug Res Rev 2023; 15(2): 105-21.
[http://dx.doi.org/10.2174/2589977515666221101153730] [PMID: 36321239]

[42] Nwabudike LC, Tatu AL. Using complementary and alternative medicine for the treatment of psoriasis: a step in the right direction. JAMA Dermatol 2019; 155(5): 636-7.
[http://dx.doi.org/10.1001/jamadermatol.2019.0106] [PMID: 30865237]

[43] Herman A, Herman A. Topically used herbal products for the treatment of psoriasis: mechanism of action, drug delivery, clinical studies. Planta Med 2016; 82(17): 1447-55.
[http://dx.doi.org/10.1055/s-0042-115177] [PMID: 27574899]

[44] Maleš Ž, Drvar DL, Duka I, Žužul K. Application of medicinal plants in several dermatovenerological entities. Acta Pharm 2019; 69(4): 525-31.
[http://dx.doi.org/10.2478/acph-2019-0045] [PMID: 31639095]

[45] Agrawal U, Gupta M, Vyas SP. Capsaicin delivery into the skin with lipidic nanoparticles for the treatment of psoriasis. Artif Cells Nanomed Biotechnol 2015; 43(1): 33-9.
[http://dx.doi.org/10.3109/21691401.2013.832683] [PMID: 24040836]

[46] Khatoon K, Ali A, Ahmad FJ, *et al.* Novel nanoemulsion gel containing triple natural bio-actives combination of curcumin, thymoquinone, and resveratrol improves psoriasis therapy: *In vitro* and *in vivo* studies. Drug Deliv Transl Res 2021; 11(3): 1245-60.
[http://dx.doi.org/10.1007/s13346-020-00852-y] [PMID: 32965640]

[47] Dhingra AK, Rathi V, Chopra B. Resveratrol. Naturally Occurring Chemicals Against Alzheimer's Disease. 1st ed. San Diego: Academic Press 2021; pp. 33-42.
[http://dx.doi.org/10.1016/B978-0-12-819212-2.00037-2]

[48] Lai CY, Su YW, Lin KI, Hsu LC, Chuang TH. Natural modulators of endosomal toll-like receptor-mediated psoriatic skin inflammation. J Immunol Res 2017; 2017: 1-15.
[http://dx.doi.org/10.1155/2017/7807313] [PMID: 28894754]

[49] Oliveira A, Monteiro V, Navegantes-Lima K, *et al.* Resveratrol role in autoimmune disease—A mini-review. Nutrients 2017; 9(12): 1306.
[http://dx.doi.org/10.3390/nu9121306] [PMID: 29194364]

[50] Shehzad A, Wahid F, Lee YS. Curcumin in cancer chemoprevention: molecular targets, pharmacokinetics, bioavailability, and clinical trials. Arch Pharm (Weinheim) 2010; 343(9): 489-99.
[http://dx.doi.org/10.1002/ardp.200900319] [PMID: 20726007]

[51] Kanai M, Yoshimura K, Asada M, *et al.* A phase I/II study of gemcitabine-based chemotherapy plus curcumin for patients with gemcitabine-resistant pancreatic cancer. Cancer Chemother Pharmacol

2011; 68(1): 157-64.
[http://dx.doi.org/10.1007/s00280-010-1470-2] [PMID: 20859741]

[52] Wu ST, Sun JC, Lee K, Sun YM. Docking prediction for tumor necrosis factor-α and five herbal inhibitors. Int J Eng Sci Technol 2010; 2: 4263-70.
[http://dx.doi.org/10.2174/157018012799079707]

[53] Kurd SK, Smith N, VanVoorhees A, *et al.* Oral curcumin in the treatment of moderate to severe psoriasis vulgaris: A prospective clinical trial. J Am Acad Dermatol 2008; 58(4): 625-31.
[http://dx.doi.org/10.1016/j.jaad.2007.12.035] [PMID: 18249471]

[54] Nowak-Perlak M, Szpadel K, Jabłońska I, Pizon M, Woźniak M. Promising strategies in plant-derived treatments of psoriasis—update of *in vitro*, *in vivo*, and clinical trials studies. Molecules 2022; 27(3): 591.
[http://dx.doi.org/10.3390/molecules27030591] [PMID: 35163855]

[55] Varma SR, Sivaprakasam TO, Mishra A, Prabhu S, M R, P R. Imiquimod-induced psoriasis-like inflammation in differentiated Human keratinocytes: Its evaluation using curcumin. Eur J Pharmacol 2017; 813: 33-41.
[http://dx.doi.org/10.1016/j.ejphar.2017.07.040] [PMID: 28736282]

[56] Li YL, Du ZY, Li PH, *et al.* Aromatic-turmerone ameliorates imiquimod-induced psoriasis-like inflammation of BALB/c mice. Int Immunopharmacol 2018; 64: 319-25.
[http://dx.doi.org/10.1016/j.intimp.2018.09.015] [PMID: 30243067]

[57] Li Y, Zhang G, Chen M, *et al.* Rutaecarpine inhibited imiquimod-induced psoriasis-like dermatitis *via* inhibiting the NF-κB and TLR7 pathways in mice. Biomed Pharmacother 2019; 109: 1876-83.
[http://dx.doi.org/10.1016/j.biopha.2018.10.062] [PMID: 30551443]

[58] Zhang Y, Xia Q, Li Y, *et al.* CD44 assists the topical anti-psoriatic efficacy of curcumin-loaded hyaluronan modified ethosomes: a new strategy for clustering drug in inflammatory skin. Theranostics 2019; 9(1): 48-64.
[http://dx.doi.org/10.7150/thno.29715] [PMID: 30662553]

[59] Arora N, Shah K, Pandey-Rai S. Inhibition of imiquimod-induced psoriasis-like dermatitis in mice by herbal extracts from some Indian medicinal plants. Protoplasma 2016; 253(2): 503-15.
[http://dx.doi.org/10.1007/s00709-015-0829-y] [PMID: 26016607]

[60] Wu D, Zhang M, Li N, *et al.* PSORI-CM02 alleviates IMQ-induced mouse dermatitis *via* differentially regulating pro- and anti-inflammatory cytokines targeting of Th2 specific transcript factor GATA3. Biomed Pharmacother 2019; 110: 265-74.
[http://dx.doi.org/10.1016/j.biopha.2018.11.092] [PMID: 30513504]

[61] Torricelli C, Fortino V, Capurro E, *et al.* Rottlerin inhibits the nuclear factor κB/Cyclin-D1 cascade in MCF-7 breast cancer cells. Life Sci 2008; 82(11-12): 638-43.
[http://dx.doi.org/10.1016/j.lfs.2007.12.020] [PMID: 18261747]

[62] Putic A, Stecher L, Prinz H, Müller K. Structure–activity relationship studies of acridones as potential antipsoriatic agents. 2. Synthesis and antiproliferative activity of 10-substituted hydroxy-10H-acridn-9-ones against human keratinocyte growth. Eur J Med Chem 2010; 45(11): 5345-52.
[http://dx.doi.org/10.1016/j.ejmech.2010.08.059] [PMID: 20850910]

[63] Min M, Yan BX, Wang P, *et al.* Rottlerin as a therapeutic approach in psoriasis: Evidence from *in vitro* and *in vivo* studies. PLoS One 2017; 12(12): e0190051.
[http://dx.doi.org/10.1371/journal.pone.0190051] [PMID: 29272319]

[64] Grewal S, Tiwary N, Malik G, *et al.* Decoding therapeutic applications of quercetin: Recent advancements in nanotechnological strategies. Pharm Nanotechnol 2024; 12.
[PMID: 38317469]

[65] Shivani SG, Singh G, Narwal S, Chopra B, Dhingra AK. Quercetin-based nanoformulation: A potential approach for cancer treatment. Anticancer Agents Med Chem 2023; 23(18): 1983-2007.

[http://dx.doi.org/10.2174/1871520623666230817101926] [PMID: 37592797]

[66] Devi V, Deswal G, Dass R, Chopra B, Kriplani P, Grewal AS, *et al.* Therapeutic potential and clinical effectiveness of quercetin: A dietary supplement. Recent Adv Food Nutr Agric. 2024; p. 15. [http://dx.doi.org/10.2174/012772574X269376231107095831] [PMID: 38258783]

[67] Ma YC, Mani A, Cai Y, *et al.* An effective identification and quantification method for *Ginkgo biloba* flavonol glycosides with targeted evaluation of adulterated products. Phytomedicine 2016; 23(4): 377-87.
[http://dx.doi.org/10.1016/j.phymed.2016.02.003] [PMID: 27002408]

[68] Koyu H, Haznedaroglu MZ. Investigation of impact of storage conditions on *Hypericum perforatum* L. dried total extract. Yao Wu Shi Pin Fen Xi 2015; 23(3): 545-51.
[PMID: 28911714]

[69] Xiong H, Xu Y, Tan G, *et al.* Glycyrrhizin ameliorates imiquimod-induced psoriasis-like skin lesions in BALB/c mice and inhibits TNF-α-induced ICAM-1 expression *via* NF-κB/MAPK in HaCaT cells. Cell Physiol Biochem 2015; 35(4): 1335-46.
[http://dx.doi.org/10.1159/000373955] [PMID: 25720416]

[70] Kiekow CJ, Figueiró F, Dietrich F, *et al.* Quercetin derivative induces cell death in glioma cells by modulating NF-κB nuclear translocation and caspase-3 activation. Eur J Pharm Sci 2016; 84: 116-22. [http://dx.doi.org/10.1016/j.ejps.2016.01.019] [PMID: 26802551]

[71] Chen H, Lu C, Liu H, *et al.* Quercetin ameliorates imiquimod-induced psoriasis-like skin inflammation in mice *via* the NF-κB pathway. Int Immunopharmacol 2017; 48: 110-7. [http://dx.doi.org/10.1016/j.intimp.2017.04.022] [PMID: 28499194]

[72] Ross JA, Kasum CM. Dietary flavonoids: bioavailability, metabolic effects, and safety. Annu Rev Nutr 2002; 22(1): 19-34.
[http://dx.doi.org/10.1146/annurev.nutr.22.111401.144957] [PMID: 12055336]

[73] Kang HK, Ecklund D, Liu M, Datta SK. Apigenin, a non-mutagenic dietary flavonoid, suppresses lupus by inhibiting autoantigen presentation for expansion of autoreactive Th1 and Th17 cells. Arthritis Res Ther 2009; 11(2): R59.
[http://dx.doi.org/10.1186/ar2682] [PMID: 19405952]

[74] Mirzoeva S, Tong X, Bridgeman BB, Plebanek MP, Volpert OV. Apigenin inhibits UVB-induced skin carcinogenesis: The role of thrombospondin-1 as an anti-inflammatory factor. Neoplasia 2018; 20(9): 930-42.
[http://dx.doi.org/10.1016/j.neo.2018.07.005] [PMID: 30118999]

[75] Chen AY, Chen YC. A review of the dietary flavonoid, kaempferol on human health and cancer chemoprevention. Food Chem 2013; 138(4): 2099-107.
[http://dx.doi.org/10.1016/j.foodchem.2012.11.139] [PMID: 23497863]

[76] Liu C, Liu H, Lu C, *et al.* Kaempferol attenuates imiquimod-induced psoriatic skin inflammation in a mouse model. Clin Exp Immunol 2019; 198(3): 403-15.
[http://dx.doi.org/10.1111/cei.13363] [PMID: 31407330]

[77] Wang A, Wei J, Lu C, *et al.* Genistein suppresses psoriasis-related inflammation through a STAT3–NF-κB-dependent mechanism in keratinocytes. Int Immunopharmacol 2019; 69: 270-8. [http://dx.doi.org/10.1016/j.intimp.2019.01.054] [PMID: 30743203]

[78] Polkowski K, Mazurek AP. Biological properties of genistein. A review of *in vitro* and *in vivo* data. Acta Pol Pharm 2000; 57(2): 135-55.
[PMID: 10934794]

[79] Smolińska E, Moskot M, Jakóbkiewicz-Banecka J, *et al.* Molecular action of isoflavone genistein in the human epithelial cell line HaCaT. PLoS One 2018; 13(2): e0192297.
[http://dx.doi.org/10.1371/journal.pone.0192297] [PMID: 29444128]

[80] Ganeshpurkar A, Saluja AK. The pharmacological potential of rutin. Saudi Pharm J 2017; 25(2): 149-

64.
[http://dx.doi.org/10.1016/j.jsps.2016.04.025] [PMID: 28344465]

[81] Dhanabal SP, Muruganantham N, Basavaraj KH, Wadhwani A, Shamasundar NM. Antipsoriatic activity of extracts and fractions obtained from *Memecylon malabaricum* leaves. J Pharm Pharmacol 2012; 64(10): 1501-9.
[http://dx.doi.org/10.1111/j.2042-7158.2012.01528.x] [PMID: 22943181]

[82] Salehi B, Fokou PVT, Sharifi-Rad M, *et al.* The therapeutic potential of naringenin: A review of clinical trials. Pharmaceuticals (Basel) 2019; 12(1): 11.
[http://dx.doi.org/10.3390/ph12010011] [PMID: 30634637]

[83] Verri WA, Vicentini FTMC, Baracat MM, Georgetti SR, Cardoso RDR, Cunha TM, *et al.* Flavonoids as anti-inflammatory and analgesic drugs: Mechanisms of action and perspectives in the development of pharmaceutical forms. Bioactive Natural Products. Amsterdam: Elsevier 2012; pp. 297-330.
[http://dx.doi.org/10.1016/B978-0-444-53836-9.00026-8]

[84] Liu Y, Su WW, Wang S, Li PB. Naringin inhibits chemokine production in an LPS-induced RAW 264.7 macrophage cell line. Mol Med Rep 2012; 6(6): 1343-50.
[http://dx.doi.org/10.3892/mmr.2012.1072] [PMID: 22965302]

[85] Deenonpoe R, Prayong P, Thippamom N, Meephansan J, Na-Bangchang K. Anti-inflammatory effect of naringin and sericin combination on Human Peripheral Blood Mononuclear Cells (hPBMCs) from patient with psoriasis. BMC Complement Altern Med 2019; 19(1): 168.
[http://dx.doi.org/10.1186/s12906-019-2535-3] [PMID: 31291937]

[86] Winiarska-Mieczan A, Mieczan T, Wójcik G. Importance of redox equilibrium in the pathogenesis of psoriasis: Impact of antioxidant-rich diet. Nutrients 2020; 12(6): 1841.
[http://dx.doi.org/10.3390/nu12061841] [PMID: 32575706]

[87] Zhang S, Liu X, Mei L, Wang H, Fang F. Epigallocatechin-3-gallate (EGCG) inhibits imiquimod-induced psoriasis-like inflammation of BALB/c mice. BMC Complement Altern Med 2016; 16(1): 334.
[http://dx.doi.org/10.1186/s12906-016-1325-4] [PMID: 27581210]

[88] Chamcheu JC, Pal HC, Siddiqui IA, *et al.* Prodifferentiation, anti-inflammatory and antiproliferative effects of delphinidin, a dietary anthocyanidin, in a full-thickness three-dimensional reconstituted human skin model of psoriasis. Skin Pharmacol Physiol 2015; 28(4): 177-88.
[http://dx.doi.org/10.1159/000368445] [PMID: 25620035]

[89] Shih CM, Hsieh CK, Huang CY, *et al.* Lycopene inhibits IMQ-induced psoriasis-like inflammation by inhibiting ICAM-1 production in mice. Polymers (Basel) 2020; 12(7): 1521.
[http://dx.doi.org/10.3390/polym12071521] [PMID: 32659890]

[90] Nguyen UT, Nguyen LTH, Kim BA, Choi MJ, Yang IJ, Shin HM. Natural compound mixture, containing emodin, genipin, chlorogenic acid, cimigenoside, and ginsenoside Rb1, ameliorates psoriasis-like skin lesions by suppressing inflammation and proliferation in keratinocytes. Evid Based Complement Alternat Med 2020; 2020(1): 9416962.
[http://dx.doi.org/10.1155/2020/9416962] [PMID: 33149756]

CHAPTER 7

Liposome-based Pharmacotherapy for the Management of Psoriasis

Manish Kumar[1,*], **Shubhi**[2], **Bhuwanendra Singh**[3], **Anuradha**[4], **Abhishek Tiwari**[5] and **Varsha Tiwari**[5]

[1] *Department of Pharmaceutics, ISF College of Pharmacy, Moga 142001, Punjab, India*

[2] *Department of Quality Assurance, ISF College of Pharmacy, Moga 142001, Punjab, India*

[3] *Department of Pharmacognosy, S.D College of Pharmacy & Vocational Studies, Muzaffarnagar 251001, Uttar Pradesh, India*

[4] *Bharat Institute of Technology, NH58 Bypass, Partapur, Meerut, Mahroli 250103, Uttar Pradesh, India*

[5] *Pharmacy Academy, IFTM University, Lodhipur-Rajput, Delhi Road, Moradabad 244102, Uttar Pradesh, India*

Abstract: The chronic inflammatory skin disease, psoriasis, affects a large number of people globally. It is typified by immune system malfunction that results in a range of symptoms. The primary goal of conventional drug delivery methods for psoriasis treatment is to alleviate symptoms; however, these methods frequently fall short due to their poor safety and efficacy, low bioavailability, and limited effectiveness. Consequently, there has been an increase in interest in creating innovative drug delivery systems that might overcome these drawbacks. Liposomes, transferosomes, ethosomes, niosomes, emulsomes, dendrimers, hydrogels, nanoparticles, and others are examples of these novel drug delivery methods. Through modifications to pharmacokinetic and physiological factors, these formulations aim to enhance the therapeutic effects of medications. Liposomes are one of these systems that are the most promising for delivering medications to treat psoriasis. Liposomes are lipid bilayer-based tiny vesicles that can enhance the penetration of medications through the stratum corneum, the outermost layer of the skin. When applied topically, this increased penetration can improve the delivery of medications into or through the skin. Improved therapeutic results are a result of liposomes' many benefits, which include longer drug release and enhanced stability. The potential of liposomes as a drug delivery mechanism for treating psoriasis is the main topic of this chapter. By encapsulating anti-psoriatic medications inside liposomes, researchers aim to enhance treatment efficiency and target areas affected by psoriasis. Treating psoriasis with liposomes has the potential to enhance patient outcomes by overcoming the limitations of traditional drug delivery methods. In conclusion, the development of innovative medication delivery methods, such as liposomes, offers a viable strategy for managing

* **Corresponding author Manish Kumar:** Department of Pharmaceutics, ISF College of Pharmacy, Moga 142001, Punjab, India; E-mail: manish_singh17@rediffmail.com

psoriasis. Through the utilisation of liposomes' distinct characteristics, such as their enhanced drug penetration and extended release, scientists aim to augment the therapeutic outcomes of pharmaceuticals and improve the overall treatment of psoriasis.

Keywords: Drug delivery, Innovative formulations, Liposomes, Pharmacotherapy, Psoriasis, Skin Disease, Targeted therapy, Topical delivery.

INTRODUCTION

Psoriasis is a skin condition typified by the production of red, thicker plaques coated in silver-white scales, indicating autoimmune T-cell activity. The research shows that the precise cause of psoriasis is still uncertain. Psoriasis can now be treated with a variety of antipsoriatic medications, but these treatments are primarily aimed at relieving symptoms and can have serious side effects. Topical treatments, phototherapy, and systemic interventions are among the available treatments, but none of them offer a permanent cure. Researchers are actively investigating the potential of various colloidal carriers within drug delivery systems to overcome the limitations of current therapies, which include safety concerns, inefficiency, and unfavourable cosmetic outcomes. These limitations underscore the need for enhanced drug delivery systems in the treatment of psoriasis [1]. Different types of carriers, including ethosomes, liposomes, niosomes, transferosomes, solid lipid nanoparticles, microspheres, micelles, dendrimers, and other innovative platforms, are being investigated. Carriers offer opportunities to develop more effective therapeutic regimens for psoriasis by addressing the shortcomings of current treatments. By utilizing these advanced drug delivery systems, researchers aim to improve drug efficacy, minimize side effects, and ultimately enhance patient outcomes. Each carrier has its unique properties and benefits, which are being explored to optimize the delivery of the drug to the affected areas of the skin. The exploration of these novel drug delivery systems holds promise for revolutionizing the treatment of psoriasis. It offers the potential to deliver antipsoriatic drugs more efficiently, enhance drug stability and release, and improve patient adherence during prolonged use. Through these advancements, researchers aim to deliver improved outcomes for individuals with psoriasis and alleviate the challenges associated with conventional therapies [2]. Research on novel drug delivery methods for treating psoriasis is currently underway, with a focus on colloidal carriers. Using carriers, such as ethosomes, liposomes, niosomes, transferosomes, solid lipid nanoparticles, microspheres, micelles, dendrimers, and others, scientists aim to overcome the limitations of existing treatments and achieve better outcomes for patients with psoriasis. These developments could significantly alter the way this chronic skin condition is treated, offering safer and more efficient alternatives.

Alec D. Bangham made the initial discovery of liposomes at the University of Cambridge's Babraham Institute in the 1960s. These lipid-based structures consist of one or more concentric lipid bilayers enclosing an aqueous compartment. Liposomes were once made entirely of natural lipids; however, nowadays they can also include surfactants and a mixture of synthetic and natural lipids. They are remarkable in that they can contain lipophilic and hydrophilic substances in their lipid membrane and watery core. Liposomes are spherical in shape and can have a size range of several micrometers to a few nanometers. However, the diameter of liposomes employed in medicine is usually between 50 and 450 nm. Over the past 50 years, liposomes have been the subject of much investigation due to their similarities to cellular membranes and their ability to incorporate different molecules [3]. They are widely valued for their benefits in biology and technology as the best delivery vehicles for biologically active compounds in both *in vitro* [lab settings] and *in vivo* [living creatures] contexts. Indeed, liposomes are considered the most effective medication delivery technology available today.

Significant advancements have been made in the field of liposome research within the past 20 years. While some liposome-based biomedical applications are currently undergoing clinical studies or are about to enter the market, others have already received approval for general use. Hence, the emphasis is on critical elements that are essential for the creation of liposomal compositions intended for medicinal use. This chapter describes how the size, surface charge, and lipid organization of liposomes, as well as the physicochemical parameters of their membranes and component makeup, affect their efficacy. It also examines how these physicochemical characteristics impact liposome stability in the circulation, their ability to enter various types of tissues, their interaction with cells, and ultimately, their final destination in the body. The overview focuses on methods that have been developed to overcome the drawbacks of early-generation liposomes, which have been crucial in facilitating the transition from laboratory research to clinical trials or commercialization. Liposomes are versatile, lipid-based structures that have garnered significant attention in the scientific community [4]. They offer numerous advantages as drug delivery systems and have shown promising results in various biomedical applications. Understanding the physicochemical properties of liposomes and their impact on efficacy, stability, tissue targeting, and cellular interactions is vital for the development of improved therapeutic liposomal formulations.

TYPES OF PSORIASIS

The degree of inflammation, the location of the rash, the persistence of a patient's medical issues, and other clinical considerations are some of the variables that determine the classification of psoriasis into different categories. These categories encompass several types of psoriasis, including guttate, pustular, erythrodermic, and plaque psoriasis, all of which are distinct chronic skin diseases. The most prevalent type of psoriasis vulgaris, or chronic plaque psoriasis, is characterized by the progressive formation of small papules that eventually coalesce to form plaques on the skin. Guttate psoriasis, in contrast, is triggered by an immune response that can be exacerbated by a Streptococcal infection, presenting as small, pink, raised bumps that later develop into flaky patches.

Erythrodermic psoriasis is a severe form of psoriasis that can result in significant protein and fluid loss, disrupting the body's normal balance. Patients with this severe condition may require hospitalization due to complications like staphylococcal infections, pustulosis, joint issues [arthropathy], and growth retardation [5]. Pustular psoriasis, another severe variant, is characterized by the presence of pus-filled lesions primarily identified on the palms and soles of the feet. However, they can also spread across the body. Although these lesions usually have minimal systemic effects, managing them can be challenging. Generalized pustular psoriasis is a more severe form of the disease, characterized by symptoms, such as fever, fatigue, and electrolyte disturbances, which can increase patients' susceptibility to infections. This type of psoriasis often recurs frequently, necessitating careful management to address symptoms and prevent complications.

Categorization According to Prevalence

Plaque Psoriasis

Plaque psoriasis, also known as psoriasis vulgaris, accounts for approximately 90% of all psoriasis cases and is the most common type. Plaques develop because of lesions and peripheral spreading [6]. Reddish, round plaques covered in dry scales that have a silvery-white appearance are among the distinctive clinical symptoms. Although plaque psoriasis can affect any part of the body, the elbows, knees, scalp, and trunk are common areas where it appears symmetrically.

Guttate Psoriasis

Approximately 8% of psoriasis cases are classified as guttate psoriasis. "*Gutta*" is a Latin word that inspired the name. Multiple tiny, pink, scaly patches, ranging in size from 3 to 5 mm, are the hallmark of guttate psoriasis. These patches are often found on the legs, upper arms, and chest. Teens and young people are the main demographic that it impacts. Upper respiratory tract infections, such as streptococcal infections, account for around 66% of newly diagnosed instances of guttate psoriasis. It is widely recognized that the guttate psoriasis rash typically appears within 2-4 days following a bacterial infection [7]. This form of psoriasis can develop into plaque psoriasis or become chronic on its own if treatment is not received.

Pustular Psoriasis

Scarlet psoriasis affects approximately 3% of people with psoriasis and is a relatively uncommon condition. This kind is also known as Von Zumbusch psoriasis. It also has systemic effects on the body and is typified by extensive skin inflammation [8]. Common histological features of pustular psoriasis include redness and sterile pustules, which are caused by neutrophils entering the stratum spinosum. Acrodermatitis continua of Hallopeau and pustulosis palmaris et plantaris are examples of localized forms of pustular psoriasis. Pustular psoriasis manifests as high fever, weakness, an elevated neutrophil count, and obvious skin abnormalities. A particular change in the interleukin 36 receptor antagonist [IL36RN] sequence, formerly known as a mutation, has been linked to generalized pustular psoriasis. Factors like pregnancy, infection, hypocalcaemia, and steroid tapering might cause this disease.

Erythrodermic Psoriasis

Erythrodermic psoriasis is a rare yet serious variant of psoriasis that affects approximately 2% to 3% of individuals with the condition. Patients suffering from this form typically exhibit significant coverage of at least 75% of their body with overlapping redness, scales, or skin shedding. This manifestation is considered a critical situation in dermatology due to its association with electrolyte imbalances and excessive skin peeling, both of which have the potential to be life-threatening. Erythrodermic psoriasis is characterized by a severe form of the disease, with redness and inflammation affecting over 90% of the body's surface [9]. It can appear in any form of psoriasis and requires immediate medical intervention.

Categorization According to Anatomical Locations

Nail Psoriasis

Psoriasis frequently extends to the nails, affecting a significant portion of individuals at a rate ranging from 10% to 82%. Five to ten percent of people have nail psoriasis alone, meaning they do not have any skin involvement. It is believed that nail psoriasis serves as a separate predictor of the advancement of Psoriatic Arthritis [PsA] [10]. Sadly, there are not many effective treatment choices for nail psoriasis, and those that are sometimes useless. Pitting of the nails is the most noticeable feature. However, onycholysis—the separation of the nail's proximal end from its nail bed—is the most common nail deformity associated with psoriasis.

Inverse Psoriasis

Flexural psoriasis, another name for inverse psoriasis, can affect the inner folds of the flexor surfaces and the perineal, inframammary, axillary, inguinal, and intergluteal regions [11]. The disease is more commonly found on the outer surfaces of the elbows and knees. It is characterized by a plaque form of psoriasis due to the accumulation of moisture in these regions.

Palmoplantar

Non-pustular palmoplantar psoriasis manifests as painful cracks and thick scaly skin. To minimize its occurrence, it is advisable to refrain from applying emollients during the day to prevent unnecessary irritation and friction. Additionally, avoiding substances that may cause irritation is also recommended.

Scalp Psoriasis

Psoriasis often affects the scalp more than any other area of the body. When psoriasis occurs along the hairline, it can significantly impact a person's life due to its visibility. Finding the right medication, dealing with the challenges of applying topical treatments, and making informed treatment decisions have all been important considerations when managing psoriasis on the scalp.

PATHOGENESIS OF PSORIASIS

Physically, psoriasis is characterized by a significant alteration in the keratinocyte transformation process, which leads to the development of scaly patches. The creation of new cells in the epidermis' basal layer is the first step in this transition. After that, these cells move in the direction of the outer layer, congregating around the stratum corneum, or keratin, and losing their organelles in the process. These cells fill with keratin as they reach the stratum corneum, giving the skin its defensive qualities. As part of the shedding and renewal cycle of the epidermis, basal layer keratinocytes normally divide every two weeks, and it takes four weeks for new cells to form.

On the other hand, the cell cycle quickens in skin affected by psoriasis, resulting in cell division every 1.5 days and keratinocytes reaching the stratum corneum in four days [12]. This quick speed prevents the cells from properly developing and maturing, giving the epidermis its distinctive scaly look and making it three to five times thicker than normal. Neutrophil clusters in the skin's outermost layer, along with a notable concentration of T-cells and dendritic cells in the subcutaneous layer, are histological indicators of psoriasis. Notable characteristics also include the presence of mononuclear leukocytes, which induce the elongation or hyperproliferation of blood vessels in the papillary dermal area, resulting in the redness of psoriatic lesions due to widespread blood vessel dilatation. Furthermore, due to the adhesion of neutrophils, monocytes, and lymphocytes, endothelial cells in psoriatic lesions exhibit traits similar to those observed in lymph node vessels. In psoriatic lesions, the presence of intracellular adhesion molecule-1 [ICAM-1 or CD54], vascular cell adhesion molecule-1 [VCAM-1 or CD106], and E-selectin [CD62E] during staining, which indicates the adherence of lymphocytes, monocytes, and neutrophils, is indicative of the activation of cells in the endothelial layer.

Histology, Keratinocytes, Proliferation and Abnormal Differentiation

As the predominant cell type in the epidermis, keratinocytes play a crucial role. They play several roles in the skin's healing process. Re-epithelialization, the process by which keratinocytes migrate, proliferate, and differentiate to repair the epidermal barrier, is one of their main responsibilities. A number of substances found in the wound, including growth hormones, cytokines, chemokines, and Matrix Metalloproteinases [MMPs], affect how keratinocytes shift between these different states [13]. Researchers are still working to pinpoint the exact cause of psoriasis. Histological results of psoriasis patients show acanthosis, characterized by an overabundance of keratinocytes, or epidermal cells, in the skin. It has been noted that the desquamation [or keratinocyte differentiation] process is accelerated to 3–4 days instead of the customary 4-6 weeks. This is demonstrated by the presence of keratinocytes' nuclei and the scaly appearance caused by the absence of the cornified layer. Cell-to-cell and cytokine interactions play a crucial role in the physiopathology of psoriasis. Psoriasis-related aberrant keratinocytes display deregulation of several genes, including those encoding β1 integrins and insulin-like growth factor receptor-1 [14]. Furthermore, because typical corneocytes are absent in psoriasis, the epidermal barrier is structurally defective. The cohesiveness of the stratum corneum, which depends on the interactions between corneocytes, is hampered by this shortage.

Modifications in the Vascular System

Keratinocytes produce Vascular Endothelial Growth Factor (VEGF) and platelet-derived growth factor (PDGF), which stimulate the formation and expansion of blood vessels. These growth factors activate endothelial cells, prompting them to release mediators, such as Keratinocyte Growth Factor (KGF), which in turn promotes keratinocyte proliferation. Additionally, they cause dermal capillaries to dilate, facilitating the passage of immune cells from the bloodstream. As a result, neutrophils and lymphocytes cross the vascular endothelium and infiltrate the skin. This migration is enabled by the upregulation of specific adhesion molecules on the surface of endothelial cells, including VCAM-1 (vascular cell adhesion molecule-1 or CD106), ICAM-1 (intercellular adhesion molecule-1 or CD54), and E-selectin (CD62E). These adhesion molecules serve as binding sites that attract and retain immune cells at sites of inflammation.

Infiltration of Inflammatory Cells in Skin and Cytokine Production

Immune cells heavily infiltrate the dermis and epidermis of psoriasis patients, releasing proinflammatory cytokines that exacerbate and prolong the inflammatory reaction. These immune cells include Langerhans cells [16], CD4+ T cells, and dendritic cells (which function as phagocytes and antigen-presenting cells), including CD11c+ Myeloid Dendritic Cells [MDCs]. These cells exhibit aberrant dermal invasion, exacerbating the inflammatory milieu present in psoriatic lesions. In addition, CD8+ T lymphocytes, Langerhans cells, and CD11c+ myeloid dendritic cells are clearly visible in the epidermis of psoriatic lesions. Interestingly, the horny layer of the skin contains a sizable percentage of neutrophils. T cells, specifically CD4+ and CD8+ subsets, are essential to the pathophysiology of psoriasis from its onset through the maintenance of the inflammatory cascade. Studies have repeatedly shown that T lymphocytes play a pivotal role in psoriasis, particularly in their activation upon encountering antigens presented by antigen-presenting cells, which are primarily dendritic cells within skin lesions. This activation occurs through interactions involving class I (CD8+) or class II (CD4+) major histocompatibility complex molecules.

Psoriasis Treatment Management

The absence of an optimal medication molecule makes effective management of psoriasis a substantial issue, even with the large assortment of therapeutic drugs available for the condition. A few major obstacles that affect psoriasis therapy are listed below:

- **Lack of an Efficient Drug Delivery Mechanism:** The successful administration of anti-psoriatic drugs is impeded by obstacles arising from the unfavourable effects of therapeutic compounds or their inadequate absorption into conventional carriers. Differences in the physicochemical properties of the active medication and the carrier lead to variations in therapeutic effectiveness and absorption. Novel colloidal delivery carriers have emerged as a promising approach to addressing these issues. These carriers offer numerous benefits, including shielding encapsulated medications from environmental and internal influences, regulating drug release to maintain therapeutic levels in the body for prolonged periods, and passively or actively delivering medications to targeted action sites [17]. By facilitating multiple channels of contact with target cells, this focused method reduces toxicity in non-target areas and enhances overall therapeutic efficacy. Essentially, these novel colloidal carriers provide a viable alternative to traditional pharmaceutical delivery methods, mitigating the adverse effects of active medication ingredients while enhancing therapeutic outcomes.

- **Lack of Suitable Animal Models:** Psoriasis predominantly affects humans, complicating the search for appropriate animal models that can accurately replicate the histopathological and immunogenic characteristics observed in human psoriasis. Although several immunogenetic models have been developed, none comprehensively capture all the unique features and limitations of the disease. Commonly used models, such as the spontaneous mutation model, the xenotransplantation model, and the transgenic model, have certain drawbacks. For instance, the spontaneous mutation model lacks significant immune responses; the xenotransplantation model may exhibit histological disparities; and the transgenic model, which focuses on the alteration of single genes, fails to reflect the multigenetic nature of psoriasis.

Addressing these challenges is crucial for enhancing psoriasis treatment strategies and developing more effective therapies for individuals affected by this chronic skin condition. Innovations in drug delivery technology and the development of animal models are essential for advancing our understanding of psoriasis and improving patient outcomes in the realm of treatment and management.

PHYSIOCHEMISTRY OF LIPOSOMES

The physicochemical characteristics of liposomes' membranes, including their component makeup, size, surface charge, and lipid arrangement, all affect how well they function as drug carriers. Phospholipids are amphiphilic molecules having two polar hydrophobic chains and a hydrophilic head that make up the majority of liposomes. Because they are amphipathic, phospholipids tend to form membranes in aqueous solutions. These membranes are made of two lipid layers with hydrophobic chains facing each other. This creates an inner lipophilic compartment that acts as an impermeable barrier to both inward and outward permeability. Van der Waals forces and hydrophobic interactions are two examples of interaction forces that support the development and stability of these lipid bilayers. Hydrogen bonds and polar interactions between water molecules and the lipid heads further stabilize the membrane organization. These interactions are regulated by nature, concentration, temperature, and shape [18]. In the formulation process, ions or molecules present can be encapsulated within these membranes. Liposomes are categorized based on preparation method, size, and lamellarity. Unilamellar vesicles [ULVs], consisting of a single lipid bilayer suitable for encapsulating hydrophilic drugs, typically range from 50 to 250 nm.

In contrast, multilamellar vesicles [MLVs], with multiple concentric lipid bilayers organized like onion layers, are better for entrapping lipid-soluble drugs and range from 1 to 5 μm. ULVs and MLVs are believed to have different release kinetics due to their structural differences, with MLVs generally having a greater entrapped volume and forming more easily at larger diameters, resulting in slower release rates compared to ULVs.

Second-generation liposomes were developed as a result of ongoing research interest in liposome properties, including stability, pharmacokinetics, and therapeutic efficacy. To improve these liposomes, alterations in lipid composition, size, and vesicle charge have been investigated. For example, adding cholesterol to the liposomes' lipid bilayer reduces permeability and facilitates the packing of phospholipids in a denser manner. In addition, cholesterol can be used for a variety of purposes to bind other molecules to liposomes, such as DNA or polyethylene glycol [PEG] [19]. Furthermore, the incorporation of hydrophilic carbohydrates or polymers, including PEG and monosialoganglioside [GM1], into the liposome composition extends its *in vivo* circulation duration by decreasing reticuloendothelial system uptake. Liposomes can be selectively targeted with ligands or monoclonal antibodies by modifying the terminal of the PEG molecule. These developments facilitate the development of liposome-based drug delivery systems that are more effective and targeted.

Methodology for the Preparation of Liposomes

There are various methods for preparing liposomes:

- The physicochemical characteristics of both the liposome's constituent components and the drug to be loaded are two primary factors considered in liposome preparation.
- The toxicity and concentration of the loaded substance must be carefully evaluated.
- The liposomal dispersion medium affects the preparation process.
- Extra procedures are required for applying and delivering liposomes.
- The ideal liposome size and half-life are critical for practical use.
- Costs, reproducibility, scalability for large-scale production, and adherence to good manufacturing practices are important considerations.

The Bangham method, also known as the thin-film hydration method, is one of the methods often employed for liposome production. Lipids are dissolved in an organic solvent using this approach. The solvent is then evaporated, and the resulting lipid film is dispersed in an aqueous medium. The medication to be ensnared may be present in the lipid film for lipophilic medications or in the aqueous medium for hydrophilic pharmaceuticals. However, the method often yields large and non-uniform multilamellar vesicles [MLVs], requiring additional processes like sonication or extrusion to produce homogeneous small unilamellar vesicles [ULVs]. Moreover, the encapsulation efficiency for water-soluble drugs is typically low, ranging from 5% to 15% [5]. In comparison to thin-film hydration, other approaches, such as reverse-phase evaporation and solvent-injection procedures, offer superior encapsulation efficiency by directly hydrating lipids from organic solvents to create MLVs and ULVs, respectively [20]. While post-formation processing techniques, such as sonication, extrusion, and high-pressure homogenization, are frequently used to control the size, lamellarity, and homogeneity of liposomes, the detergent-depletion method and the dehydration-rehydration technique offer alternatives for liposome preparation, each with varying benefits in terms of simplicity and efficiency.

Sonication is one method that helps reduce vesicle size. Other methods used to reduce liposome size further and improve its characteristics for drug delivery applications include membrane extrusion and high-pressure homogenization. More recent approaches, such as microfluidic-based methods, which provide exact control over liposome synthesis, have been added to the repertoire of liposome preparation techniques. These microfluidic technologies offer significant opportunities for rapid and efficient liposomal drug manufacture by enabling real-time, continuous-flow synthesis of liposomes with high drug loadings and increased efficiency. Techniques for monitoring liposome properties, including size, shape, and lamellarity, are essential for ensuring their effectiveness in drug delivery applications [21]. For the investigation of liposome size and distribution, various techniques, including dynamic light scattering, electron microscopy, and size-exclusion chromatography, are frequently employed. These analytical instruments offer crucial insights into liposome characteristics that are required for their efficient use in drug delivery and biological applications.

Thin Film Hydration Method

To achieve the desired drug loading and increase the lipid content, blank liposomes were first prepared. At a 65:35 ratio of lipids, blank liposomes with a fixed molar ratio of cholesterol and DOTAP were made with different lipid concentrations [2 mg/ml, 6 mg/ml, 10 mg/ml, and 15 mg/ml]. Furthermore, liposomes containing 30 mg/mL were also generated, as shown in the figure below. Essentially, cholesterol and DOTAP were dissolved, and the solvent, along with chloroform, was evaporated using a rotary evaporator at 37 degrees Celsius. Subsequently, the film was hydrated with Millipore water to disperse the liposomes [22]. After obtaining the formulation, ultrasonication was carried out using a 40% amplitude, on-off pulse sonicator at varying durations [20s:10s] to achieve a consistent liposome dispersion. An ice bath was utilized during sonication.

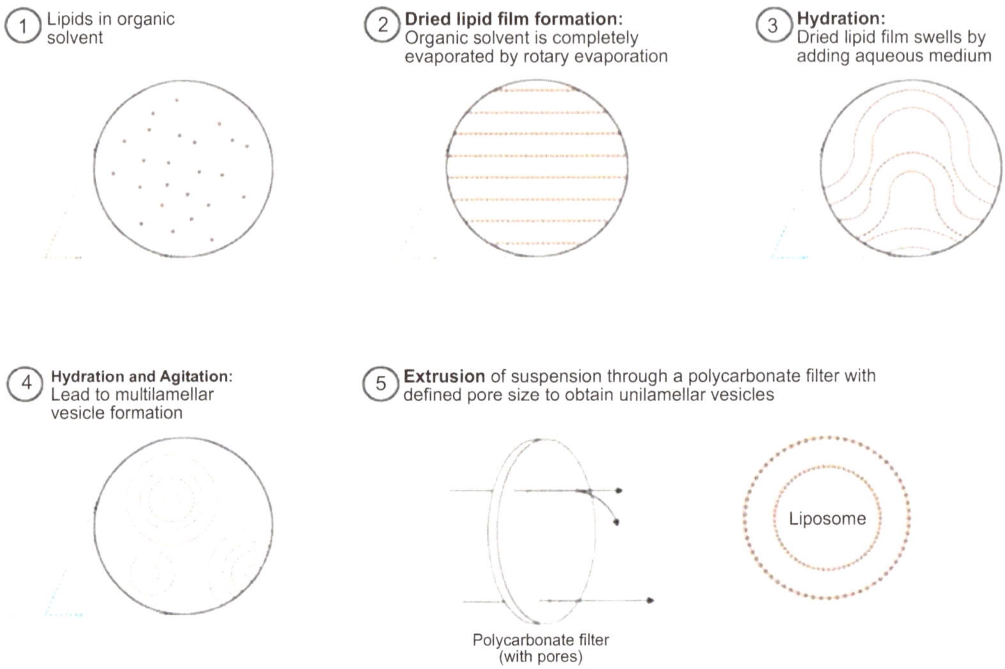

Fig. (1). Liposome preparation.

Ethanol Injection Method

The medicine was injected into the liposomes using an optimal composition after the lipid concentration of the blank liposomes was optimized. Lipids were dissolved in ethanol and then added to the external aqueous phase to produce liposomes for the ethanol injection liposome preparation method. The ethanol was removed by evaporating it in a rotary evaporator while under vacuum. In order to achieve a homogeneous liposome dispersion, the remaining lubricant in the prepared liposomal dispersion was subsequently exposed to size reduction using on-off pulse [20s:10s] at 40% amplitude using an ultrasonicator for varied time intervals [23]. To stop the sound waves from producing heat during sonication, an ice bath was used. Similar to how blank liposomes were made, drug-loaded liposomes were made by adding the drug during the ethanol phase. The other processes were then carried out in the same manner.

Reverse Phase Evaporation Method

As stated in the other two methods, blank liposomes were refined and then drug-loaded. Lipids were dissolved in chloroform to make liposomes. After adding the aqueous phase to the organic phase [millipore water], the mixture was sonicated for 10 minutes using a bath sonicator to produce a milky consistency [24]. The milky solution was then stored for evaporation of chloroform at normal temperature. After obtaining the liposome dispersion, probe sonication was performed with ultra sonicators set to 40% amplitude and on-off pulse [20s:10s] at different time intervals to achieve a uniform liposome dispersion. Sonication was carried out with an ice bath to prevent overheating.

Preparation of Drug-Loaded Liposomes

Drug-loaded liposomes were produced *via* ethanol injection and thin film hydration techniques. To create CYC-loaded liposomes, drug loading varied between 5 and 15% w/w in both methods. Drug-loaded liposomes had their polydispersity index, entrapment efficiency, and particle size adjusted.

Preparation of Drug-Loaded Liposomal Gels

CYC plain gel [CYC D gel] and CYC liposomal gel [CYC L gel], each containing 0.45% w/w CYC, were produced using 1% w/v carbopol 934 [25]. About 200 mg of Carbopol was mixed with 20 mL of CYC liposomal dispersion to form the CYC L gel. To make plain gels, CYC was dissolved in 20 mL of Milli-Q water, and the resulting dispersion was then added to the Carbopol gel foundation. Both gels were neutralized with triethanolamine to a pH of six. A full day was spent in storage prior to using the gels.

Pharmacokinetics of Liposomes

The number of factors that influence a drug's final destination may include the target cell's cytoplasm or extracellular fluid. These factors include the specific structural characteristics of the drug molecule, the method of release, and the composition of the carrier in which it is transported. To put it another way, a drug's molecular architecture refers to the specific arrangement of its atoms and functional groups. These factors have a significant impact on the drug's fate within the body, and comprehending them is essential to figuring out how well the drug works to achieve its intended goal. This architecture plays a critical role in determining how the drug interacts with its target and how it is recognized and internalized by the target cell. Certain structural features may enhance or hinder the drug's ability to penetrate cellular barriers and reach its intended site of action [26]. The mechanism of release refers to the process by which the drug is liberated from its carrier or delivery system. Different methods can be employed, including gradual diffusion, controlled release, and rapid release. The release mechanism significantly influences the drug's availability and distribution within the body. The drug's ability to penetrate the target cell's cytoplasm or stay in the extracellular fluid can be ascertained.

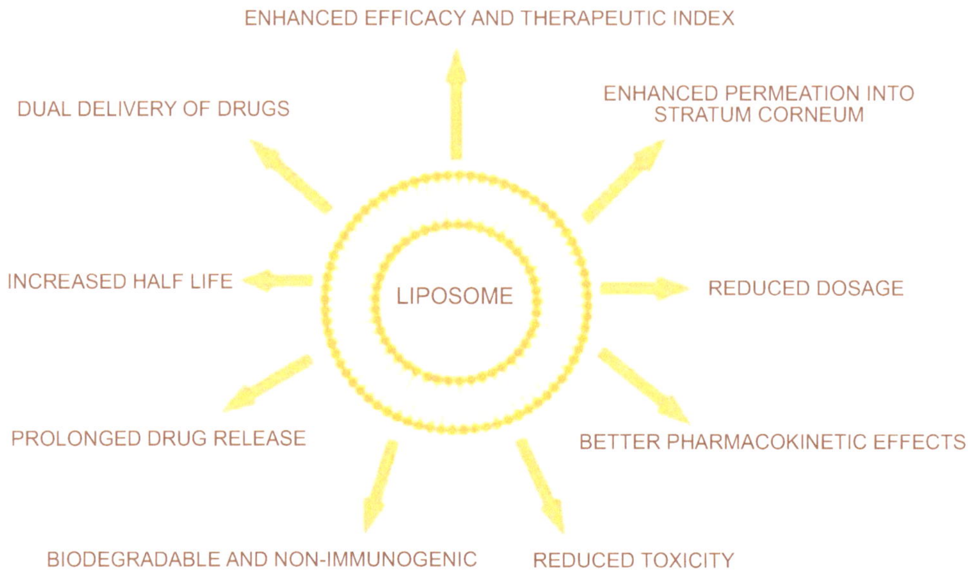

Fig. (2). Significant features of Liposome drug delivery.

The drug's fate is also influenced by the composition of the carrier, which can be any of several delivery mechanisms, including proteins, liposomes, and nanoparticles. The medicine is transported to its intended location *via* the carrier. The properties of drugs, such as stability, solubility, and cellular absorption, can be influenced by the composition of the carrier [27]. Furthermore, the carrier may have an impact on the drug's overall pharmacokinetics and biodistribution, influencing whether it penetrates the cytoplasm or stays in the extracellular fluid. Numerous factors influence a drug's ultimate destiny, including whether it enters the target cell's cytoplasm or extracellular fluid. These consist of the carrier's makeup, the drug's molecular structure, and the release mechanism. Comprehending these variables facilitates the development of more efficient medication delivery mechanisms and enhances treatment results [28]. There are multiple methods for removing liposomes from the body. One way is when certain proteins in the blood bind to the surface of the liposomes, which are then recognized by a system in the body called the reticuloendothelial system [also known as RES]. This recognition leads to the release of the content contained within the liposomes in the liver, where special cells called Kupffer cells break it down. Another way liposomes are eliminated is when they are broken down by certain cells called macrophages in the spleen. Additionally, when liposomes accumulate in specific tissues, they undergo metabolism and eventually get eliminated.

Over time, conventional liposomes have faced several challenges, which have had a significant impact on pharmacology. One significant drawback is that they are quickly captured by the RES, which causes them to primarily accumulate in the liver and spleen. This happens because these organs contain numerous phagocytic cells and have a rich blood supply, as mentioned in Figure 2 above. While this is beneficial for treating localized infections, during chemotherapy, it can hinder the normal functioning of macrophages. Moreover, liposomal drugs can become trapped in organs, such as the spleen and liver, resulting in a delayed clearance of lipophilic anticancer agents from the bloodstream. Researchers have employed several techniques to develop a new generation of liposomes that overcome these limitations [29]. The most effective method, first introduced in the early 1990s, involved adding a material known as PEGylation to the liposome surface. Because of this alteration, liposomes are no longer detectable by macrophages, which significantly increases their stability and duration of circulation. The ability of these altered liposomes, dubbed "Stealth liposomes," to elude the immune system results in a noticeably longer blood circulation duration.

PEG, or polyethylene glycol, is a polymer with several advantageous characteristics, including low toxicity, biocompatibility, oil and water solubility, and effective bodily excretion. The FDA has given it approval for internal use in the biomedical industry. PEG chains provide liposomes with a layer of defence that keeps them from interacting with mononuclear phagocytic system cells. These chains cover the liposomes' surface to create a hydrophilic layer [30]. This layer prevents different substances or compounds in the bloodstream from affecting liposomes through a process called "steric hindrance." Moreover, PEG on the surface of the liposome can increase its size in a fluid environment, thereby slowing down the rate at which the body eliminates it. Both the particle's volume and the molecule's size affect clearance.

The unique property of PEG-modified liposomes is their resistance to complement components and phagocytic cell engulfment. Furthermore, by extending circulation time and avoiding the reticuloendothelial system, PEG promotes the creation of small, homogeneous particles, inhibits clumping, and improves the Enhanced Permeability and Retention (EPR) effect. Comparing PEGylated Stealth liposomes to regular liposomes reveals important practical ramifications of these phenomena [31]. With a prolonged half-life, stealth liposomes limit dispersion within healthy tissues, reduce systemic plasma clearance, and remain in the bloodstream for extended periods. They may, therefore, more effectively target particular sites and attain a significantly greater drug concentration over an extended period of time [as seen by the area under the curve].

When the half-lives of PEGylated and non-PEGylated liposomes are compared, the advantages of PEGylation become evident. PEGylation is an effective method for enhancing drug accumulation at target sites, as it extends the liposome half-life from a few hours to approximately 45 hours [32, 33]. Nevertheless, because PEG creates steric hindrance, its presence can impede cellular uptake even while it lengthens the circulation time. While there are therapeutic benefits associated with liposome-based medicines approved by the FDA, these therapies do not actively target specific cells. Instead, these treatments rely on passive accumulation *via* the EPR effect. To put it another way, these nanomedicines can only release pharmaceuticals passively at the target region; they cannot release drugs actively.

In certain situations, such as with cisplatin-loaded liposomes, the simple release of medications may not function optimally or yield the desired outcome. To overcome these limitations, a more specific and advanced method known as active targeting can be employed using ligand-mediated strategies. The aim is to develop liposome platforms that exhibit enhanced biodistribution, pharmacokinetics, and active targeting capabilities. These targeted liposomes can be tailored to meet different needs and can utilize various ligands, such as peptides, carbohydrates, glycoproteins, receptor ligands, monoclonal antibodies, and growth factors, by selectively recognizing antigens or receptors on the surface of target cells. Ligand-targeted liposomes can enhance the accumulation of liposomal drugs specifically at target sites while minimizing the impact on healthy cells. With the employment of this selective targeting approach, lower doses of medication can be used to achieve the desired cytotoxic effect, resulting in a superior therapeutic index characterized by increased drug efficacy and fewer side effects [33]. Several comprehensive evaluations have indicated that ligand-targeted liposomes offer greater effectiveness compared to passively targeted liposomes due to improved targeting and intracellular uptake. However, these targeted liposome systems also introduce new challenges, such as inhibited diffusion and penetration into the target tissue, the potential for immune responses, and the risk of targeting deactivation caused by non-specific binding of serum proteins. Consequently, the consistent success of ligand-targeted liposome systems in preclinical settings varies, necessitating further studies to address concerns related to efficiency.

Characterization of liposomes:

PDI, Particle Size, and Zeta Potential

The Malvern Zeta sizer Nano device was used to measure the zeta potential of drug-loaded liposomes. The zeta potential is the electric potential difference between the liposome's surface and the surrounding fluid; this difference provides information about the liposomes' stability and charge properties. The drug-loaded liposomes were diluted at a 1:10 ratio with Millipore water to determine the zeta potential. This dilution helps ensure accurate measurements and reduces any interference from other components in the sample. The diluted liposome samples were then analysed in triplicate to obtain reliable data.

Electrophoretic light scattering is used by the Malvern Zeta sizer Nano to ascertain the liposomes' zeta potential [34]. Using an electric field to the liposome suspension and tracking the particles' migratory speed in response to the applied field are the steps involved in this technique. Researchers can determine the stability of the liposomes and the probability of flocculation or aggregation by measuring the zeta potential, which is computed using the velocity data.

Additionally, zeta potential provides insights into the surface charge of the liposome, which can affect interactions with biological systems and cellular uptake. It is worth noting that the zeta potential determination was specifically carried out for the drug-loaded liposomes, indicating the effect of the encapsulated drug on the electrical charge of the liposome surface. This information is crucial for understanding the behaviour and potential applications of the liposomes in drug delivery systems.

Entrapment Efficiency

The entrapment efficiency of CYC was assessed circumstantially. In order to achieve this, freshly generated liposomal dispersion containing CYC was combined with Millipore water and then put into centrifuge tubes [more precisely, Amicon Ultra 4 10000 MWCO tubes manufactured by Millipore, an American business]. Next, the tubes were centrifuged for 25 minutes at 4°C at 6000 revolutions per minute [35]. Using the methods described in section 2.2, the CYC contained in the filtrate was analysed. The amount of CYC that was trapped was calculated by deducting the amount of free CYC from the total amount of CYC included in the liposomal dispersion.

Scanning Electron Microscopy

With a scanning electron microscope, the surface characteristics of the liposomes were investigated. We used the Quanta 250 microscope, manufactured by FEI in the USA, and operated it in high-vacuum mode. After letting the liposome sample air dry and positioning it on a sample stub, we used a 5 kV voltage to take pictures.

FTIR-ATR Interaction Study

The interactions between medications and excipients in the 4000–500 cm^{-1} range were investigated using an FTIR-ATR spectrometer [Perkin Elmer, USA] [36]. A small quantity of the sample was placed on the surface of the crystal and compressed to begin acquiring the spectra. CYC (pure drug), a physical mixture of CYC and lipids (PM 1), CYC-loaded liposomes (CYC L), and blank liposomes were also processed. Drug-lipid and drug-drug compatibility were determined by comparing the obtained spectra.

Liposome Stability

Optimized liposome dispersions were stored for thirty days at temperatures between 2 and 8 °C and at room temperature. At specified time intervals (0, 15, and 30 days), samples were collected and analyzed. The stability of the liposomal dispersion was assessed using the dynamic light scattering method, which measured particle size, polydispersity index (PDI), and zeta potential. At each time point, the zeta potential of the samples was also evaluated.

A NEW MEDICATION DELIVERY SYSTEM FOR PSORIASIS TREATMENT

The primary goals of conventional medication delivery systems are to improve patients' quality of life by alleviating psoriasis symptoms and preventing the condition from worsening. Sometimes systemic medicine, phototherapy, and topical therapy are combined to increase therapeutic success. The Stratum Corneum [SC], which keeps the medication from passing through the layers of skin to reach the target tissues, has been regarded as a crucial barrier in transdermal drug delivery systems. Maximum penetration through SC should be possible with the optimum drug delivery mechanism, but irreversible changes to the skin barrier should be prevented.

Percutaneous absorption varies based on age, condition, location, and other variables [37]. Skin damage and inflammation could happen if the medication has a harmful nature. The skin's first-pass metabolic system is one barrier to topical dispersion, as the medication's instability and short half-life render conventional drug delivery methods ineffective. Since there is no known treatment for recurrent psoriasis, the patient must endure therapies for the remainder of their lives, which comes at a substantial financial cost. The shortcomings of conventional drug delivery systems led to the development of Novel Drug Delivery Systems [NDDS], which include liposomes, transferosomes, ethosomes, niosomes, invasomes, microemulsions, endosomes, dendrimers, hydrogel, nanoparticles, *etc.*

Furthermore, it has been demonstrated that nanostructures can impact the immune system, facilitating faster absorption and preventing drug degradation biochemically [38]. As a result, they may be beneficial in the treatment of autoimmune diseases, such as psoriasis. In an effort to develop a psoriasis treatment that is both safe and effective, extensive research is being conducted on novel carriers. Improved biocompatibility, higher drug concentration at the target site, and enhanced drug encapsulation efficiency are just a few advantages of novel carriers. These qualities, therefore, result in reduced dosages and shorter dosing intervals, which enhance efficacy and patient compliance. A significant amount of research has been conducted and continues to be conducted on various nanotechnology-based treatments for dermatological issues.

Possible Transporter for Topical Administration: Liposomes

The word “liposome” comes from the Greek words “*Lipos*,” meaning fat, and “*Soma*,” meaning body. Liposomes are microscopic, closed vesicles made up of one or more concentrically arranged phospholipid bilayers and one or more narrow diameter phospholipid bilayers that surround an equal number of watery compartments. Phospholipid molecules can self-assemble in aquatic environments due to their amphiphilic nature, which makes them suitable for delivering both hydrophilic and lipophilic drugs. Since liposomes can be used to target the release of specific medications, they are important alternatives. This capability is widely employed to enhance the therapeutic profile and mitigate the adverse effects associated with various medications. Liposomes are categorized into five types based on how they function and are delivered into cells: Immunological liposomes, cationic liposomes, conventional liposomes, pH-sensitive liposomes, and long-circulating liposomes [39]. Liposomes are available in a range of diameters, from 0.025 μm to 2.5 μm, and with varying degrees of lamellarity, or the quantity of bilayers. Both size and lamellarity influence the amount of medication encapsulated in the liposomes, and the size of the vesicle affects the duration of the liposomes' circulation.

Depending on their size and number of bilayers, liposomes can be divided into two groups:

i. Multilamellar vesicles [MLV]
ii. Unilamellar vesicles.

Unilamellar vesicles are further divided into two categories:

a. Small unilamellar vesicles (SUVs) (b) Large unilamellar vesicles (LUVs)
   Among other physical properties, the components of liposomes control their size, charge, lamellarity, permeability, and thermodynamic phase. Their electrostatic characteristics have an impact on liposome stability. Numerous factors, including biocompatibility, penetrability, diffusivity, shielding effect, increased half-life, reduced immunogenic response, extended systemic circulation, and improved efficacy and safety, are contributing to the growing need for liposomes as a drug delivery vehicle.

The lipid composition of liposomes is comparable to that of intercellular lamellar membranes and keratinocytes. This characteristic facilitates the penetration of liposomes through the stratum corneum and into deeper epidermal layers [40].

Greater and more sustained drug release in the dermis and epidermis is a result of decreased drug clearance from the epidermis. Liposomes are considered exclusive and unique because they function as an organic solvent to solubilize poorly soluble drugs, a local depot for sustained drug release, a penetration enhancer to achieve higher localized drug concentrations, and a rate-limiting membrane barrier that moderates systemic absorption. Liposomes tend to localize in the stratum corneum, which promotes increased drug accumulation in the skin.

Psoriasis Prodigy: Liposomal Drug Delivery Innovation

Liposomes possess a range of unique characteristics that make them promising drug delivery systems. One of their most notable advantages is their biocompatibility and natural biodegradability, which allows for safe use in the body [41]. By encapsulating drugs within their protective lipid bilayer, liposomes shield the drugs from enzymatic degradation, chemical inactivation, and immune system clearance. This protective capability enhances the drug's stability and efficacy by preventing premature breakdown before reaching the target tissue. As a result, liposomes help concentrate the active form of the medication at the site of action, thereby increasing its potency, particularly in targeting and killing cancer cells.

At the same time, healthy tissues receive only a small amount of the drug while it circulates in the bloodstream, which reduces negative or unwanted side effects. Using liposomes as drug carriers provides excellent control over both the timing and location of drug distribution in the body. This control is especially important for drugs with a narrow therapeutic range, where even slight deviations from the correct dosage can cause harmful side effects. Liposomes help maintain these drugs within the therapeutic range, ensuring they work effectively and minimize adverse effects, such as those seen in psoriasis. However, it is essential to note that the addition of non-natural substances to liposomes can potentially increase toxicity, as illustrated in Figure 3. Therefore, careful testing is crucial when modifying liposomes for drug delivery. Overall, liposomes offer numerous advantages as drug carriers, as they are biocompatible, protect drugs from degradation, enhance drug efficacy, and help reduce side effects. Ongoing research in this area may lead to significant improvements in the diagnosis and treatment of various diseases, particularly psoriasis. The immune system's T cells are responsible for the inflammation that characterizes psoriasis [42]. Along with hormonal and immunological factors, psoriasis is believed to be influenced by a combination of genetic, environmental, and epigenetic variables. The Major Histocompatibility Complex (MHC) comprises ten distinct human leukocyte antigen (HLA) alleles that are associated with an increased risk of developing psoriasis. Other genetic loci are also implicated. It remains unclear whether the triggering antigens originate from the body itself, the environment, or a combination of both. This autoimmune disorder accelerates the life cycle of skin cells, resulting in an abnormal increase in keratinocyte production due to the infiltration of inflammatory cells in the skin.

Psoriasis is mostly controlled by antigen-presenting cells [APCs], such as specific dendritic cells called Langerhans cells. They utilize lymphatic channels to transport HLA antigens associated with psoriasis from the skin's surface to lymph nodes, with the assistance of inflammatory cytokines, such as TNF-α and IL-1β. These APCs in the lymph nodes expose naïve T cells to antigens, which stimulate T-cell proliferation in the dermis of the skin, thereby regulating the immune response [43]. Th1 and Th17 cells are activated when dermal dendritic cells release pro-inflammatory cytokines, such as IL-12 and IL-23.

Other types of inflammatory dendritic cells also secrete cytokines, such as TNF-α, IL-18, and IL-23. This procedure changes CD45RA+ CLA− naïve T cells into CD45RO+ CLA− effector memory T cells. Intradermal T-cell proliferation drives memory CD45RO+ CLA-positive T cells, Th1 and Th17 cells, and other cells through blood vessels from the dermis to the epidermis. Natural killer T cells present antigens directly to keratinocytes in the epidermis. IFN-γ is produced by Th1 cells triggered by IL-18 and IL-23, whereas IL-17 and IL-22 are produced by Th17 cells. The IL-23/IL-17 axis mediates the invasion of skin-resident innate lymphocytes. IFN-γ and IL-22 activate keratinocytes, resulting in the increased thickness of the epidermis observed in plaque psoriasis [44]. Moreover, this activation enhances the synthesis of IL-17, which in turn stimulates keratinocyte proliferation and the secretion of chemokines.

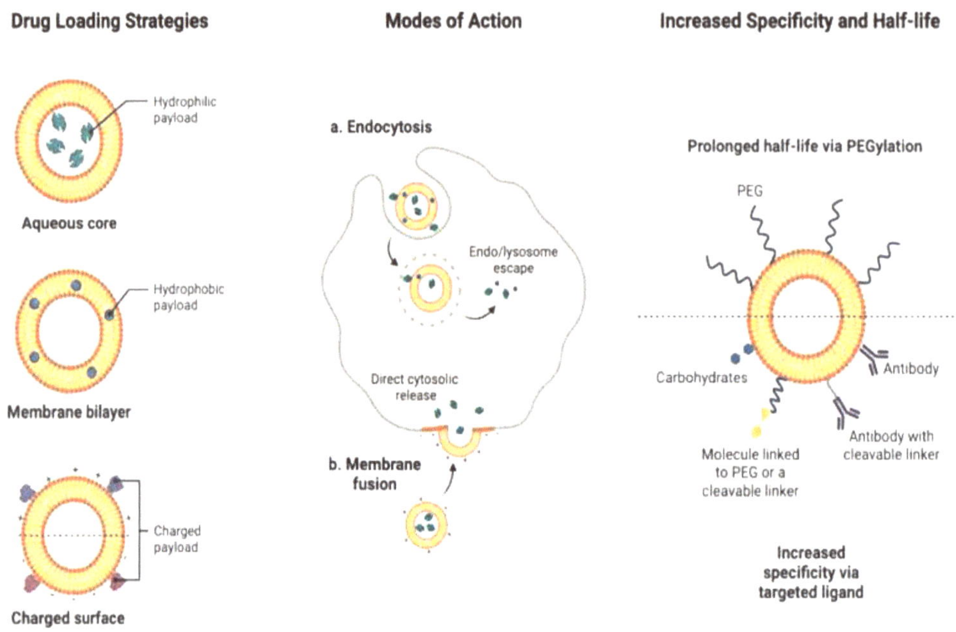

Fig. (3). Liposome base drug delivery.

Future Potential Uses of Lipid-Based Liposomes in Pharmaceuticals

The rise of nanotechnology in pharmaceutical applications is driving a significant increase in market value, which is expected to reach approximately US$334 billion in 2025, compared to previous years. This growth will drive extensive research in nanomedicine over the next two decades, with a focus on material design to meet clinical needs, particularly in the treatment of conditions, such as psoriasis [45]. Lipid-based liposomes are gaining prominence in psoriasis treatment due to their adaptability and the ability to customize lipid components, such as cardanol, sugar-based surfactants, glycolipids, and biosurfactants. These nanoparticles can form different structures based on their Critical Packing Parameter (CPP), which determines their success in preparing lipid-based nanoparticles, such as niosomes or nanoemulsions.

Numerous lipid-based nanoparticles have been effective in encapsulating antipsoriatic medications, including betamethasone, tretinoin, retinoic acid, psoralens, methotrexate, cyclosporine, and bexarotene. Due to their adaptability, lipid-based nanoparticles hold great potential for use in clinical research and drug development. Currently, despite ClinicalTrials.gov being an extensive database for clinical trials, there are no authorized nanodrugs for psoriasis. Only one psoriasis nanodrug, identified as NCT03348462, is being studied in clinical trials. Phase 4 studies using anthralin nanoformulations encapsulated in liposomes and ethosomes have yielded encouraging results [46]. Pharmaceutical companies, mostly small and medium-sized enterprises (SMEs), are currently conducting phase II clinical studies for marketable nanodrugs. Challenges include a lack of regulations governing nanotechnology, insufficient research on nanoparticle interactions with tissues, and the need for additional safety assessments of nanoparticles. The delivery of nanotherapeutics could be enhanced by cutting-edge technologies, such as Artificial Intelligence (AI) and machine learning, which can better understand the physicochemical and biological characteristics of nanoparticle medications and improve their efficacy and safety. Clinical trials must follow thorough investigations into the cytotoxicity and biological effects of nanomedicines.

CONCLUSION

Millions of individuals worldwide suffer from psoriasis, a recurrent, chronic inflammatory skin disease that requires specialized care to prevent it from becoming severe. Since the epidemiology of psoriasis is not fully understood, topical treatments, such as emollients and corticosteroids are commonly used, although they are not always effective. For the treatment of mild to moderate psoriasis, standard dosage forms often require high doses over an extended period. In contrast, novel drug delivery methods are preferred for their superior local effects and reduced toxicity. Among these innovative delivery methods, lipid nanocarriers offer several benefits, including increased therapeutic efficacy and safety. Due to the improved targeting ability and enhanced penetrability of anti-psoriatic medications, these nanocarriers perform better than conventional formulations.

Moreover, liposomes have been shown to be effective lipid nanocarriers for the treatment of psoriasis in numerous lab-scale animal models. Research from several studies suggests that incorporating anti-psoriatic medications into liposomes improves their effectiveness and reduces unfavorable effects. Therapeutic efficacy may be enhanced by improving drug targeting at the molecular level. Comprehensive clinical research has also been conducted to investigate the delivery of active compounds in both oral and topical therapies. Given the rationale behind the therapy, which includes lowering the risk of drug toxicity with long-term administration, greater attention should be given to improved permeability and retention, as well as the use of safe and tolerable natural excipients in liposomal carrier system research.

Depending on recent discoveries on the pathophysiology of the condition, different drug targeting strategies may potentially be employed to treat psoriasis. These developments may ultimately lead to improved understanding of dermal medicine. Liposome-based nanocarrier therapy is a promising approach for treating psoriasis. However, the success of any drug delivery system ultimately depends on the completion of clinical trials using reliable animal models and the scientific validation of the drug's therapeutic potential. Therefore, extensive clinical trials are necessary for liposome-based drug delivery systems to effectively treat psoriasis.

REFERENCES

[1] Bahadur S, Sharma M. Liposome based drug delivery for the management of psoriasis-A comprehensive review. Curr Pharm Biotechnol 2023; 24(11): 1383-96. [http://dx.doi.org/10.2174/1389201024666221213144228] [PMID: 36518042]

[2] Zhu B, Jing M, Yu Q, Ge X, Yuan F, Shi L. Treatments in psoriasis: from standard pharmacotherapy to nanotechnology therapy. Advances in Dermatology and Allergology/Postępy Dermatologii i Alergologii. 2022; 39(3): 460-71. [http://dx.doi.org/10.5114/ada.2021.108445]

[3] van Alem CMA, Metselaar JM, van Kooten C, Rotmans JI. Recent advances in liposomal-based anti-inflammatory therapy. Pharmaceutics 2021; 13(7): 1004. [http://dx.doi.org/10.3390/pharmaceutics13071004] [PMID: 34371695]

[4] Alam M, Rizwanullah M, Mir SR, Amin S. Promising prospects of lipid-based topical nanocarriers for the treatment of psoriasis. OpenNano 2023; 10: 100123. [http://dx.doi.org/10.1016/j.onano.2023.100123]

[5] Saleem S, Iqubal MK, Garg S, Ali J, Baboota S. Trends in nanotechnology-based delivery systems for dermal targeting of drugs: an enticing approach to offset psoriasis. Expert Opin Drug Deliv 2020; 17(6): 817-38. [http://dx.doi.org/10.1080/17425247.2020.1758665] [PMID: 32315216]

[6] Pradhan M, Alexander A, Singh MR, *et al.* Understanding the prospective of nano-formulations towards the treatment of psoriasis. Biomed Pharmacother 2018; 107: 447-63. [http://dx.doi.org/10.1016/j.biopha.2018.07.156] [PMID: 30103117]

[7] Rahman M, Akhter S, Ahmad J, Ahmad MZ, Beg S, Ahmad FJ. Nanomedicine-based drug targeting for psoriasis: potentials and emerging trends in nanoscale pharmacotherapy. Expert Opin Drug Deliv 2015; 12(4): 635-52. [http://dx.doi.org/10.1517/17425247.2015.982088] [PMID: 25439967]

[8] Jyothi SL, Krishna KL, Ameena Shirin VK, Sankar R, Pramod K, Gangadharappa HV. Drug delivery systems for the treatment of psoriasis: Current status and prospects. J Drug Deliv Sci Technol 2021; 62: 102364. [http://dx.doi.org/10.1016/j.jddst.2021.102364]

[9] Doppalapudi S, Jain A, Bulbake U, Khan W. Nanotherapeutics: Emerging trends in management of psoriasis. Pharm Nanotechnol 2016; 4(4): 267-83. [http://dx.doi.org/10.2174/2211738504666161014091932]

[10] Zhao Z, Liu T, Zhu S, *et al.* Natural medicine combined with nanobased topical delivery systems: a new strategy to treat psoriasis. Drug Deliv Transl Res 2022; 12(6): 1326-38. [http://dx.doi.org/10.1007/s13346-021-01031-3] [PMID: 34287767]

[11] Chime A, Onyishi IV. Lipid-Based Drug Delivery Systems (LDDS): Recent advances and applications of lipids in drug delivery. Afr J Pharm Pharmacol 2013; 7(48): 3034-59.

[http://dx.doi.org/10.5897/AJPPX2013.0004]

[12] Chudasma MP, Shah SA, Qureshi MHN, *et al.* Brief insight on nanovesicular liposomes as drug-delivery carriers for medical applications. Journal of Exploratory Research in Pharmacology 2023; 8(3): 222-236.
[http://dx.doi.org/10.14218/JERP.2022.00086]

[13] Siler-Marinkovic S. Liposomes as drug delivery systems in dermal and transdermal drug delivery. Percutaneous Penetration Enhancers Chemical Methods in Penetration Enhancement: Nanocarriers. 2016: 15-38.
[http://dx.doi.org/10.1007/978-3-662-47862-2_2]

[14] Vovesná A, Zhigunov A, Balouch M, Zbytovská J. Ceramide liposomes for skin barrier recovery: A novel formulation based on natural skin lipids. Int J Pharm 2021; 596: 120264.
[http://dx.doi.org/10.1016/j.ijpharm.2021.120264] [PMID: 33486027]

[15] Torchilin V, Weissig V. Liposomes: a practical approach. Oxford University Press 2003.
[http://dx.doi.org/10.1093/oso/9780199636556.001.0001]

[16] Arias JL. Liposomes in drug delivery: a patent review (2007 – present). Expert Opin Ther Pat 2013; 23(11): 1399-414.
[http://dx.doi.org/10.1517/13543776.2013.828035] [PMID: 23957267]

[17] Walunj M, Doppalapudi S, Bulbake U, Khan W. Preparation, characterization, and *in vivo* evaluation of cyclosporine cationic liposomes for the treatment of psoriasis. J Liposome Res 2020; 30(1): 68-79.
[http://dx.doi.org/10.1080/08982104.2019.1593449] [PMID: 30897993]

[18] Zhang YT, Shen LN, Wu ZH, Zhao JH, Feng NP. Comparison of ethosomes and liposomes for skin delivery of psoralen for psoriasis therapy. Int J Pharm 2014; 471(1-2): 449-52.
[http://dx.doi.org/10.1016/j.ijpharm.2014.06.001] [PMID: 24907596]

[19] Allaw M, Manca ML, Castangia I, Manconi M. From plants to phospholipid vesicles: A comprehensive review on the incorporation of phytochemicals into phospholipid vesicles designed for skin applications with special focus on scalability and in vitro and *in vivo* efficacy. J Drug Deliv Sci Technol 2022; 67: 103049.
[http://dx.doi.org/10.1016/j.jddst.2021.103049]

[20] Perrett S, Golding M, Williams WP. A simple method for the preparation of liposomes for pharmaceutical applications: characterization of the liposomes. J Pharm Pharmacol 1991; 43(3): 154-61.
[http://dx.doi.org/10.1111/j.2042-7158.1991.tb06657.x] [PMID: 1675270]

[21] Lichtenberg D, Barenholz Y. Liposomes: preparation, characterization, and preservation. Methods Biochem Anal 1988; 33: 337-462.
[http://dx.doi.org/10.1002/9780470110546.ch7] [PMID: 3282152]

[22] Varona S, Martín Á, Cocero MJ. Liposomal incorporation of lavandin essential oil by a thin-film hydration method and by particles from gas-saturated solutions. Ind Eng Chem Res 2011; 50(4): 2088-97.
[http://dx.doi.org/10.1021/ie102016r]

[23] Charcosset C, Juban A, Valour JP, Urbaniak S, Fessi H. Preparation of liposomes at large scale using the ethanol injection method: Effect of scale-up and injection devices. Chem Eng Res Des 2015; 94: 508-15.
[http://dx.doi.org/10.1016/j.cherd.2014.09.008]

[24] Otake K, Shimomura T, Goto T, *et al.* Preparation of liposomes using an improved supercritical reverse phase evaporation method. Langmuir 2006; 22(6): 2543-50.
[http://dx.doi.org/10.1021/la051654u] [PMID: 16519453]

[25] Mourtas S, Fotopoulou S, Duraj S, Sfika V, Tsakiroglou C, Antimisiaris SG. Liposomal drugs dispersed in hydrogels. Colloids Surf B Biointerfaces 2007; 55(2): 212-21.

[http://dx.doi.org/10.1016/j.colsurfb.2006.12.005] [PMID: 17223020]

[26] Allen TM, Hansen CB, de Menezes DEL. Pharmacokinetics of long-circulating liposomes. Adv Drug Deliv Rev 1995; 16(2-3): 267-84. [http://dx.doi.org/10.1016/0169-409X(95)00029-7]

[27] Song G, Wu H, Yoshino K, Zamboni WC. Factors affecting the pharmacokinetics and pharmacodynamics of liposomal drugs. J Liposome Res 2012; 22(3): 177-92. [http://dx.doi.org/10.3109/08982104.2012.655285] [PMID: 22332871]

[28] Qian S, Li C, Zuo Z. Pharmacokinetics and disposition of various drug loaded liposomes. Curr Drug Metab 2012; 13(4): 372-95. [http://dx.doi.org/10.2174/138920012800166562] [PMID: 22443534]

[29] Immordino ML, Brusa P, Rocco F, Arpicco S, Ceruti M, Cattel L. Preparation, characterization, cytotoxicity and pharmacokinetics of liposomes containing lipophilic gemcitabine prodrugs. J Control Release 2004; 100(3): 331-46. [http://dx.doi.org/10.1016/j.jconrel.2004.09.001] [PMID: 15567500]

[30] Sato Y, Kiwada H, Kato Y. Effects of dose and vesicle size on the pharmacokinetics of liposomes. Chem Pharm Bull (Tokyo) 1986; 34(10): 4244-52. [http://dx.doi.org/10.1248/cpb.34.4244] [PMID: 3829156]

[31] Fielding RM. Liposomal drug delivery. Advantages and limitations from a clinical pharmacokinetic and therapeutic perspective. Clin Pharmacokinet 1991; 21(3): 155-64. [http://dx.doi.org/10.2165/00003088-199121030-00001] [PMID: 1764868]

[32] Large DE, Abdelmessih RG, Fink EA, Auguste DT. Liposome composition in drug delivery design, synthesis, characterization, and clinical application. Adv Drug Deliv Rev 2021; 176: 113851. [http://dx.doi.org/10.1016/j.addr.2021.113851] [PMID: 34224787]

[33] De Gier J, Mandersloot JG, Van Deenen LLM. Lipid composition and permeability of liposomes. Biochim Biophys Acta Biomembr 1968; 150(4): 666-75. [http://dx.doi.org/10.1016/0005-2736(68)90056-4]

[34] Vemuri S, Rhodes CT. Preparation and characterization of liposomes as therapeutic delivery systems: a review. Pharm Acta Helv 1995; 70(2): 95-111. [http://dx.doi.org/10.1016/0031-6865(95)00010-7] [PMID: 7651973]

[35] Taylor TM, Gaysinsky S, Davidson PM, Bruce BD, Weiss J. Characterization of antimicrobial-bearing liposomes by ζ-potential, vesicle size, and encapsulation efficiency. Food Biophys 2007; 2(1): 1-9. [http://dx.doi.org/10.1007/s11483-007-9023-x]

[36] Pašalić L, Maleš P, Čikoš A, Pem B, Bakarić D. The rise of FTIR spectroscopy in the characterization of asymmetric lipid membranes. Spectrochim Acta A Mol Biomol Spectrosc 2024; 305: 123488. [http://dx.doi.org/10.1016/j.saa.2023.123488] [PMID: 37813090]

[37] Katare O, Raza K, Singh B, Dogra S. Novel drug delivery systems in topical treatment of psoriasis: Rigors and vigors. Indian J Dermatol Venereol Leprol 2010; 76(6): 612-21. [http://dx.doi.org/10.4103/0378-6323.72451] [PMID: 21079304]

[38] Dhandapani NV, Thapa A, Sandip G, Shrestha A, Shrestha N, Bhattarai RS. Liposomes as novel drug delivery system: A comprehensive review. Int J Res Pharm Sci(Madurai, India) 2013; 4: 187.

[39] Touitou E, Junginger HE, Weiner ND, Nagai T, Mezei M. Liposomes as carriers for topical and transdermal delivery. J Pharm Sci 1994; 83(9): 1189-203. [http://dx.doi.org/10.1002/jps.2600830902] [PMID: 7830230]

[40] Pierre MBR, dos Santos Miranda Costa I. Liposomal systems as drug delivery vehicles for dermal and transdermal applications. Arch Dermatol Res 2011; 303(9): 607-21. [http://dx.doi.org/10.1007/s00403-011-1166-4] [PMID: 21805180]

[41] Shah S, Dhawan V, Holm R, Nagarsenker MS, Perrie Y. Liposomes: Advancements and innovation in

the manufacturing process. Adv Drug Deliv Rev 2020; 154-155: 102-22.
[http://dx.doi.org/10.1016/j.addr.2020.07.002] [PMID: 32650041]

[42] Kumar KS, Bhowmik D, Deb L. Recent trends in liposomes used as novel drug delivery system. Pharma Innov 2012; 1 (1, Part A): 29.

[43] Krishnamachari Y, Salem AK. Innovative strategies for co-delivering antigens and CpG oligonucleotides. Adv Drug Deliv Rev 2009; 61(3): 205-17.
[http://dx.doi.org/10.1016/j.addr.2008.12.013] [PMID: 19272328]

[44] Kraft JC, Freeling JP, Wang Z, Ho RJY. Emerging research and clinical development trends of liposome and lipid nanoparticle drug delivery systems. J Pharm Sci 2014; 103(1): 29-52.
[http://dx.doi.org/10.1002/jps.23773] [PMID: 24338748]

[45] Mohd Nordin UU, Ahmad N, Salim N, Mohd Yusof NS. Lipid-based nanoparticles for psoriasis treatment: a review on conventional treatments, recent works, and future prospects. RSC Advances 2021; 11(46): 29080-101.
[http://dx.doi.org/10.1039/D1RA06087B] [PMID: 35478537]

[46] Teixeira MC, Carbone C, Souto EB. Beyond liposomes: Recent advances on lipid based nanostructures for poorly soluble/poorly permeable drug delivery. Prog Lipid Res 2017; 68: 1-11.
[http://dx.doi.org/10.1016/j.plipres.2017.07.001] [PMID: 28778472]

CHAPTER 8

Niosomes-Based Pharmacotherapy for the Management of Psoriasis

Vishnu Mittal[1,*], **Anjali Sharma**[2], **Abhinav Singhal**[2], **Pushkar Upadhyay**[2] and **Devkant Sharma**[3]

[1] *Adesh Institute of Pharmacy and Biomedical Sciences, Adesh University, Bathinda 151101, Punjab, India*

[2] *Department of Pharmaceutics, Guru Gobind Singh College of Pharmacy, Yamunanagar 135001, Haryana, India*

[3] *Department of Pharmaceutics, Ch. DeviLal College of Pharmacy, Jagadhai 135003, Haryana, India*

Abstract: Background: Psoriasis is a long-term autoimmune disease that causes skin cells to develop quickly, resulting in thick, red, scaly areas on the skin's surface. The itchiness and pain associated with these patches can significantly impact the quality of life for those affected. The primary objectives of psoriasis therapy are to reduce inflammation, inhibit excessive skin cell growth, and alleviate symptoms.

Objective: Despite ongoing research efforts, patient satisfaction with existing topical therapies for psoriasis remains limited. There is a pressing need to enhance the safety, efficacy, and comfort of topical therapies by developing innovative drug delivery and carrier systems.

Method: Using niosomes, which are non-ionic surfactant-based vesicles that can encapsulate both hydrophilic and hydrophobic medications, is one intriguing strategy. The pharmaceutical industry has shown considerable interest in niosomes due to their potential to reduce toxicity and enhance therapeutic efficacy. With low toxicity and optimal targeting efficacy, these vesicles provide a unique method of delivering a variety of therapeutic agents, including chemical drugs, protein-based therapies, and genetic materials.

Results: Studies have reported that niosomes can increase drug bioavailability and stability, making them a viable option for drug delivery in the treatment of psoriasis. Compared to conventional topical treatments, niosomes offer improved stability during formulation and storage, which may lead to enhanced therapeutic outcomes and increased patient satisfaction.

* **Corresponding author Vishnu Mittal:** Adesh Institute of Pharmacy and Biomedical Sciences, Adesh University, Bathinda 151101, Punjab, India; E-mail: vishnumittal720@gmail.com

Anjali Sharma, Prerna Sharma, Roy Rillera Marzo & Ahmed A. Al Karmalawy (Eds.)

Conclusion: The use of niosomes represents a promising approach to enhancing topical therapy in the management of psoriasis. Their capacity to minimize toxicity and encapsulate a variety of medications, including hydrophilic and hydrophobic agents, makes them a desirable choice for improving the comfort, safety, and efficacy of psoriasis therapy. Continued research and development in this field could significantly advance the treatment of psoriasis and other dermatological conditions.

Keywords: Drug delivery system, Nanotechnology, Niosomes, Pharmacotherapy, Psoriasis.

INTRODUCTION

Psoriasis is an autoimmune disease that is influenced by both genetics and environmental factors. It causes inflammation and activates keratinocytes, leading to their proliferation and differentiation. Psoriasis affects approximately 2% of the global population, and significant progress has been made in its diagnosis and treatment. However, epidemiological data are available for only 19% of countries. Although psoriasis affects fewer than 1% of youth worldwide, regional differences exist in its incidence [1]. East Asia has the lowest frequency of psoriasis at 0.12%, whereas Western countries have an average incidence of around 2%. Norway has the greatest prevalence of psoriasis, accounting for 1.98% of its population. Although it may appear anywhere on the skin, psoriasis is categorized as an epithelial disorder characterized by red, scaly patches that are usually seen on the elbows, knees, scalp, and lower back. Other side effects include psychological diseases, cardiometabolic problems, and psoriatic arthritis [2].

To initiate and sustain the inflammatory state, including epigenetic modifications, targeting keratinocytes is crucial in psoriasis therapy regimens. Human keratinocytes, which proliferate up to 10 times faster than normal epithelial cells, are a hallmark of psoriasis. In response to injury, HaCaT generates distal antigens that stimulate dendritic cells at the primary level. Keratinocyte cells use pattern recognition receptors to identify tissue damage and external or pathogenic contaminants. Bacteriocins and inflammatory cytokines are among the secondary intermediates produced when HaCaT is activated. Due to their antibacterial, antispasmodic, antiproliferative, and antioxidant properties, Intrinsically Therapeutic Nanoparticles (ITNPs) are effective in treating a range of diseases. The field of psoriasis therapy has seen a revolutionary change since the FDA approved etanercept in 2004. Research has reported that different kinds of NPs may encapsulate different APIs. The best nano-based treatments for psoriasis, however, are liposomes and nanocapsules [3]. Lipid-based nanostructures, combined with anti-psoriatic drugs, improve skin permeability and reduce psoriasis symptoms. Furthermore, due to their large porous structure, which promotes durability, extended dispersion, and percutaneous absorption, these treatments are more effective in treating psoriasis lesions. Colloidal carriers, such as lipoprotein nanostructures (NLCs) and solid lipid nanoparticles (SLNPs), facilitate the transport and dispersion of bioactive substances. NLCs and SLNPs are also efficient choices for targeted medication delivery.

The current method for treating superficial psoriasis is to ensure that the NPs remain on the afflicted region for an extended period by maintaining the nanomaterial composition during API release. Psoriasis, particularly in its advanced stages, is closely associated with inflammatory diseases, metabolic syndrome, and cardiovascular conditions [4]. Topical medications are used in short-term therapy for moderate to severe psoriasis and mild psoriasis. Innovative psoriasis treatments, such as siRNAs and targeted therapies for cutaneous (skin) and mucosal manifestations, are increasingly focused on genetic variations underlying the disease's etiology. Several studies have reported that although different APIs can be added to various lipid nanostructures, liposomes and nanoemulsions are the most effective carriers for psoriasis treatments. Anti-psoriatic agents delivered *via* SLNPs reduce the symptoms of psoriasis while increasing skin permeability. Nowadays, psoriasis may be successfully and safely treated using nanoformulations [5].

PATHOPHYSIOLOGY OF PSORIASIS

Pustular psoriasis, including localized forms, such as Palmoplantar Pustulosis (PPP), is a severe autoimmune condition characterized by abnormal epithelial stratification, inflammatory cell infiltrates, and a predominant Th1 and Th17 immune response. There is growing recognition that psoriasis is a systemic clinical issue rather than just a skin condition. This illness causes skin abnormalities and promotes the proliferation of HaCaT cells by activating pathogenic T lymphocytes and innate immune cells. While T cells play a central role in the development of Palmoplantar Pustulosis (PPP), an autoimmune disease, the role of B cells has only recently gained attention. Although T cell activation contributes significantly to PPP pathology, it does not fully explain all aspects of the disease [6]. Additionally, interactions between platelets and lymphocytes have been observed in psoriatic mouse models and other inflammatory conditions; however, their role within psoriatic lesions in human patients remains unclear [7].

An immune-competent skin model of inflammatory lesions has demonstrated a slow initiation of epithelial differentiation, hyperproliferation of basal keratinocytes, increased production of pro-inflammatory cytokines, and alterations in the expression of key transcriptional regulators. This highlights the importance of incorporating cutaneous chemicals into T cells to develop a functional prototype for PPP. Psoriasis development is driven by the malfunctioning of both innate and adaptive immune systems, which have also been linked to elevated insulin sensitivity, atherosclerosis, and increased coagulation. Plaque, erythrodermic, guttate, and pustular psoriasis are the four primary types of psoriasis, distinguished by their distinct diagnostic features [8]. Abnormalities in the skin's innate and adaptive immune systems are what cause and prolong psoriatic inflammation. In certain situations, autoinflammatory persistence involves activation of innate immune responses through surface receptors and cytokines, while in others, T cells trigger autoimmune reactions. As a result, psoriasis displays inflammatory characteristics typical of autoimmune diseases, with both pathways overlapping and amplifying each other [9].

Types of Psoriasis

Plaque Psoriasis

Plaque psoriasis is the most common form of the condition, affecting approximately 70–85% of patients. It typically involves areas, such as the lower back, scalp, wrists, and knees. Common triggers include radiation exposure, alcohol consumption, psychological stress, certain medications, infections, skin trauma (such as dermal scraping), and smoking.

Flexural Psoriasis

Flexural psoriasis, also known as inverse psoriasis, commonly appears in skin folds, such as the breasts, groin, armpits, and around the buttocks and genital areas. It affects approximately 20% of people with psoriasis. Causes include increased sensitivity to sweat and friction, as well as yeast overgrowth [10].

Guttate Psoriasis

Guttate psoriasis is characterized by small, drop-shaped lesions that commonly appear on the scalp, limbs, and body. These lesions are often triggered by microbial infections, particularly streptococcal infections. Other causes include various microbial infections, certain medications, sun damage, psychological stress, alcohol use, and skin injuries such as cuts, blisters, and insect bites.

Nail Psoriasis

Nail psoriasis can affect both fingernails and toenails, leading to discoloration and irregular nail formation. Symptoms include color changes, tiny pits, horizontal lines across the nails, white patches on the nail plate, thickening of the skin beneath the nails, and nail loosening. The causes involve a combination of immunological, environmental, and hereditary factors [11].

Psoriatic arthritis

It is a kind of psoriasis that causes inflammation in the joints of both adults and children. Symptoms include red, swollen, tender, warm, and stiff joints. It is also associated with increased risks of cardiovascular events, such as myocardial infarction, stroke, and atherosclerosis. Common triggers include burns or other skin trauma, certain medications, alcohol consumption, irritants, and smoking.

Erythrodermic Psoriasis

It is characterized by recurrent, severe erythema of the skin and a buildup of scales in layers, as opposed to small flakes, followed by an elevated heart rate, temperature changes, and skin reddening. Common causes include the use of corticosteroids, burns, psychological distress, alcoholism, diseases, and allergies.

Pustular Psoriasis

It is characterized by skin redness, followed by scaling and pustule formation, often accompanied by discomfort or sensitivity to light. Common triggers include severe trauma, infections, steroid use or withdrawal, excessive UV exposure, pregnancy, and abrupt discontinuation of systemic medications or potent topical agents [12].

CONVENTIONAL TOPICAL TREATMENT

The pharmacokinetics of an active corticosteroid may be greatly altered by the vehicle employed in its formulation, which can also have an unfavorable effect. Due to this, the development of a suitable corticosteroid carrier is a major focus of both pharmaceutical and dermatological research. Clobetasol is more effective when added to a spray vehicle than when used in other types of vehicles, according to numerous studies. Nonetheless, a more odourless and convenient vehicle may enhance patient compliance, which might account for the higher efficacy. Although retinoids, or vitamin A derivatives administered topically, have been demonstrated in multiple trials to have anti-psoriatic properties, they are not often used as first-line treatments for psoriasis. They work well for treating psoriasis on the face and in skin folds, where the skin is thinner and more sensitive, such as in inverted psoriasis [13, 14]. Topical retinoids, such as acitretin and tazarotene, regulate keratinocyte differentiation and proliferation, helping to normalize the growth and shedding of epidermal cells. Studies have also shown that while increasing the concentration of the active ingredient enhances efficacy, it simultaneously raises the risk of side effects. Topical retinoids offer many benefits; however, when treatment is initiated, they may cause side effects such as skin irritation, photosensitivity, redness, and peeling, which can limit their use in psoriasis (PSO) [15]. While these medications are commonly used to treat atopic dermatitis (eczema), they are sometimes employed for psoriasis treatment, particularly in sensitive areas like the face and genitalia, where conventional therapies may be less effective [16]. This cautious use is partly because topical calcineurin inhibitors, often preferred in these areas, have a higher potential for side effects due to their enhanced percutaneous penetration [17].

Coal Tar

Since ancient times, coal tar has been used to treat psoriasis, particularly scalp psoriasis; however, its use has declined in recent years, unlike in other tropical countries where it remains more common. This is likely due to its unappealing traits, which include offensive stains on clothing and unpleasant odors, especially in individuals whose hair is not black. Polycyclic aromatic hydrocarbon, one of the hundreds of chemicals found in the tar, has been studied the most because it possesses psoriasis-related therapeutic benefits [18]. It is suggested that the effects of coal tar are significantly influenced by the aryl hydrocarbon carbazole. However, both physicians and patients have growing concerns about coal tar because of its hundreds of unidentified components. Due to potential carcinogenic risks, its use for cosmetic purposes is also banned in Canada and the European Union [19].

Dithranol

Studies on human keratinocyte (HaCaT) cells demonstrate that dithranol (also known as anthralin) is one of the oldest treatments for plaque psoriasis, primarily acting through the suppression of keratinocyte proliferation and the induction of keratinocyte death. However, despite extensive research, little is known about the direct or indirect effects of dithranol on the inflammatory response associated with psoriasis [20]. Further findings suggest that, to suppress psoriatic activity, the primary target may not be immune cells but rather the keratinocytes of the epidermis [21].

Retinoids

Retinoids are byproducts of vitamin A, also known as vitamers. The FDA has approved only acitretin and tazarotene as retinoids for the treatment of psoriasis. Tazarotene is used topically, while acitretin is taken orally. Since tazarotene reduces irritation and topical corticosteroids possess anti-inflammatory properties that enhance the therapeutic benefits for psoriasis, the efficacy of tazarotene in combination with corticosteroids has been extensively studied [22].

Calcineurin Inhibitors

Topical calcineurin inhibitors, also known as immunosuppressants, such as pimecrolimus and tacrolimus, are first-line therapy for inverse psoriasis (body fold area) when used long-term. They possess anti-inflammatory and immunomodulatory properties that inhibit T-cell activation and cytokine production by blocking calcineurin phosphatase. Genital psoriasis may also be treated with tacrolimus, a medication well-tolerated in adults and suitable for those with steroid allergies. On the other hand, there are some side effects, such as slight burning and itching, which may occur when the treatment first begins. Although less effective as a treatment, pimecrolimus has also been used to treat comparable psoriasis symptoms, including pediatric facial psoriasis [23].

Salicylic Acid

Strong keratolytic salicylic acid is often used topically in conjunction with corticosteroids and calcineurin inhibitors. It is believed that the drug is more effectively absorbed into psoriasis plaques when used with calcineurin inhibitors. When taking salicylic acid alone to treat scalp psoriasis, telogen hair may suddenly shed; however, discontinuing the drug may resolve this issue. Moreover, it is not recommended to apply salicylic acid to large areas of the body's surface at concentrations greater than 10%. The primary motivation for this is to prevent potential adverse effects, such as nausea, frontal headaches, and burns to the oral mucosa. Previous research has shown that salicylic acid, when combined with a corticosteroid, calcineurin inhibitor, and vitamin D analogue, exhibits potent penetration-enhancing effects, increasing skin penetration and sustaining a release profile [24].

Vitamin D Analogues

Two synthetic vitamin D analogs, calcitriol and calcipotriol, are commonly used in psoriasis treatment. Vitamin D, produced in the skin upon sunlight exposure, suppresses the production of potent inflammatory cytokines, including IL-2, IL-6, and IFN-γ, which are involved in psoriasis pathogenesis [25 - 27].

CHALLENGES IN TOPICAL FORMULATION

Anti-psoriatic medications are challenging to use in treating psoriasis due to several factors that impact the medication's effectiveness and the patient's compliance. One of the biggest obstacles to using drugs to their fullest therapeutic potential is drug dispersion through the skin. This problem is exacerbated by the condition's extreme symptoms, which include discomfort and hyperkeratosis. Two psoriasis-related skin characteristics that may limit the absorption of active ingredients into the deeper skin layers are elevated cholesterol and reduced ceramide levels. Moreover, inadequate hydration stimuli, such as epidermal water, considerably limit the uptake of medications [28, 29]. The unique characteristics of the affected region must be considered while selecting a distribution plan [30]. Long-term use of anti-psoriatic medications, particularly potent corticosteroids, may cause skin irritation, itching, or dryness, which can reduce adherence and lead to treatment discontinuation. Moreover, systemic side effects may occur from the topical administration of drugs to individuals with compromised skin integrity or to significant areas of the body where the pharmaceuticals may be absorbed into the circulation. Psoriatic skin is often stiff or lacks a usual moisturizing component; therefore, the moisture content of stratum corneum is a crucial factor in determining absorption of medications through skin [31].

NANOTECHNOLOGY

The study of nanotechnology focuses on polymer drug delivery systems, which aim to transport medications within a nanoscale framework. They are referred to as "drug nanocarriers," even though they may be larger than 100 nanometers. Due to its ability to boost pharmacological effectiveness and permit targeted distribution, this approach is beneficial to the medical community [32]. Nanotechnology has numerous applications, but its greatest benefits are found in the fields of science, engineering, and technology. Nanomedicine, a subspecialty of medicine, utilizes nanotechnology to diagnose, treat, and prevent diseases. There are various types of nanomedicines, including nanoparticles, nanocarriers, and nanodevices. Their unique properties make them valuable for both diagnostic and therapeutic purposes [33]. Nanotechnology has always piqued the curiosity of researchers, particularly in the administration of medications and other related sectors. Nanotechnology offers several advantages over traditional medication delivery methods in the medical field. Engineered nanoparticles may be used to deliver medication directly to the targeted site. They can also be used to enhance therapeutic effectiveness, minimize systemic adverse effects, and provide controlled or sustained release [34].

CURRENT NANOTECHNOLOGY-BASED APPROACHES

Many technologies have been developed recently to enhance the safety and effectiveness of topical medication treatments. Moreover, innovative drug carriers have enabled the incorporation of new compounds into topical psoriasis treatments. Consequently, non-vascular drug delivery methods such as foams, gels, and nanoparticles, along with vesicular delivery technologies including liposomes, transfersomes, niosomes, and proniosomes, have been developed [35, 36].

NIOSOMES

When dealing with a material in its bulk form, it is impossible to attain the unique properties exhibited by its nanoparticle form. Numerous businesses have proposed leveraging these unique features, with the cosmetics industry being one of the most promising sectors to do so [37]. Niosomes have been utilized to enhance the functionality of various products, including hair care products, anti-aging creams, and moisturizers. Many leading cosmetics brands now include at least one "nano-enhanced" product in their lines. The use of nanoemulsions and nanocrystals in skincare is steadily increasing in popularity. These materials are typically bio-organic and present minimal toxicological concerns. The application of nanobiomaterials in cosmetics offers several advantages, including improved efficacy, enhanced transparency, unique texture, protection of active ingredients, and increased consumer compliance [38]. Fig. (**1**) illustrates the nano-interventions in topical delivery for psoriasis.

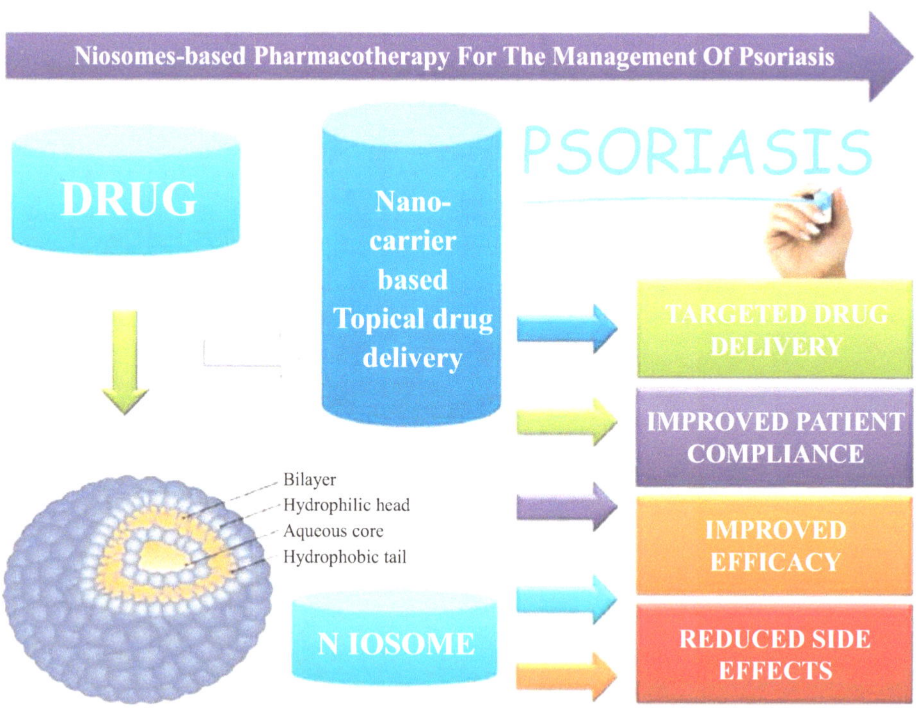

Fig. (1). Nano intervention in topical delivery for psoriasis.

These carriers are beneficial for topical delivery because they may reduce systemic absorption while extending the resident duration of active chemicals in the stratum corneum and epidermis. They are still favored over liposomes. Niosomes are a type of vesicular nanocarrier that may replace lipid-solid carriers, such as liposomes [39, 40]. They are also comparatively non-toxic, biodegradable, stable, and reasonably priced. The instability, rapid disintegration, bioavailability, and insolubility of several medications or natural chemicals may be resolved using niosomes. When it comes to the targeted administration of antibacterial, anticancer, anti-inflammatory, and antioxidant agents, niosomes may be very effective delivery vehicles. The purpose of this chapter is to provide a summary of their makeup, the most popular methods of formulation, and their most recent use as delivery systems in cancer treatment [41].

Niosomes provide the following benefits over liposomes:

- Compared to phospholipid, the surfactant in niosomes is more chemically stable.
- Ambient conditions may be used for both preparation and storage.
- There are no issues with purity when they are utilized as intended.
- It is inexpensive to create them.

Compared to liposomes, niosomes have a few advantages, but they also have some disadvantages. One of them is the lack of components that are generally acknowledged to be safe (GRAS), such as the phospholipid present in liposomes. Furthermore, they cause more irritation than liposomes [42, 43]. The pharmaceutical administration of niosomes is precise, controlled, and long-lasting due to their structure, which confines the hydrophilic drug to the bilayer matrix and hydrophobic moiety to the core watery compartment. Niosomes may be administered orally, intravenously, topically, or internally. The structure of niosomes is determined by thermodynamic parameters, including entropy, free-energy fluctuation, and enthalpy contributions from forces, such as hydrophobic interactions, electrostatic forces, hydrogen bonding, and van der Waals forces. Niosomes are formed through the self-assembly of non-ionic surfactants. It has been demonstrated that this self-assembly process is influenced by geometric factors, including lipid chain length, aqueous interlayer thickness, membrane symmetry, and chain confinement [44].

Composition of Niosomes

The composition of niosomes influences their formulation, pharmacokinetic behavior, and application in cancer treatment. The primary building blocks of niosomes include charge-inducing substances, cholesterol, and non-ionic surfactants, all of which are typically non-toxic and biocompatible [45, 46]. As non-ionic surfactants have an amphiphilic structure, they are the main component of niosome formulations. Since they require no particular handling or storage conditions and exhibit higher stability, low toxicity, and biocompatibility compared to other surfactant molecules (positive, negative, and amphoteric), non-ionic surfactants are preferred. Literature sources state that the phase transition temperature, chemical structure, HLB value, and critical packing parameter of non-ionic surfactants are the primary factors influencing niosome manufacturing. These factors affect the interactions between the surfactant molecules, which in turn restrict bilayer acyl chain mobility and enhance membrane cohesion. As a result, changes in the fluidity of the bilayer chains impact vesicle stability and can lead to a lower phase transition temperature [47]. Adding charged molecules to niosome formulations increases the surface charge density, preventing vesicle fusion or aggregation and thereby improving the stability of the resulting vesicles. The three charged substances most often used in the creation of niosomes are stearyl amine, phosphatidic acid, and decyl phosphate. Phosphate buffer is often used because it may help with niosome production and the loading of natural or therapeutic substances. Niosome formulation also requires a hydration medium [48].

Niosome in Psoriasis Management

Niosomes, which are vesicles composed primarily of non-ionic surfactants and cholesterol, have these two substances as their main components. They have the ability to bind hydrophilic or lipophilic medicines in vesicular bilayer membranes. Niosomes can also exhibit osmotic activity. An analogue of vitamin A, actiretin, has anti-inflammatory and antipsoriatic properties. To avoid serious side effects, systemic acitretin treatment must be administered under close laboratory supervision [49]. Niosomes with a diameter of approximately 370 nanometers were loaded with acitretin. Regarding drug deposition in the layers of live skin, the *ex vivo* permeability profile of the nanosized acitretin-loaded niosomal gel outperformed that of the conventional acitretin gel. In HaCaT cell culture, activated carbon-loaded nano-niosomes showed enhanced antiproliferative activity [50]. Improved tolerability and much reduced skin irritation were two benefits of the formulation. Research has also been conducted on the use of niosome technology in the treatment of PUVA with 8-MOP. The entrapment efficiency of niosomes was remarkable, ranging from 83% to 90%. Over a six-month period, excellent physical stability was observed at various temperatures. Using rhodamine-loaded niosomal hydrogels rather than rhodamine 123 hydrogel, the *in vivo* investigation employed confocal laser scanning microscopy to examine the skin penetration of niosomes. Research on the *in vitro* deposition and penetration of the drug in rat skin showed that 8-MOP accumulated and penetrated more readily after eight hours [51, 52]. Proniosomes are compact, liquid-crystalline hybrids of niosomes that turn into niosomes when hydrated. By aggregating, fusing, and leaking, they provide physical stability. Research on drug release *via* cellulose membranes and rat skin demonstrated that tazarotene, included in various formulations, was released over an extended period. The rates of medication penetration and retention *in vitro* vary between formulations. For *in vivo* research, a male albino NMRI mouse was used as the tail model. It was found that PNG formulations based on Span 60 enhanced medication accumulation in the skin and decreased parakeratosis in the skin's horny layer [53].

Non-ionic surfactants are essential for the vesicular drug delivery system known as niosomes. These systems offer several advantages, including the ability to incorporate both hydrophilic and hydrophobic medications, as well as reduced toxicity, improved compatibility, and enhanced biodegradation [54]. Their expense, susceptibility to oxidation, and chemical instability are some of their main disadvantages, which are gradually making liposomes a more popular option. Niosomes' structure, which encloses the hydrophilic drug in a bilayer matrix and the hydrophobic moiety in the core aqueous compartment, enables targeted, regulated, and prolonged drug administration [55]. Niosomes may be used topically, intravenously, or orally. Niosomes are self-assembling structures based on non-ionic surfactants [56]. In response to the numerous shortcomings of available psoriasis therapies, including their high cost, withdrawal rebound, and numerous side effects, Meng *et al.* developed celastrol-loaded niosomes. Celastrol niosomes demonstrated higher *in vitro* permeability as compared to traditional medicine. Furthermore, in *in vivo* investigations, these niosomes were found to lessen scaling and redness on the back skin of animal models with psoriasis. According to research, the skin penetration and water solubility of celastrol were enhanced when it was encapsulated in niosomes, resulting in a stronger anti-inflammatory effect in mice. Moreover, Pandey *et al.* developed a niosome gel that enhanced the permeability and deposition of cyclosporine, thereby facilitating effective local psoriasis therapy. *Ex vivo* permeability tests on rat skin showed that, after 24 hours, niosomes displayed permeability rates of 50.57%, which exceeded the permeability rate of a standard cyclosporine solution, which was 10.13% [57, 68].

Pentoxifylline may be used to treat psoriasis and is believed to lessen the negative effects of cyclosporine. Given this, Bhardwaj *et al.* optimized niosomes containing pentoxifylline and cyclosporine using the thin film hydration process [58]. The niosomes significantly affected the drug's penetration, as the majority of the medication remained in the stratum corneum, with very little able to cross the skin. Goat skin was utilized for an *ex vivo* study. Even with the low percentage of drug penetration, niosomes permitted significantly more medication than solution to get through the skin [59 - 61]. In the *ex vivo* permeation study, niosomes performed much better than the solution in terms of medicine penetration through the goat skin. The mice treated with cyclosporine niosomes exhibited significantly improved skin conditions compared to those given the drug dispersion, as indicated by histology and the PASI score. Furthermore, after three months of storage stability testing at 40 °C and room temperature, niosomes remained stable. These findings suggest that cyclosporine-containing non-ionic surfactant vesicles may improve psoriasis therapy while mitigating the adverse effects of systemic administration [62]. The features of the niosomes mentioned earlier are presented in Table 1, and Table 2 lists the numerous herbal niosomes used to treat psoriasis.

Table 1. Recently formulated niosomes containing anti-psoriatic agents [63 - 67]

Bioactive Substance	Excipients	Preparation Method	Particle size (nm) Polydispersity Index Zeta Potential (mV)	Encapsulation Efficiency	Result of the *In Vivo/Ex Vivo* Experiments
Celastrol	Cholesterol, Span 20, Span 60, Chloroform, Methanol, Carbopol 974	Thin-film hydration, sonication techniques	147.4 ± 5.6 0.258 ± 0.02 −48.9 ± 1.1	N/A	Reduced cytokine levels and lowered erythema and cutaneous scaling in the mouse model
Cyclosporine	Cholesterol, Span 60, Chloroform, Carbopol 970 Methanol	Thin-film hydration	100.0 ± 0.8 to 284.5 ± 1.6 0.12 ± 0.02 to 0.31 ± 0.04 −32.2 ± 0.9 to 57.0 ± 0.9	88.23 to 96.5	Greater penetration as compared to cyclosporine suspension; a noteworthy reduction in PASI scores; a 59-fold rise in cyclosporine deposition in stratum corneum and epidermis/ dermis layers
Cyclosporine Pentoxifylline	Cholesterol, Tween 80, Span 80, Chloroform, Methanol	Thin-film hydration	-179 -0.285 -37.5	-75.03	Enhanced penetration of pentoxifylline and cyclosporine; significant amelioration in mice's skin condition as measured by PASI and histology scores

(Table 1) cont.....

Bioactive Substance	Excipients	Preparation Method	Particle size (nm) Polydispersity Index Zeta Potential (mV)	Encapsulation Efficiency	Result of the *In Vivo/Ex Vivo* Experiments
Pentoxifylline	Cholesterol, Tween 80, Soya-lacithin, Chloroform, Methanol	Thin-film hydration	69.52 to 1340.7 0.019 to 0.338 22.7 to 38.6	21.98 to 77.23	Decreased inflammation of stratum corneum and epidermis; a drop in PASI scores
Cyclosporine	Cholesterol, Span 60, Chloroform, Methanol	Thin-film hydration	61.96 ± 0.91 to 193.7 ± 0.23 0.101 ± 0.024 to 0.587 ± 0.098 −20.7 to 31.6	80.53 ± 1.18 to 98.19 ± 0.94	Deeper and larger accumulation; mice's skin health improved based on histology and PASI scores in comparison to drug dispersion

Table 2. Biological source, family, common name, and tamil name of herbal niosomes [69 - 74]

Biological Source	Source Family	Common Name	Tamil Name
Nerium oleander	Apocynaceae	Aralli	Aralli
Salvia kronenburgii	Lamiaceae	Garden sage	Chimaikkarppuram
Myrtus communis	Myrtaceae	Myrtle	Kulinaval
Hypericum perforatum	Hypericaceae	St. John's wort	Vettai Pakku
Lawsonia inermis	Lythraceae	Henna	Marudaani

EXPERT OPINION

Professional opinion indicates that niosome-based medicine is a potentially viable therapeutic approach for treating psoriasis. Niosomes are nano-sized vesicles composed of non-ionic surfactant, showing potential for topical drug delivery to treat psoriasis and other dermatological conditions. Their ability to efficiently penetrate the skin and encapsulate drugs makes them attractive for focused therapy. Studies have reported that niosomes enhance the dispersion of anti-psoriatic drugs, leading to fewer side effects and more efficacy. They are also suitable for long-term treatment as they are stable and biocompatible. Despite the encouraging outcomes, further research is necessary to fully understand the therapeutic potential of niosome formulations in the management of psoriasis and to maximize their use [75].

FUTURE PERSPECTIVES AND CHALLENGES

Psoriasis is a persistent autoimmune skin condition that affects people worldwide and is very difficult to treat. By avoiding issues with conventional methods, innovative pharmaceutical delivery systems provide a viable solution [76]. Niosome-based pharmacotherapy in the future offers both challenges and promising prospects for treating psoriasis. Niosomes have considerable promise as a pharmaceutical delivery system, as they can encapsulate and transport drugs to the skin areas affected by psoriasis. More research is required to develop niosome formulations for the treatment of psoriasis. Future studies may be able to mix several anti-psoriatic drugs with niosomes to reduce adverse effects and boost their efficacy. In addition, research on the biocompatibility and long-term durability of niosomes is necessary to ensure their safe and effective use in chronic conditions, such as psoriasis. Niosome-based medications need to be made broadly accessible and affordably priced by addressing cost and scalability concerns with the production process. Despite these challenges, the use of niosomes in psoriasis therapy has great promise for improved patient outcomes and treatment management [77]. Many studies have examined this issue over the past few decades, with a focus primarily on lipidic and polymeric nanoparticles. Several studies have demonstrated that niosomes can target specific cells or tissues to facilitate targeted drug administration, accelerate the rate at which medications enter the body, and release chemicals in a controlled and sustained manner [78].

CONCLUSION

In conclusion, niosome-based drugs hold great potential in the treatment of psoriasis. Research indicates that niosomes have the potential to enhance treatment outcomes by efficiently encapsulating and delivering anti-psoriatic medications to the affected skin regions. The capacity of niosomes to effectively penetrate the skin and target the inflammatory area is a promising method for treating the intricate pathophysiology of psoriasis. While further research is required to optimize niosome formulations and guarantee their long-term stability and safety, there are significant potential advantages in terms of improved drug administration and reduced side effects. Pharmacotherapy based on niosomes is an intriguing approach to treating psoriasis, as it generally offers patients hope for improved therapeutic options and an enhanced quality of life.

REFERENCES

[1] Grän F, Kerstan A, Serfling E, Goebeler M, Muhammad K. Current developments in the immunology of psoriasis. Yale J Biol Med 2020; 93(1): 97-110.
[PMID: 32226340]

[2] Parisi R, Iskandar IYK, Kontopantelis E, Augustin M, Griffiths CEM, Ashcroft DM. National,

regional, and worldwide epidemiology of psoriasis: systematic analysis and modelling study. BMJ 2020; 369: m1590.
[http://dx.doi.org/10.1136/bmj.m1590] [PMID: 32467098]

[3] Liang SE, Cohen JM, Ho RS. Psoriasis and suicidality: A review of the literature. Dermatol Ther 2019; 32(1): e12771.
[http://dx.doi.org/10.1111/dth.12771] [PMID: 30315629]

[4] Armstrong AW, Puig L, Joshi A, *et al.* Comparison of biologics and oral treatments for plaque psoriasis: A meta-analysis. JAMA Dermatol 2020; 156(3): 258-69.
[http://dx.doi.org/10.1001/jamadermatol.2019.4029] [PMID: 32022825]

[5] Menter A, Strober BE, Kaplan DH, *et al.* Joint AAD-NPF guidelines of care for the management and treatment of psoriasis with biologics. J Am Acad Dermatol 2019; 80(4): 1029-72.
[http://dx.doi.org/10.1016/j.jaad.2018.11.057] [PMID: 30772098]

[6] Kumari S, Goyal A, Garg M, Antonescu A, Sindhu RK. Lyotropic liquid crystal system for drug delivery of astaxanthin: Physical characterization and enhanced antioxidant potential. Crystals (Basel) 2023; 13(1): 142.
[http://dx.doi.org/10.3390/cryst13010142]

[7] Gaspar-Pintiliescu A, Stanciuc AM, Craciunescu O. Natural composite dressings based on collagen, gelatin and plant bioactive compounds for wound healing: A review. Int J Biol Macromol 2019; 138: 854-65.
[http://dx.doi.org/10.1016/j.ijbiomac.2019.07.155] [PMID: 31351963]

[8] Shrivastav S, Sindhu R, Kumar S, Kumar P. Anti-psoriatic and phytochemical evaluation of Thespesia populnea bark extracts. Int J Pharm Pharm Sci 2009; 1: 176-85.

[9] Florek AG, Wang CJ, Armstrong AW. Treatment preferences and treatment satisfaction among psoriasis patients: a systematic review. Arch Dermatol Res 2018; 310(4): 271-319.
[http://dx.doi.org/10.1007/s00403-018-1808-x] [PMID: 29442137]

[10] Augustin M, Mrowietz U, Bonnekoh B, *et al.* Topical long-term therapy of psoriasis with vitamin D_3 analogues, corticosteroids and their two compound formulations: position paper on evidence and use in daily practice. J Dtsch Dermatol Ges 2014; 12(8): 667-82.
[http://dx.doi.org/10.1111/ddg.12396] [PMID: 25039309]

[11] Norsgaard H, Kurdykowski S, Descargues P, *et al.* Calcipotriol counteracts betamethasone-induced decrease in extracellular matrix components related to skin atrophy. Arch Dermatol Res 2014; 306(8): 719-29.
[http://dx.doi.org/10.1007/s00403-014-1485-3] [PMID: 25027750]

[12] Schoepe S, Schäcke H, May E, Asadullah K. Glucocorticoid therapy-induced skin atrophy. Exp Dermatol 2006; 15(6): 406-20.
[http://dx.doi.org/10.1111/j.0906-6705.2006.00435.x] [PMID: 16689857]

[13] Mahrle G, Bonnekoh B, Wevers A, Hegemann L. Anthralin: how does it act and are there more favourable derivatives? Acta Derm Venereol Suppl (Stockh) 1994; 186: 83-4.
[PMID: 8073848]

[14] Sehgal VN, Verma P, Khurana A. Anthralin/dithranol in dermatology. Int J Dermatol 2014; 53(10): e449-60.
[http://dx.doi.org/10.1111/j.1365-4632.2012.05611.x] [PMID: 25208745]

[15] Kadian V, Kumar S, Saini K, Kakkar V, Rao R. Dithranol: An insight into its novel delivery cargos for psoriasis management. Curr Drug Res Rev 2021; 12(2): 82-96.
[http://dx.doi.org/10.2174/2589977512666200525154954] [PMID: 32484107]

[16] Chat VS, Kearns DG, Uppal SK, Han G, Wu JJ. Management of psoriasis with topicals: Applying the 2020 AAD-NPF guidelines of care to clinical practice. Cutis 2022; 110(2 Suppl) (Suppl.): 8-14.
[http://dx.doi.org/10.12788/cutis.0573] [PMID: 36219602]

[17] Yamamoto T, Matsuuchi M, Irimajiri J, Otoyama K, Nishioka K. Topical anthralin for psoriasis vulgaris: evaluation of 70 Japanese patients. J Dermatol 2000; 27(7): 482-5. [http://dx.doi.org/10.1111/j.1346-8138.2000.tb02212.x] [PMID: 10935350]

[18] Dogra S, Kaur I. Childhood psoriasis. Indian J Dermatol Venereol Leprol 2010; 76(4): 357-65. [http://dx.doi.org/10.4103/0378-6323.66580] [PMID: 20657115]

[19] Elmets CA, Korman NJ, Prater EF, *et al.* Joint AAD–NPF guidelines of care for the management and treatment of psoriasis with topical therapy and alternative medicine modalities for psoriasis severity measures. J Am Acad Dermatol 2021; 84(2): 432-70. [http://dx.doi.org/10.1016/j.jaad.2020.07.087] [PMID: 32738429]

[20] Yadav K, Soni A, Singh D, Singh MR. Polymers in topical delivery of anti-psoriatic medications and other topical agents in overcoming the barriers of conventional treatment strategies. Prog Biomater 2021; 10(1): 1-17. [http://dx.doi.org/10.1007/s40204-021-00154-7] [PMID: 33738750]

[21] Chandrashekara S. The treatment strategies of autoimmune disease may need a different approach from conventional protocol: A review. Indian J Pharmacol 2012; 44(6): 665-71. [http://dx.doi.org/10.4103/0253-7613.103235] [PMID: 23248391]

[22] Pradhan M, Alexander A, Singh MR, *et al.* Understanding the prospective of nano-formulations towards the treatment of psoriasis. Biomed Pharmacother 2018; 107: 447-63. [http://dx.doi.org/10.1016/j.biopha.2018.07.156] [PMID: 30103117]

[23] Khadka P, Ro J, Kim H, *et al.* Pharmaceutical particle technologies: An approach to improve drug solubility, dissolution and bioavailability. Asian Journal of Pharmaceutical Sciences 2014; 9(6): 304-16. [http://dx.doi.org/10.1016/j.ajps.2014.05.005]

[24] Monteiro RC, Nikam VN, Dandakeri S, Bhat R. Transepidermal water loss in psoriasis: A case-control study. Indian Dermatol Online J 2019; 10(3): 267-71. [http://dx.doi.org/10.4103/idoj.IDOJ_180_18] [PMID: 31149569]

[25] Bhalani DV, Nutan B, Kumar A, Singh Chandel AK. Bioavailability enhancement techniques for poorly aqueous soluble drugs and therapeutics. Biomedicines 2022; 10(9): 2055. [http://dx.doi.org/10.3390/biomedicines10092055] [PMID: 36140156]

[26] Ruela ALM, Perissinato AG, Lino MES, Mudrik PS, Pereira GR. Evaluation of skin absorption of drugs from topical and transdermal formulations. Braz J Pharm Sci 2016; 52(3): 527-44. [http://dx.doi.org/10.1590/s1984-82502016000300018]

[27] Pascher F. Systemic reactions to topically applied drugs. Int J Dermatol 1978; 17(10): 768-75. [http://dx.doi.org/10.1111/j.1365-4362.1978.tb05977.x] [PMID: 730430]

[28] Shetty K, Sherje AP. Nano intervention in topical delivery of corticosteroid for psoriasis and atopic dermatitis—a systematic review. J Mater Sci Mater Med 2021; 32(8): 88. [http://dx.doi.org/10.1007/s10856-021-06558-y] [PMID: 34331599]

[29] Akhtar N, Verma A, Pathak K. Exploring preclinical and clinical effectiveness of nanoformulations in the treatment of atopic dermatitis: Safety aspects and patent reviews. Bull Fac Pharm Cairo Univ 2017; 55(1): 1-10. [http://dx.doi.org/10.1016/j.bfopcu.2016.12.003]

[30] Piperno A, Sciortino MT, Giusto E, Montesi M, Panseri S, Scala A. Recent advances and challenges in gene delivery mediated by polyester-based nanoparticles. Int J Nanomedicine 2021; 16: 5981-6002. [http://dx.doi.org/10.2147/IJN.S321329] [PMID: 34511901]

[31] Nohynek GJ, Dufour EK, Roberts MS. Nanotechnology, cosmetics and the skin: is there a health risk? Skin Pharmacol Physiol 2008; 21(3): 136-49. [http://dx.doi.org/10.1159/000131078] [PMID: 18523411]

[32] Sindrilaru A, Filip A, Scharffetter-Kochanek K, Crisan D. How can nanoparticle-based technologies revolutionize the topical therapy in psoriasis? Exp Dermatol 2020; 29(11): 1097-103. [http://dx.doi.org/10.1111/exd.14149] [PMID: 32657487]

[33] Cevc G. Lipid vesicles and other colloids as drug carriers on the skin. Adv Drug Deliv Rev 2004; 56(5): 675-711. [http://dx.doi.org/10.1016/j.addr.2003.10.028] [PMID: 15019752]

[34] Alam M, Rizwanullah M, Mir SR, Amin S. Promising prospects of lipid-based topical nanocarriers for the treatment of psoriasis. OpenNano 2023; 10: 100123. [http://dx.doi.org/10.1016/j.onano.2023.100123]

[35] Schäferkorting M, Mehnert W, Korting H. Lipid nanoparticles for improved topical application of drugs for skin diseases. Adv Drug Deliv Rev 2007; 59(6): 427-43. [http://dx.doi.org/10.1016/j.addr.2007.04.006] [PMID: 17544165]

[36] Gupta SK, Kuila P, Jana PK. GAR: An energy efficient GA-based routing for wireless sensor networks. Distributed Computing and Internet Technology. Berlin/Heidelberg, Germany: Springer 2013; pp. 267-77. [http://dx.doi.org/10.1007/978-3-642-36071-8_21]

[37] Azeem A, Anwer MK, Talegaonkar S. Niosomes in sustained and targeted drug delivery: some recent advances. J Drug Target 2009; 17(9): 671-89. [http://dx.doi.org/10.3109/10611860903079454] [PMID: 19845484]

[38] Muzzalupo R, Mazzotta E. Do niosomes have a place in the field of drug delivery?. Expert opinion on drug delivery. 2019 Nov 2;16(11):1145-7.

[39] Aparajay P, Dev A. Functionalized niosomes as a smart delivery device in cancer and fungal infection. Eur J Pharm Sci 2022; 168: 106052. [http://dx.doi.org/10.1016/j.ejps.2021.106052] [PMID: 34740786]

[40] Gharbavi M, Amani J, Kheiri-Manjili H, Danafar H, Sharafi A. Niosome: A promising nanocarrier for natural drug delivery through blood-brain barrier. Adv Pharmacol Sci 2018; 2018: 1-15. [http://dx.doi.org/10.1155/2018/6847971] [PMID: 30651728]

[41] Momekova DB, Gugleva VE, Petrov PD. Nanoarchitectonics of multifunctional niosomes for advanced drug delivery. ACS Omega 2021; 6(49): 33265-73. [http://dx.doi.org/10.1021/acsomega.1c05083] [PMID: 34926878]

[42] Abdelkader H, Alani AWG, Alany RG. Recent advances in non-ionic surfactant vesicles (niosomes): self-assembly, fabrication, characterization, drug delivery applications and limitations. Drug Deliv 2014; 21(2): 87-100. [http://dx.doi.org/10.3109/10717544.2013.838077] [PMID: 24156390]

[43] Izhar MP, Hafeez A, Kushwaha P, Simrah . Drug delivery through niosomes: A comprehensive review with therapeutic applications. J Cluster Sci 2023; 34(5): 2257-73. [http://dx.doi.org/10.1007/s10876-023-02423-w]

[44] Shah N, Prajapati R, Gohil D, Sadhu P, Patel S. Niosomes: A promising novel nano carrier for drug delivery. J Pharm Res Int 2021; 33: 53-66. [http://dx.doi.org/10.9734/jpri/2021/v33i48B33260]

[45] Chen S, Hanning S, Falconer J, Locke M, Wen J. Recent advances in non-ionic surfactant vesicles (niosomes): Fabrication, characterization, pharmaceutical and cosmetic applications. Eur J Pharm Biopharm 2019; 144: 18-39. [http://dx.doi.org/10.1016/j.ejpb.2019.08.015] [PMID: 31446046]

[46] Somjid S, Krongsuk S, Johns JR. Cholesterol concentration effect on the bilayer properties and phase formation of niosome bilayers: A molecular dynamics simulation study. J Mol Liq 2018; 256: 591-8. [http://dx.doi.org/10.1016/j.molliq.2018.02.077]

[47] Ge X, Wei M, He S, Yuan WE. Advances of Non-Ionic Surfactant Vesicles (Niosomes) and their application in drug delivery. Pharmaceutics 2019; 11(2): 55.
[http://dx.doi.org/10.3390/pharmaceutics11020055] [PMID: 30700021]

[48] Junyaprasert VB, Teeranachaideekul V, Supaperm T. Effect of charged and non-ionic membrane additives on physicochemical properties and stability of niosomes. AAPS PharmSciTech 2008; 9(3): 851-9.
[http://dx.doi.org/10.1208/s12249-008-9121-1] [PMID: 18636334]

[49] Kumar GP, Rajeshwarrao P. Nonionic surfactant vesicular systems for effective drug delivery—an overview. Acta Pharm Sin B 2011; 1(4): 208-19.
[http://dx.doi.org/10.1016/j.apsb.2011.09.002]

[50] Witika BA, Bassey KE, Demana PH, Siwe-Noundou X, Poka MS. Current advances in specialised niosomal drug delivery: Manufacture, characterization and drug delivery applications. Int J Mol Sci 2022; 23(17): 9668.
[http://dx.doi.org/10.3390/ijms23179668] [PMID: 36077066]

[51] García-Manrique P, Machado ND, Fernández MA, Blanco-López MC, Matos M, Gutiérrez G. Effect of drug molecular weight on niosomes size and encapsulation efficiency. Colloids Surf B Biointerfaces 2020; 186: 110711.
[http://dx.doi.org/10.1016/j.colsurfb.2019.110711] [PMID: 31864114]

[52] Bartelds R, Nematollahi MH, Pols T, *et al.* Niosomes, an alternative for liposomal delivery. PLoS One 2018; 13(4): e0194179.
[http://dx.doi.org/10.1371/journal.pone.0194179] [PMID: 29649223]

[53] Abu Hashim I, Abo El-Magd N, El-Sheakh A, Hamed M, Abd El-Gawad AEG. Pivotal role of Acitretin nanovesicular gel for effective treatment of psoriasis: *ex vivo–in vivo* evaluation study. Int J Nanomedicine 2018; 13: 1059-79.
[http://dx.doi.org/10.2147/IJN.S156412] [PMID: 29503541]

[54] Kassem AA, Abd El-Alim SH, Asfour MH. Enhancement of 8-methoxypsoralen topical delivery *via* nanosized niosomal vesicles: Formulation development, *in vitro* and *in vivo* evaluation of skin deposition. Int J Pharm 2017; 517(1-2): 256-68.
[http://dx.doi.org/10.1016/j.ijpharm.2016.12.018] [PMID: 27956194]

[55] Ahmad MZ, Mohammed AA, Mokhtar Ibrahim M. Technology overview and drug delivery application of proniosome. Pharm Dev Technol 2017; 22(3): 302-11.
[http://dx.doi.org/10.3109/10837450.2015.1135344] [PMID: 26794727]

[56] Prasad V, Chaurasia S. Performance evaluation of non-ionic surfactant based tazarotene encapsulated proniosomal gel for the treatment of psoriasis. Mater Sci Eng C 2017; 79: 168-76.
[http://dx.doi.org/10.1016/j.msec.2017.05.036] [PMID: 28629004]

[57] Bhardwaj P, Tripathi P, Gupta R, Pandey S. Niosomes: A review on niosomal research in the last decade. J Drug Deliv Sci Technol 2020; 56: 101581.
[http://dx.doi.org/10.1016/j.jddst.2020.101581]

[58] Rajera R, Nagpal K, Singh SK, Mishra DN. Niosomes: a controlled and novel drug delivery system. Biol Pharm Bull 2011; 34(7): 945-53.
[http://dx.doi.org/10.1248/bpb.34.945] [PMID: 21719996]

[59] Ruckmani K, Sankar V. Formulation and optimization of Zidovudine niosomes. AAPS PharmSciTech 2010; 11(3): 1119-27.
[http://dx.doi.org/10.1208/s12249-010-9480-2] [PMID: 20635228]

[60] Yasamineh S, Yasamineh P, Ghafouri Kalajahi H, *et al.* A state-of-the-art review on the recent advances of niosomes as a targeted drug delivery system. Int J Pharm 2022; 624: 121878.
[http://dx.doi.org/10.1016/j.ijpharm.2022.121878] [PMID: 35636629]

[61] Marianecci C, Di Marzio L, Rinaldi F, *et al.* Niosomes from 80s to present: The state of the art. Adv

Colloid Interface Sci 2014; 205: 187-206.
[http://dx.doi.org/10.1016/j.cis.2013.11.018] [PMID: 24369107]

[62] Kaputlu İ, Şadan G, Karayalçin B, Boz A. Beneficial effects of pentoxifylline on cyclosporine-induced nephrotoxicity. Clin Exp Pharmacol Physiol 1997; 24(5): 365-9.
[http://dx.doi.org/10.1111/j.1440-1681.1997.tb01203.x] [PMID: 9143789]

[63] Meng S, Sun L, Wang L, *et al.* Loading of water-insoluble celastrol into niosome hydrogels for improved topical permeation and anti-psoriasis activity. Colloids Surf B Biointerfaces 2019; 182: 110352.
[http://dx.doi.org/10.1016/j.colsurfb.2019.110352] [PMID: 31306831]

[64] Pandey SS, Shah KM, Maulvi FA, *et al.* Topical delivery of cyclosporine loaded tailored niosomal nanocarriers for improved skin penetration and deposition in psoriasis: Optimization, *ex vivo* and animal studies. J Drug Deliv Sci Technol 2021; 63: 102441.
[http://dx.doi.org/10.1016/j.jddst.2021.102441]

[65] Bhardwaj P, Tripathi P, Pandey S, Gupta R, Khar RK, Patil PR. Improved dermal delivery of pentoxifylline niosomes for the management of psoriasis: Development, optimization and *in-vivo* studies in imiquimod induced psoriatic plaque model. J Drug Deliv Sci Technol 2022; 75: 103643.
[http://dx.doi.org/10.1016/j.jddst.2022.103643]

[66] Bhardwaj P, Tripathi P, Pandey S, Chaurasia D, Ramchandra Patil P. Tailored non-ionic surfactant vesicles of cyclosporine for the treatment of psoriasis: formulation, *ex-vivo* and *in-vivo* investigation-application of box-behnken design. Advanced Materials Science and Technology 2023; 5(2): 0.
[http://dx.doi.org/10.37155/2717-526X-0502-2]

[67] Qiu F, Xi L, Chen S, Zhao Y, Wang Z, Zheng Y. Celastrol niosome hydrogel has anti-inflammatory effect on skin keratinocytes and circulation without systemic drug exposure in psoriasis mice. International Journal of Nanomedicine. 2021 Sep 4:6171-82.

[68] Tomar S, Kalia A. Recent advances in topical niosomal delivery for the treatment of psoriasis. World J Pharm Sci 2015; 4(5): 669-85.

[69] Pradhan M, Singh D, Singh MR. Novel colloidal carriers for psoriasis: Current issues, mechanistic insight and novel delivery approaches. J Control Release 2013; 170(3): 380-95.
[http://dx.doi.org/10.1016/j.jconrel.2013.05.020] [PMID: 23770117]

[70] Singh MR, Nag MK, Patel S, Daharwal SJ, Singh D. Novel approaches for dermal and transdermal Delivery of herbal drugs. Res J Pharmacogn Phytochem 2013; 5(6): 271-9.

[71] Salim N, Ahmad N, Musa SH, Hashim R, Tadros TF, Basri M. Nanoemulsion as a topical delivery system of antipsoriatic drugs. Royal Society of Chemistry 2016; pp. 1-56.

[72] Singh A, Bedi N. Psoriasis: History, present and future prospects. Curr Trends Biotechnol Pharm 2013; 7(3): 808-24.

[73] Dhole VM, Shelgavkar DD, Rathore VK, Pande SD. Development and characterization of topical drug delivery system containing Niosomes. World J Pharm Res 2014; 5: 881-91.

[74] Trivedi K, Ravikumar P. Topical formulations in psoriasis management: An overview. Indo Am J Pharm Res 2016; 6(11): 6895-904.

[75] Bodnár K, Fehér P, Ujhelyi Z, Bácskay I, Józsa L. Recent approaches for the topical treatment of psoriasis using nanoparticles. Pharmaceutics 2024; 16(4): 449.
[http://dx.doi.org/10.3390/pharmaceutics16040449] [PMID: 38675110]

[76] Begines B, Ortiz T, Pérez-Aranda M, *et al.* Polymeric nanoparticles for drug delivery: recent developments and future prospects. Nanomaterials (Basel) 2020; 10(7): 1403.
[http://dx.doi.org/10.3390/nano10071403] [PMID: 32707641]

[77] Mohd Nordin UU, Ahmad N, Salim N, Mohd Yusof NS. Lipid-based nanoparticles for psoriasis treatment: a review on conventional treatments, recent works, and future prospects. RSC Advances

2021; 11(46): 29080-101.
[http://dx.doi.org/10.1039/D1RA06087B] [PMID: 35478537]

[78] Liu L, Zhao W, Ma Q, *et al.* Functional nano-systems for transdermal drug delivery and skin therapy. Nanoscale Adv 2023; 5(6): 1527-58.
[http://dx.doi.org/10.1039/D2NA00530A] [PMID: 36926556]

CHAPTER 9

Nanostructured Lipid-Based Pharmacotherapy for the Management of Psoriasis

Manish Kumar[1,*], **Dev Kashyup**[1], **Nidhi Arora**[2], **Ajay Kumar**[3] and **Dileep Kumar**[4]

[1] *Department of Pharmaceutics, ISF College of Pharmacy, Moga 142001, Punjab, India*

[2] *Department of Pharmacy, Chandigarh Pharmacy College, Chandigarh Group of Colleges, Jhanjeri 140307, Punjab, India*

[3] *Department of Pharmacology, Sardar Patel College of Pharmacy, Gorakhpur 2730113, Uttar Pradesh, India*

[4] *Department of Entomology and Nematology, UC Davis Comprehensive Cancer Center, University of California Davis, One Shields Avenue, Davis, California 95616, USA*

Abstract: Psoriasis, a chronic autoimmune skin disorder, poses a significant therapeutic challenge due to its complex Etiology and variable clinical manifestations. This abstract highlights recent advancements in novel carrier systems that revolutionize psoriasis management and pharmacotherapy. These innovative carriers aim to improve drug delivery, enhance therapeutic efficacy, and mitigate the adverse effects of conventional treatments. Psoriasis is characterised by hyperproliferation of keratinocytes, inflammation, and immune dysregulation. Conventional treatments often involve topical corticosteroids, phototherapy, or systemic immunosuppressants, each with its limitations, such as variable efficacy and side effects. The emergence of novel carrier systems, including liposomes, nanoparticles, and microneedle arrays, provides a promising avenue for addressing these challenges. Advanced drug delivery systems enable the precise delivery and management of the release of therapeutic agents, enhancing their penetration into the affected skin layers. Liposomal formulations, for instance, offer improved drug stability and sustained release, minimizing the need for frequent applications and reducing side effects. Nanoparticles provide a platform for encapsulating various drugs, offering enhanced solubility and bioavailability. Moreover, the integration of personalized medicine approaches into carrier design allows for tailored treatment regimens based on individual patient characteristics. This shift towards precision medicine holds the potential to optimize therapeutic outcomes and minimize adverse reactions.

* **Corresponding author Manish Kumar:** Department of Pharmaceutics, ISF College of Pharmacy, Moga 142001, Punjab, India; E-mail: manish_singh17@rediffmail.com

Anjali Sharma, Prerna Sharma, Roy Rillera Marzo & Ahmed A. Al Karmalawy (Eds.)

Keywords: Autoimmune skin disorders, Carriersystems, Drug delivery, Innovative formulations, Nanomedicine, Pharmacotherapy, Psoriasis, Personalized medicine, Targeted therapy, Topical treatments.

INTRODUCTION

Psoriasis, a skin disorder driven by autoimmune T-cell activity, manifests as red, thickened plaques covered by a silver-white scale, characterized by repeated episodes of inflammation and excessive skin thickening. Despite its prevalence, the exact origin of psoriasis remains unidentified. Contemporary treatments employ a diverse range of antipsoriatic drugs with varying mechanisms and administration routes [1]. However, many conventional therapies focus on symptom suppression and often yield notable side effects. Presently, treatment modalities include topical applications, phototherapy, and systemic interventions, yet none of these approaches guarantees a complete cure for the condition [2]. These methods are not only unsafe and inefficient but also contribute to unfavourable cosmetic outcomes and the associated side effects, resulting in less-than-ideal patient outcomes and poor adherence during prolonged use. A critical challenge in achieving effective therapy lies in the absence of a perfect carrier for antipsoriatic drug delivery. To address this limitation, researchers are actively exploring the potential of various types of colloidal carriers that are utilized within the drug delivery system. Some commonly used carriers are ethosomes, spherical lipid structures like liposomes, niosomes, transferosomes, solid lipid nanoparticles, microspheres, micelles, dendrimers, and other innovative platforms. The aim is to establish more effective therapeutic regimens by utilizing these distinct drug delivery systems, addressing the shortcomings of current treatments, and ultimately offering improved outcomes for individuals dealing with psoriasis [3].

Types of Psoriasis

Psoriasis is categorized into four types based on various factors, such as the extent of inflammation, rash localization, acute or persistent health conditions in patients, and various clinical factors. Various forms of psoriasis exist, such as plaque, guttate, pustular, and erythrodermic forms of the chronic skin condition. The prevalent form is chronic plaque psoriasis, also known as psoriasis vulgaris, characterized by the development of lesions from small papules that aggregate to form plaques [4]. Guttate psoriasis, on the other hand, results from an immune response that can be exacerbated by a *Streptococcal* infection. This begins with tiny pink raised bumps that periodically become flaky. Erythrodermic psoriasis is a type of psoriasis that can cause significant loss of protein and fluids, which can disrupt the body's normal balance (homeostasis). This severe form represents an advancement of existing psoriasis and often necessitates hospitalization due to complications like increased sophisticated conditions, such as *staphylococcal* infections, pustulosis, arthropathy, and growth retardation can manifest [5]. Pustular psoriasis, a severe variant, refers to the appearance of pus-filled lesions on the surface of the skin, typically confined to the palms and soles, but potentially spreading to other areas. Although these lesions have minimal systemic effects, they can be challenging to manage. Frequently, generalized pustular psoriasis is accompanied by symptoms, such as fever and malaise, along with complications that include fluid retention, disturbances in electrolyte levels, and susceptibility to infection. This type of psoriasis is characterized by frequent recurrence, requiring vigilant and aggressive management [6].

Pathogenesis of Psoriasis

The physical expression of psoriasis at a biological level arises from a profound alteration in the process of keratinocyte transformation, resulting in the creation of scaly patches. The process initiates as fresh cells are produced within the basal layer of the epidermis and move towards the outer layer, collecting around keratin, known as the stratum corneum, while losing their organelles. These cells become filled with keratin upon reaching the stratum corneum, providing protective benefits to the skin. Under normal conditions, keratinocytes within cells in the basal layer undergo division approximately every two weeks, during the shedding and renewal cycle of the epidermis. New cells span approximately four weeks [7]. However, in the skin affected by psoriasis, there is an expedited cell cycle, leading to cell division every 1.5 days, and keratinocytes migrate to the stratum corneum within 4 days. This rapid pace results in inadequate development and maturation of cells, contributing to the characteristic scaly appearance of an epidermis that has a thickness, *i.e.*, 3 to 5 times greater than normal. Psoriasis is further characterized by histological markers, including neutrophil clusters present in the outer skin layer, and significant quantities of T-cells and dendritic cells are found within the subcutaneous layer [8]. Noteworthy features also include a significant presence of mononuclear leukocytes, which results in the alteration of blood vessels within the papillary dermal region into elongated or excessively proliferative forms, resulting in the redness of psoriatic lesions, attributable to considerable dilation of these blood vessels. Additionally, endothelial cells in psoriatic lesions exhibit characteristics resembling those of vessels with elevated endothelial characteristics typically found within lymph nodes, attributed to the attachment comprising lymphocytes, monocytes, and neutrophils. Activation of cells present in the endothelial layer is evident in psoriatic lesions, the existence of intracellular adhesion molecule-1 (ICAM-1 or CD54), vascular cell adhesion molecule-1 (VCAM-1 or CD106), and E-selectin (CD62E) during staining signifies the adherence of lymphocytes, monocytes, and neutrophils [9].

Challenges in Psoriasis Treatment

Despite the availability of numerous therapeutic agents, treating psoriasis remains a formidable challenge primarily because an ideal drug molecule has not yet been identified [10]. The significant hurdles in addressing psoriasis treatment are expounded upon below.

Absence of an effective vehicle for transporting anti-psoriatic medications: The effective administration of antipsoriatic treatment drugs faces challenges due to the intrinsic adverse effects of the drug compounds or their inadequate integration into traditional carriers. Significant issues arise from variations in drug absorption and effectiveness, which arise from the physicochemical attributes of both the carrier and the active drug. To address these challenges, novel colloidal delivery carriers emerge as a promising option [11]. These carriers offer several advantages, including securing the encapsulated drugs from external as well as internal factors, controlling the release of drugs to maintain the therapeutic levels within the body for prolonged periods, and the possibility of directing the drugs to specific sites of action either passively or actively. This targeted approach ensures diverse interaction pathways with the intended cells, minimizing toxicity at non-target sites and enhancing the therapeutic efficacy of the drug. In summary, these innovative colloidal carriers present a viable alternative as drug delivery vehicles, mitigating the side effects associated with active drug compounds while improving overall therapeutic effectiveness [12].

Lack of Animal Models: This menacing ailment exclusively affects humans, creating a challenge in finding suitable animal models that can faithfully replicate the histopathological and immunogenic characteristics of psoriasis as observed in humans. While several immunogenetic models have been developed, none of them fully encompasses all the distinctive features and limitations of the disease. Among the commonly employed models, the following three are frequently utilized, yet they also exhibit certain shortcomings [13].

Spontaneous Mutation Model: Within this framework, mutations arise from errors during DNA replication, the development of unprovoked lesions, and the functioning of mobile genetic elements. While the model displays features like hyperkeratosis and the creation of scales, it lacks adequate responses from T cells and neutrophils. As a consequence, it does not entirely replicate the features of psoriasis [14]. Examples of this model include homozygous sebaceous mice with the (Scd1ab/Scd1ab) genotype, mice with a flaky skin phenotype (Ttcfsn/Ttcfsn), and mice bearing mutations associated with spontaneous chronic proliferative dermatitis (Sharpincpdm/Sharpincpdm).

Xenotransplantation Model: In this method, psoriasis is induced through xenotransplantation, where a portion of psoriatic skin is grafted onto genetically modified mice; however, a drawback of this model is that it exhibits histological characteristics that are absent in psoriasis. For instance, arthymic nude mice exhibit the existence of a granular stratum, AGR129 models show the existence of underdeveloped natural killer (NK) cells, and SCID mice display a prevalence of mature NK cells. Examples of this model include mice lacking a thymus (athymic nude mice, Fraki *et al.,* 1983), mice with profoundly merged immunodeficiency (SCID) (Nickoloff *et al.,* 1995), and AGR129 models with spontaneous mutations (Boyman *et al.*, 2004) [15].

Transgenic Model: This system is created through the alteration of a solitary gene, which is inadequate given that psoriasis is a multigenetic disorder. The modification at a singular gene level does not encompass the numerous factors associated with psoriasis [16].

Novel Carriers for Psoriasis Management and Pharmacotherapy

The innovative objective of the drug delivery system is to enhance efficacy in currently available drugs for therapeutic purposes and offer a secure and effective method for administering newly formulated drugs, catering to the body's specific spatial and temporal needs. Extensive research has been devoted to devising different delivery methods to overcome the constraints linked with traditional formulations [17]. Colloidal Drug Delivery Systems (CDDS) consist of particles or vesicles that vary in size from 1 nm to 0.5 μm. Termed particulate carrier systems, these colloidal drug carriers play a vital role in ensuring the effective conveyance of enclosed medications. They efficiently capture, convey, and maintain the presence of active drugs, ensuring precise delivery to the targeted site, where they exert their effects [18]. This targeted drug delivery approach enhances drug accessibility, reduces and mitigates adverse effects, and enhances the therapeutic margin, thereby significantly minimizing systemic side effects. An ideal drug carrier in colloidal form should have specific characteristics. These factors include the ability to navigate through anatomical barriers, specific recognition of target cells through surface ligands, the stability of the drug-ligand interaction in the biological environment, and the carrier's biodegradability characterized by non-toxic properties [19]. By meeting these criteria, these highly selective strategies contribute to a substantial reduction in systemic side effects, offering a promising avenue for advancing drug delivery technologies. Innovative formulations for delivering drugs at a colloidal level have several advantages over conventional ones. They minimize drug bioavailability, thereby preventing harmful toxic effects and enhancing the effectiveness of a drug. It is therefore important to improve its accumulation in the targeted region by reducing degradation and loss. Additionally, they provide adaptability and pliability in managing drugs, resulting in enhanced adherence by patients [20]. However, key obstacles in drug delivery involve high production costs and issues related to stability and characterization. Nevertheless, nanotechnology has surfaced as a promising approach to boost the skin penetration of drugs and improve their bioavailability. Nanotechnology provides several assets, such as increased solubility, reduced dose, and exploring diverse nanocarriers like polymeric nanoparticles, solid lipid nanoparticles (SLN), nanoliposomes, and nanohydrogels, leading to improved therapeutic effects, prolonged release, and increased patient compliance [21] (Fig. **1**).

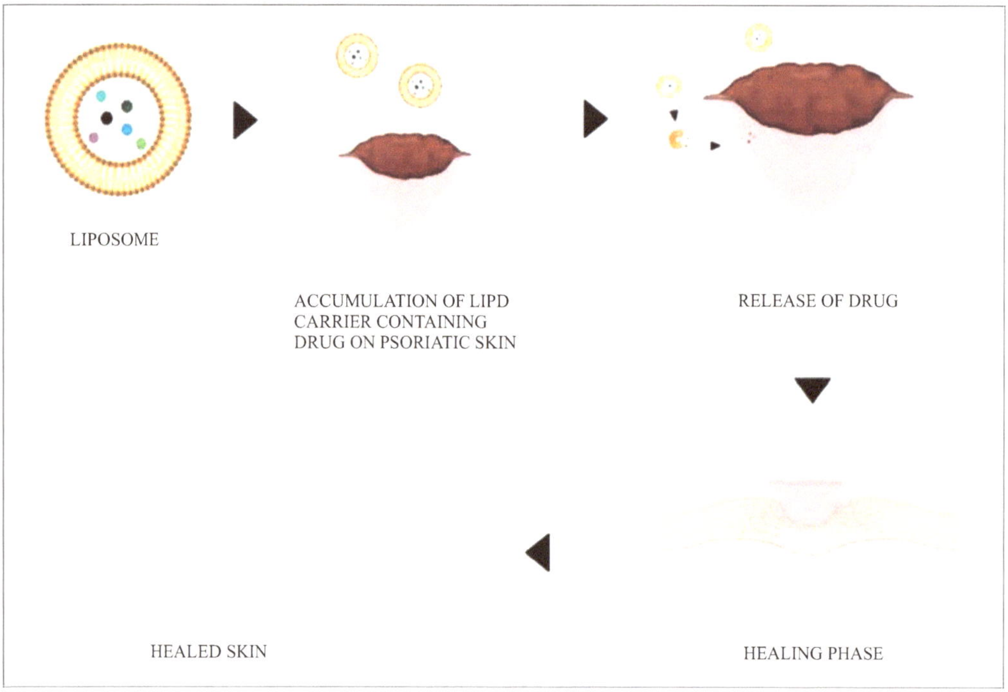

Fig. (1). Diagrammatic representation of the mechanism of drug release from lipid-based colloidal carriers.

Lipid-BasedColloidalCarriers

Colloidal carriers composed of lipid-based formulations are well-accepted because of the presence of natural lipids that are typically harmless and break down into non-toxic components within the body. Lipid-based carriers provide benefits including regulated release, stability, targetability, substantial drug capacity, biodegradability, cost-effectiveness, and the ability to convey both lipophilic and hydrophilic drugs, particularly within lipid carriers like SLN and NLC. Additionally, they share a unique advantage of resembling many compounds found naturally or in physiological processes [22]. Different categories of lipid-based carriers are being investigated as potential options and alternatives with promising outcomes for delivering topically and systemically anti-psoriatic effects. Various types of lipidic carriers are available, including transferosomes, niosomes, liposomes, ethosomes, Microemulsion, Solid Lipid Nanoparticles (SLN), and Nanostructured Lipids [23] (Fig. **2**).

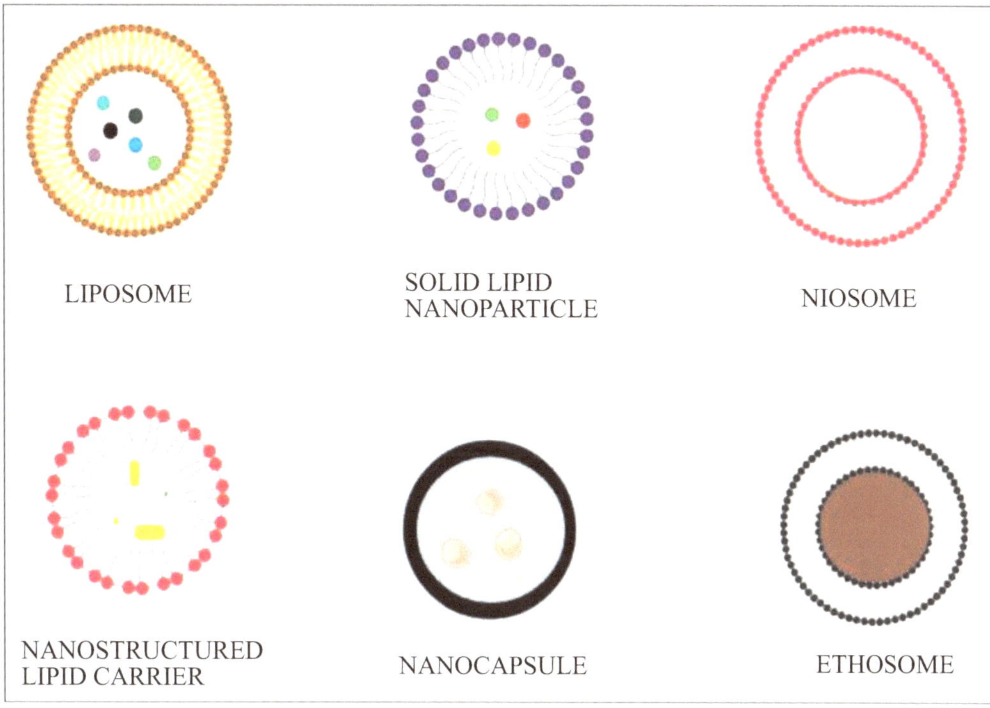

Fig. (2). Diagrammatic representation of lipid-based colloidal carriers.

Lipid-Vesicular Carriers

Liposomes:

Liposomes, tiny sacs employed for delivering drugs topically, offer customization options regarding dimensions, membrane composition, and cholesterol content. The effectiveness of drug delivery using liposomes relies on factors like size, charge, fluidity, and the type and concentration of surfactants. Surfactants play a crucial role by disrupting liposome bilayers and facilitating drug penetration into the skin [24]. PEGylated liposomes, commonly utilized for systemic and transdermal drug delivery, are particularly noteworthy. Calcipotriol, a potent psoriasis treatment, is a compound similar to vitamin D3 that inhibits the growth of skin cells called keratinocytes located within the skin's epidermal layer.

PEGylated liposomes can target calcipotriol to the deeper epidermal layer by binding it to the vitamin D receptor [25]. The hydrophilic polymer, polyethylene glycol (PEG), enhances stability but may impact the drug release profile. Moreover, PEGylated liposomes can be actively directed to specific tissues through receptor-ligand conjugation [26].

Transferosomes:

Transferosomes, extremely pliable lipid vesicles, demonstrate an exceptional ability to permeate undamaged skin, offering a needle-free method for delivering therapeutic agents. In contrast to conventional liposomes, which typically have limited transdermal effects and primarily induce localized effects, transferosomes exhibit significantly greater elasticity, enabling them to transport therapeutic effects to deeper skin layers [27]. These self-aggregating vesicles possess remarkable flexibility. When applied to non-occlusive skin, these products can struggle to penetrate the outermost layer of the skin, identified as the stratum corneum. Transferosomes, being metastable vesicles, can permeate the skin by preserving the integrity of the skin as they traverse either the intracellular lipid barrier or the openings within the stratum corneum. Their ability to reduce in size to one-tenth of their initial dimensions enables them to easily penetrate through the skin, with vesicles up to 200–300 nm in size [28]. The main components include phospholipids (such as soya phosphatidylcholine, egg phosphatidylcholine, and dipalmitoyl phosphatidylcholine), 10%–25% of incorporating a single-chain surfactant with edge-activating properties (using substances, such as sodium cholate, Tween 80, and Span-80, employing alcohol in the range of 3-10% as a solvent, and utilizing a saline phosphate buffer with a pH ranging from 6.5-7) [29].

Niosomes

The need for a cryogenic environment to handle phospholipid vesicles and the problem of lipid oxidation during storage have led to the development of non-ionic surfactants. Vesicular drug delivery systems known as Niosomes are in existence. Niosomes are small vesicles generated using non-ionic surfactants, such as alkyl or di-alkyl polyglycerol ethers, in combination with cholesterol, establishing a bilayer structure with hydrophobic tails internally and polar heads distributed on both the inside and the periphery [30]. This arrangement enables hydrophilic drugs to be entrapped in the peripheral head region while hydrophobic drugs can be trapped within the hydrophobic bilayer tail. Thus, niosomes act as an amphiphilic carrier [31]. Niosome formulation involves a diverse range of non-ionic surfactants, including polyglycerol alkyl ethers, crown ethers, ester-linked surfactants, glucosyl dialkyl ethers, polyoxyethylene alkyl ethers, and well-known brands such as Brij, Tweens, and Spans. These surfactants are gentle, non-toxic, and uncharged. While niosomes and liposomes share similar functions and physical compositions, both serving as targeted and sustained drug delivery systems, niosomes present various benefits compared to liposomes [32]. Niosomes are highly stable and attractive for industrial manufacturing due to their natural skin permeability and economic viability. Additionally, there is no requirement for specific conditions in the preparation and storage of Niosomes [33].

Novasome

Novasomes, derived from altered liposomes, akin to a form of niosomes, are produced by blending a monoester constituted of polyoxyethylene fatty acids, cholesterol, and free fatty acids in the ratio of 74/22/4. This process results in the production of particles with diameters ranging from 0.1 to 1.0 micrometers; these entities exhibit variable size measurements. These structures comprise 2 to 7 layers of shells encasing a sizable amorphous core within an unstructured compartment. This core contains a mixture of water-soluble/hydrophilic molecules along with hydrophobic materials [34]. In the context of a Novasome A cream formulation, an agent tailored for PTH (1-34) has been added, with its emphasis on targeting the Parathyroid Hormone-Related Peptide Receptors. When applied to human skin, Novasome A cream showed improved skin absorption of PTH (1-34) compared to preparations in propylene glycol or standard saline solutions. Application of PTH (1-34) demonstrated marked enhancements in the scaling, redness, and hardening of psoriatic skin lesions [35].

Ethosomes

Ethosomes serve as soft, flexible, and non-invasive carriers for drug delivery, primarily comprising components that include lipids, ethanol, and water. The unique efficacy of ethosomes can be attributed to the heightened concentration of ethanol, which leads to the disruption of the skin's lipid bilayer structure. This characteristic allows these formulations relying on ethanol vesicles to effortlessly permeate the outer layer of the skin, making them safe for use in both medicinal and beauty products [36]. Ethosomes are suitable for delivering drugs topically, as they remain concentrated in the upper stratum corneum. They have proven successful in delivering a range of drugs for skin-related issues like alopecia, dermatitis, and psoriasis through both dermal and transdermal routes [37]. In a research investigation led by Li and the team, ethosomes loaded with tacrolimus were examined and compared with classic liposomes for dermal drug delivery potential. The results indicated that tacrolimus demonstrated increased entrapment efficiency and more effective localization in the dermis when administered through ethosomes as opposed to conventional liposomes. This indicates the potential benefits of ethosomes in dermal drug delivery for conditions like psoriasis [38]. Similarly, in research led by Dubey and their collaborators, these formulations loaded with methotrexate (MTX) were created as a potential treatment for psoriasis. They noted increased sustained retention of MTX in the skin over a prolonged duration, enhancing the therapeutic effect and suggesting the utility of ethosomes in treating dermal disorders, such as psoriasis [39].

Microemulsions

Microemulsions are stable and uniform dispersion systems composed of two liquids that do not mix, stabilized by a blend of surfactant and co-surfactant molecules interacting at the interface. These particles are typically between 5 and 100 nanometers in size and can exist in various forms, such as oil-in-water (O/W) or water-in-oil (W/O). Microemulsions are recognized for their ease of production, thermodynamic stability, convenient sterilization process, and minute droplet size, collectively contributing to the uncomplicated development of drugs that exhibit improved oral bioavailability [40]. Drug liberation from microemulsions is contingent on the dynamic interaction between the drug and the surfactant, coupled with the distribution of the drug within the oil and water phases. Microemulsions have been employed for therapeutic purposes in the treatment of psoriasis and other skin disorders, with studies showing that they have the potential to enhance the delivery of drugs through the skin. They are also beneficial for formulations applied to and penetrating the skin surface, being absorbed by, and enhancing the absorption of both water-soluble and lipid-soluble drugs, unlike traditional carriers like emulsions, pure oils, and aqueous solutions [41]. Microemulsions provide numerous benefits for pharmaceutical applications, such as straightforward preparation, prolonged stability, substantial solubilization capacity for diverse drug types, and enhanced drug delivery. The research done indicates that microemulsions can improve percutaneous absorption of drugs, such as methotrexate and cyclosporine, and also improve the photostability of drugs, such as 8-methoxsalen [42].

Lipidic Particulate Carriers

Nanostructured Lipid Carrier

Nanostructured Lipid Carriers (NLCs) stand as a more sophisticated evolution of Solid Lipid Nanoparticles (SLNs), providing improved characteristics for loading drugs, controlling release patterns, and maintaining drug stability over time. The process of formulating NLCs involves combining solid lipids with lipids that lack spatial compatibility, resulting in the creation of a distinctive lipid matrix structure. This integration of both liquid and solid lipids produces a less structurally perfect crystalline arrangement with numerous imperfections, ultimately increasing the ability to incorporate drugs [43]. Solid lipids consist of triglycerides like tristearin, tripalmitin, and trimyristin, as well as fatty acids encompassing stearic acid, palmitic acid, and waxes, such as carnauba and cetyl palmitate. On the other hand, liquid lipids include materials like medium-chain triglycerides, oleic acid, and isopropyl myristate [44]. NLCs have demonstrated suitability for dermatological applications, successfully formulating drugs for the treatment of skin diseases. They emerge as favourable vehicles for the external application of drugs used to treat psoriasis, demonstrating improved penetration into the skin, minimal skin irritation, and drug compatibility [45]. Studies, exemplified by those conducted by Lin *et al.* (2010), employed Nanostructured Lipid Carriers (NLCs) to deliver calcipotriol and methotrexate simultaneously. Nam *et al.* (2007) investigated the utilization of Nanostructured Lipid Carriers (NLCs) loaded with tacrolimus for topical transdermal drug delivery. The research showed enhanced skin penetration rates in hairless mice compared to a commercially accessible dermal ointment containing tacrolimus [46]. The inclusion of fluticasone propionate into advanced NLCs incorporating polyethylene glycol (PEG) not only improved the physicochemical stability of the developed NLC but also enhanced the resistance of the compounds to photo, oxidative, and hydrolytic degradation. Additionally, these lipid nanoparticles contribute to increased skin hydration due to their occlusive properties [47].

Solid Lipid Nanoparticles

Solid Lipid Nanoparticles (SLNs) are minute structures of sizes ranging from 50 to 1000 nanometers, comprising natural lipids that solidify upon dispersion in water or surfactant solutions. These nanoparticles exhibit distinct characteristics, including an expansive surface area, which, relative to their size, enables them to carry a high drug load and release drugs gradually, leading to degradation of the lipid matrix. SLNs provide benefits like drug protection, preventing degradation, and increasing bioavailability by enhancing encapsulation efficiency and initial release through a homogenization production process [48]. The formation of SLNs involves two methods of incorporating hydrophobic drug molecules into lipids [49]. Solid lipid nanoparticles reduce drug toxicity, the need for frequent dosing, and the concentration of the drug in the bloodstream, leading to fluctuations by contributing to sustained drug release. The drug release characteristics are influenced by the deposition pattern and melting points of the lipids used [50]. Lipids that exhibit a solid state at body temperature exhibit a gradual degradation pace, rendering them valuable in the development of extended-release formulations. Two primary approaches for crafting Solid Lipid Nanoparticles (SLN) include the drug-enriched shell model, marked by an initial rapid release of the drug, followed by a slower, more gradual release, and the model where the drug is dissolved within the matrix core. The latter model leads to prolonged and sustained drug release, facilitated by an increased distance for drug diffusion from the lipid matrix core [51]. Solid Lipid Nanoparticles (SLNs) have been effectively employed in diverse cosmetic and dermatological uses. As an illustration, Shah and their collaborators employed a straightforward Emulsification-Solvent Diffusion (ESD) method to create SLNs of tretinoin, enhancing its resistance to photodegradation. The tretinoin-encapsulated SLNs exhibited substantial improvements, enhancing resistance to light-induced degradation and reducing irritation effects compared to a solution containing methanol of tretinoin [52]. In another example, Jensen and his coworkers utilized the hot high-pressure homogenization technique to develop SLNs of betamethasone 17-valerate. The SLNs loaded with the drug demonstrated significantly enhanced penetration of the drug held in both compromised and intact skin barriers, suggesting their ability to serve as a drug reservoir in the epidermis [53].

Polymeric Colloidal Carriers

Polymeric colloidal carriers are pivotal in drug delivery technology, allowing for personalized and regulated release of therapeutic agents to achieve the intended effects [54]. Made from natural or synthetic polymers, these carriers envelop drugs in micro- or nanoscale systems. This section will explore various types of polymeric colloidal carriers employed for psoriasis treatment [55].

Self-Assembled Carriers

Complex structures known as self-assembled carriers are created through the natural organization of molecular components *via* non-covalent interactions. Specific amphiphilic molecules can organize themselves at interfaces when certain solvents are present. This enables them to segregate their hydrophobic portions and prevent interaction with polar solvents [56]. Self-assembled carriers have surfaced as promising instruments in diverse therapeutic and diagnostic applications. In particular, their potential in delivering antipsoriatic drugs is explored below:

Polymeric micelles

Micelles are small, Self-assembling particles in colloidal form with sizes ranging from 5 to 100 nanometers. They possess a core that repels water and an outer shell that interacts with water and are commonly used to carry drugs that are not soluble in water. The hydrophobic centre of a micelle offers a safeguarded environment for the drug, while the hydrophilic outer layer creates a strong shield that hinders recognition and binding by opsonins, thus increasing the drug's circulation life [57]. Micellar nanocarriers offer several benefits, such as the desired attributes of medication, in terms of "high drug loading, diminished drug degradation, minimized side effects, and enhanced bioavailability." These characteristics signify a medication with a substantial concentration of active ingredients, minimal degradation, resulting in fewer adverse effects, and increased absorption by the body. There are two ways to load a drug into a micelle: by physically trapping the drug or by covalently attaching the drug to a polymer. These nanocarriers provide a compartment that can contain drugs, and their nanoscale size enables them to be taken up by cells through endocytosis, which is particularly useful in the treatment of cancer, neurodegenerative disorders, fungal infections, gene therapy, ocular drug delivery, and psoriasis [58].

Dendrimers

Dendrimers are a type of highly branched macromolecule that consists of a central unit surrounded by numerous branching surface groups. The core can hold drugs, and its size facilitates internalization [59]. Dendrimers are a class of molecules employed for drug transport. They possess numerous sites where drugs can be linked, either in the molecule's core or at its extremities. The attachment of drugs can occur through chemical bonds or electrostatic charges. The release of the drug can take place in two ways: either the bond between the drug and dendrimer is broken down by enzymes within the body, or the drug is discharged as a result of physical environmental conditions, such as pH and temperature [60].

Hydrogel

Hydrogels are networks of hydrophobic polymers that contain polymer chains that, when cross-linked either chemically or physically, can absorb substantial quantities of water without dissolving in water-based solutions [61]. Hydrogels can be categorized into three types according to the size of their pores: large-pored macroporous, small-pored microporous, and nonporous. Macroporous hydrogels are characterized by pores measuring between 0.1 and 1 μm, while microporous hydrogels feature smaller pores ranging from 100 to 1000 Å. Nonporous hydrogels are composed of larger macromolecules with dimensions spanning from 10 to 100 Å. Polymers are either obtained from natural or synthetic origins and are used for the manufacturing of hydrogels [62]. Polymers that are obtained from natural origins are used in the manufacturing of hydrogels and exhibit features such as biocompatibility, biodegradability, and biological friendliness, thereby supporting cellular activities.

On the other hand, Synthetic hydrogels showcase precisely engineered structures that can be adjusted to achieve desired degradability, functionality, and predictable release characteristics. How drugs are released from hydrogels is impacted by the approach to drug loading and the physical and chemical properties of the hydrogel structure. Pathways like diffusion, swelling followed by diffusion, or polymer degradation, are responsible for the release of drugs from hydrogels [63]. Drug incorporation into hydrogels can be achieved through two methods: loading after an initial stage/post-loading and loading at the original location, or *in situ* loading. Post-loading entails adding drugs after hydrogel formation, leading to release through diffusion or gel swelling. Conversely, in *in-situ* loading, drugs are introduced during the various phases of hydrogel manufacturing [64]. Within *in-situ* loaded systems, the liberation of drugs or other substances is influenced by various factors, encompassing diffusion, hydrogel expansion, polymer degradation, association between the polymer and the drug, and breakdown of the covalent bonds. Hydrogels are widely utilized in various medical fields, including tissue engineering, diagnostics, cell separation, and immobilization [65].

Polymeric Particulate Carriers

The following text discusses polymer matrix systems that disperse or dissolve drugs. The release of a drug can be managed through diffusion, swelling, or erosion [66]. Here are some examples of particulate carriers employed for delivering drugs in the treatment of psoriasis.

Microsphere

Microspheres, also known as microparticles, are structures characterized by a spherical polymer matrix, typically exhibiting sizes ranging from 1 to 1000 microns. These tiny particles provide a steady and sustained release of medication, resulting in improved therapeutic effects. By reducing the frequency of dosing, patient compliance is increased [67]. Microspheres can be created through diverse methods, offering applications like precision in targeting, specificity, and regulated drug release. Microspheres facilitate drug release through mechanisms triggered by osmotic pressure, diffusion through pores, or degradation of the polymer, all of which are involved in the release. Key elements affecting this release encompass the attributes of the polymer, drug amount, ratio of drug to polymer, size of the particles, and the various methods involved in preparation [68]. The drug is either integrated or dispersed within the polymer matrix during the production process of nanospheres. The polymers used for manufacturing can be categorized as biodegradable or non-biodegradable [69].

Polymeric Nanospheres

Nanoparticles are tiny particles that have a size between 10 and 1000 nanometers. Polymeric nanoparticles come in two forms: nanospheres and nanocapsules, where the drug is encapsulated within or evenly spread within the polymer matrix [70]. Polymers are categorized into two groups: non-biodegradable and biodegradable. Biodegradable polymeric nanoparticles are frequently employed for the precise and regulated delivery of medications or other bioactive substances like proteins, peptides, and genetic material. The release of drugs from nanospheres is influenced by the specific characteristics of the system, which is responsible for the drug delivery [71]. Nanospheres refer to organized matrices in which the drug is distributed uniformly within the polymer matrix. The release mechanism of the drug can be ascribed to diffusion, matrix erosion, or a combination of both, depending on the polymer or the method utilized in the manufacturing process [72]. The initial rapid release from nanospheres occurs because of drugs adhering to the surface; later on, a sustained and consistent release is allowed through the drug's diffusion within the matrix or erosion, adhering to first-order kinetics.

Capsular Carriers

Drug carriers are commonly designed in a core-shell arrangement. In this arrangement, the drug is encased within an enclosed space or storage area shielded by a membrane formed by the bonds between the polymers or a coating. The active components may exist in either a liquid or solid state, or they may be dispersed at the molecular level within the enclosed space [73]. Capsules are often utilized as carriers for medications, providing the benefit of concealing unpalatable tastes and ensuring controlled release characteristics.

Nanocapsules

Nanocapsules are a specific category of nanoparticles that include enclosing one or multiple active substances (core) inside a protective matrix(shell), creating a containment for the therapeutic substance [74]. The attention garnered by these tiny capsules is due to their protective layer, which is frequently pyrophoric and susceptible to oxidation. These capsules find application in controlled release and precise drug targeting. The choice of surfactant and the characteristics of the external coating are pivotal factors influencing dispersion stability and the initial physiological response [75]. Nanocapsules offer numerous advantages, including the gradual release of drugs, enhanced precision and efficacy of drugs, heightened drug availability in the body, and decreased drug-related toxicity. The attributes of nanocapsules and the results concerning encapsulated substances, including their release and degradation, are largely contingent upon the choice of polymer, and the specific drugs in question influence the outcome and the preparation technique [76]. The order of release patterns is as follows, based on the preparation methods: the sequence involves utilizing emulsion-diffusion and emulsification coacervation methods, followed by nanoprecipitation, polymer coating, layer-by-layer application, and concluding with double emulsification [77]. Nanocapsules demonstrate a release pattern with two phases, characterized by an initial rapid release of the drug, followed by a gradual and prolonged release. The quick burst is influenced by either drugs absorbed on the surface or the degradation of the thin polymeric membrane [78]. The drug molecules diffuse from the inner compartment to the outer compartment [79]. The control of the second phase is influenced by factors like how the release occurs, which is influenced by elements like the drug's partition coefficient, considering the relationship between the oily core and the surrounding aqueous medium, the distribution of the phases, the interplay between the drug and the polymer, and the concentration of surfactant. In cases where a notable amount of polymer is involved, multiple researchers have identified polymer erosion as the primary mechanism governing the release [80].

CONCLUSION

Psoriasis remains a significant dermatological challenge due to its complex pathophysiology and the limitations of conventional treatment options. While traditional therapies provide symptomatic relief, they often result in adverse effects and inadequate drug penetration, necessitating the development of advanced drug delivery systems. Polymeric Nanoparticles (PNPs) have emerged as a promising strategy for improving psoriasis management by offering enhanced bioavailability, controlled drug release, and targeted delivery, thereby reducing systemic toxicity and improving therapeutic outcomes. Various lipid-based and polymeric nanocarriers have demonstrated potential in overcoming the limitations of conventional formulations, ensuring better skin penetration and prolonged drug action. Despite these advancements, challenges such as formulation stability, large-scale production, and regulatory approvals remain. Future research should focus on optimizing nanocarrier formulations, evaluating their long-term safety, and exploring novel polymeric materials to enhance treatment efficacy and effectiveness. Also, the integration of nanotechnology in psoriasis therapy holds great promise for revolutionizing treatment approaches and improving patient care.

REFERENCES

[1] Dubey S, Sharma R, Mody N, Vyas SP. Novel carriers and approaches: insight for psoriasis management. InNanostructures for novel therapy 2017 Jan 1, pp. 657-684. Elsevier. [http://dx.doi.org/10.1016/B978-0-323-46142-9.00024-4]

[2] Pradhan M, Singh D, Singh MR. Novel colloidal carriers for psoriasis: Current issues, mechanistic insight and novel delivery approaches. J Control Release 2013; 170(3): 380-95. [http://dx.doi.org/10.1016/j.jconrel.2013.05.020] [PMID: 23770117]

[3] Galimova ES, Akhmetova VL, Khusnutdinova EK. Molecular genetic basis of susceptibility to

psoriasis. Russ J Genet 2008; 44(5): 513-22.
[http://dx.doi.org/10.1134/S1022795408050025]

[4] Swanbeck G, Inerot A, Martinsson T, *et al.* Age at onset and different types of psoriasis. Br J Dermatol 1995; 133(5): 768-73.
[http://dx.doi.org/10.1111/j.1365-2133.1995.tb02753.x] [PMID: 8555031]

[5] Greaves MW, Weinstein GD. Treatment of psoriasis. N Engl J Med 1995; 332(9): 581-9.
[http://dx.doi.org/10.1056/NEJM199503023320907] [PMID: 7838193]

[6] Peters BP, Weissman FG, Gill MA. Pathophysiology and treatment of psoriasis. Am J Health Syst Pharm 2000; 57(7): 645-59.
[http://dx.doi.org/10.1093/ajhp/57.7.645] [PMID: 10768819]

[7] Nickoloff BJ, Nestle FO. Recent insights into the immunopathogenesis of psoriasis provide new therapeutic opportunities. J Clin Invest 2004; 113(12): 1664-75.
[http://dx.doi.org/10.1172/JCI200422147] [PMID: 15199399]

[8] Fang JY, Fang CL, Liu CH, Su YH. Lipid nanoparticles as vehicles for topical psoralen delivery: Solid lipid nanoparticles (SLN) versus nanostructured lipid carriers (NLC). Eur J Pharm Biopharm 2008; 70(2): 633-40.
[http://dx.doi.org/10.1016/j.ejpb.2008.05.008] [PMID: 18577447]

[9] Naldi L. Epidemiology of psoriasis. Curr Drug Targets Inflamm Allergy 2004; 3(2): 121-8.
[http://dx.doi.org/10.2174/1568010043343958] [PMID: 15180464]

[10] Oji V, Luger TA. The skin in psoriasis: assessment and challenges. Clin Exp Rheumatol 2015; 33(5) (Suppl. 93): S14-9.
[PMID: 26472560]

[11] Katare O, Raza K, Singh B, Dogra S. Novel drug delivery systems in topical treatment of psoriasis: Rigors and vigors. Indian J Dermatol Venereol Leprol 2010; 76(6): 612-21.
[http://dx.doi.org/10.4103/0378-6323.72451] [PMID: 21079304]

[12] Morganti P, Ruocco E, Wolf R, Ruocco V. Percutaneous absorption and delivery systems33The opinions expressed herein are solely those of the writers and do not necessarily reflect the opinions of the institutions with which the writers are associated. Clin Dermatol 2001; 19(4): 489-501.
[http://dx.doi.org/10.1016/S0738-081X(01)00183-3] [PMID: 11535394]

[13] Schön MP. Animal models of psoriasis: a critical appraisal. Exp Dermatol 2008; 17(8): 703-12.
[http://dx.doi.org/10.1111/j.1600-0625.2008.00751.x] [PMID: 18557923]

[14] Mizutani H, Yamanaka K, Konishi H, Murakami T. Animal models of psoriasis and pustular psoriasis. Arch Dermatol Res 2003; 295(S1) (Suppl. 1): S67-8.
[http://dx.doi.org/10.1007/s00403-002-0374-3] [PMID: 12677436]

[15] Fraki JE, Briggaman RA, Lazarus GS. Transplantation of psoriatic skin onto nude mice. Journal of Investigative Dermatology. 1983 Jun 1; 80(s 6): 31-5.

[16] Zollner T, Renz H, Asadullah K. Animal models of T cell-mediated skin diseases. Springer 2005.
[http://dx.doi.org/10.1007/b138119]

[17] Mehnert W, Mäder K. Solid lipid nanoparticles. Adv Drug Deliv Rev 2012; 64: 83-101.
[http://dx.doi.org/10.1016/j.addr.2012.09.021] [PMID: 11311991]

[18] Rawat Singh M, Pradhan K, Singh D. Lipid matrix systems with emphasis on lipid microspheres: potent carriers for transcutaneous delivery of bioactives. Curr Drug Deliv 2012; 9(3): 243-54.
[http://dx.doi.org/10.2174/156720112800389124] [PMID: 22283658]

[19] Rahman M, Akhter S, Ahmad J, Ahmad MZ, Beg S, Ahmad FJ. Nanomedicine-based drug targeting for psoriasis: potentials and emerging trends in nanoscale pharmacotherapy. Expert Opin Drug Deliv 2015; 12(4): 635-52.
[http://dx.doi.org/10.1517/17425247.2015.982088] [PMID: 25439967]

[20] Danaei M, Dehghankhold M, Ataei S, Hasanzadeh Davarani F, Javanmard R, Dokhani A, *et al.* Impact of particle size and polydispersity index on the clinical applications of lipidic nanocarrier systems. Pharmaceutics.
[http://dx.doi.org/10.3390/pharmaceutics10020057] [PMID: 29772679]

[21] Patel JM. Paclitaxel Loaded Proliposome: A Novel Approach for Cancer Therapy (Doctoral dissertation, KLE University, Belagavi, Karnataka).

[22] Rawat M, Singh D, Saraf S, Saraf S. Nanocarriers: promising vehicle for bioactive drugs. Biol Pharm Bull 2006; 29(9): 1790-8.
[http://dx.doi.org/10.1248/bpb.29.1790] [PMID: 16946487]

[23] Cortesi R, Esposjto E, Luca G, Nastruzzi C. Production of lipospheres as carriers for bioactive compounds. Biomaterials 2002; 23(11): 2283-94.
[http://dx.doi.org/10.1016/S0142-9612(01)00362-3] [PMID: 12013175]

[24] Knudsen NØ, Rønholt S, Salte RD, *et al.* Calcipotriol delivery into the skin with PEGylated liposomes. Eur J Pharm Biopharm 2012; 81(3): 532-9.
[http://dx.doi.org/10.1016/j.ejpb.2012.04.005] [PMID: 22538098]

[25] Srisuk P, Thongnopnua P, Raktanonchai U, Kanokpanont S. Physico-chemical characteristics of methotrexate-entrapped oleic acid-containing deformable liposomes for in vitro transepidermal delivery targeting psoriasis treatment. Int J Pharm 2012; 427(2): 426-34.
[http://dx.doi.org/10.1016/j.ijpharm.2012.01.045] [PMID: 22310459]

[26] Yang F, Kamiya N, Goto M. Transdermal delivery of the anti-rheumatic agent methotrexate using a solid-in-oil nanocarrier. Eur J Pharm Biopharm 2012; 82(1): 158-63.
[http://dx.doi.org/10.1016/j.ejpb.2012.05.016] [PMID: 22713517]

[27] Cevc G, Blume G. Lipid vesicles penetrate into intact skin owing to the transdermal osmotic gradients and hydration force. Biochim Biophys Acta Biomembr 1992; 1104(1): 226-32.
[http://dx.doi.org/10.1016/0005-2736(92)90154-E] [PMID: 1550849]

[28] Trotta M, Peira E, Carlotti ME, Gallarate M. Deformable liposomes for dermal administration of methotrexate. Int J Pharm 2004; 270(1-2): 119-25.
[http://dx.doi.org/10.1016/j.ijpharm.2003.10.006] [PMID: 14726128]

[29] Vinod KR, Kumar MS, Anbazhagan S, *et al.* Critical issues related to transfersomes - novel vesicular system. Acta Sci Pol Technol Aliment 2012; 11(1): 67-82.
[PMID: 22230977]

[30] Madhav NV, Saini A. Niosomes: a novel drug delivery system. Int J Res Pharm Chem 2011; 1(3): 498-511.

[31] Agarwal R, Katare OP, Vyas SP. Preparation and *in vitro* evaluation of liposomal/niosomal delivery systems for antipsoriatic drug dithranol. Int J Pharm 2001; 228(1-2): 43-52.
[http://dx.doi.org/10.1016/S0378-5173(01)00810-9] [PMID: 11576767]

[32] Sankhyan A, Pawar P. Recent trends in niosome as vesicular drug delivery system. Journal of applied pharmaceutical science. 2012 Jun 30(Issue): 20-32.

[33] Lakshmi PK, Devi G, Bhaskaran S, Sacchidanand S. Niosomal methotrexate gel in the treatment of localized psoriasis: Phase I and phase II studies. Indian J Dermatol Venereol Leprol 2007; 73(3): 157-61.
[http://dx.doi.org/10.4103/0378-6323.32709] [PMID: 17558046]

[34] Abd-Elal RMA, Shamma RN, Rashed HM, Bendas ER. Trans-nasal zolmitriptan novasomes: *in-vitro* preparation, optimization and *in-vivo* evaluation of brain targeting efficiency. Drug Deliv 2016; 23(9): 3374-86.
[http://dx.doi.org/10.1080/10717544.2016.1183721] [PMID: 27128792]

[35] Agarwal SW, Kumari PV. Advances in Novasome technology-a review. Int J App Pharm 2013; 5(1):

1-4.

[36] Dubey V, Mishra D, Dutta T, Nahar M, Saraf DK, Jain NK. Dermal and transdermal delivery of an anti-psoriatic agent *via* ethanolic liposomes. J Control Release 2007; 123(2): 148-54. [http://dx.doi.org/10.1016/j.jconrel.2007.08.005] [PMID: 17884226]

[37] Manconi M, Sinico C, Caddeo C, Vila AO, Valenti D, Fadda AM. Penetration enhancer containing vesicles as carriers for dermal delivery of tretinoin. Int J Pharm 2011; 412(1-2): 37-46. [http://dx.doi.org/10.1016/j.ijpharm.2011.03.068] [PMID: 21530626]

[38] Ma H, Guo D, Fan Y, Wang J, Cheng J, Zhang X. Paeonol-loaded ethosomes as transdermal delivery carriers: design, preparation and evaluation. Molecules 2018; 23(7): 1756. [http://dx.doi.org/10.3390/molecules23071756] [PMID: 30018278]

[39] Guo F, Wang J, Ma M, Tan F, Li N. Skin targeted lipid vesicles as novel nano-carrier of ketoconazole: characterization, *in vitro* and *in vivo* evaluation. J Mater Sci Mater Med 2015; 26(4): 175. [http://dx.doi.org/10.1007/s10856-015-5487-2] [PMID: 25825320]

[40] Zhi XH, Jin L, Yang CG. Preparation and quality evaluation of methotrexate microemulsion. China Pharm 2011; 5: 433-6.

[41] Shaji J, Reddy MS. Microemulsions as drug delivery systems. Pharma times. 2004; 36(7): 17-24.

[42] Alvarez-Figueroa MJ, Blanco-Méndez J. Transdermal delivery of methotrexate: iontophoretic delivery from hydrogels and passive delivery from microemulsions. Int J Pharm 2001; 215(1-2): 57-65. [http://dx.doi.org/10.1016/S0378-5173(00)00674-8] [PMID: 11250092]

[43] How CW, Abdullah R, Abbasalipourkabir R. Physicochemical properties of nanostructured lipid carriers as colloidal carrier system stabilized with polysorbate 20 and polysorbate 80. Afr J Biotechnol 2011; 10(9): 1684-9.

[44] Xia Q, Saupe A, Müller RH, Souto EB. Nanostructured lipid carriers as novel carrier for sunscreen formulations. Int J Cosmet Sci 2007; 29(6): 473-82. [http://dx.doi.org/10.1111/j.1468-2494.2007.00410.x] [PMID: 18489386]

[45] Zhang X, Liu J, Qiao H, *et al.* Formulation optimization of dihydroartemisinin nanostructured lipid carrier using response surface methodology. Powder Technol 2010; 197(1-2): 120-8. [http://dx.doi.org/10.1016/j.powtec.2009.09.004]

[46] Pople PV, Singh KK. Development and evaluation of colloidal modified nanolipid carrier: Application to topical delivery of tacrolimus. Eur J Pharm Biopharm 2011; 79(1): 82-94. [http://dx.doi.org/10.1016/j.ejpb.2011.02.016] [PMID: 21447390]

[47] Pople PV, Singh KK. Development and evaluation of colloidal modified nanolipid carrier: Application to topical delivery of tacrolimus, Part II – *In vivo* assessment, drug targeting, efficacy, and safety in treatment for atopic dermatitis. Eur J Pharm Biopharm 2013; 84(1): 72-83. [http://dx.doi.org/10.1016/j.ejpb.2012.11.026] [PMID: 23246619]

[48] Sathali AH, Ekambaram P, Priyanka K. Solid lipid nanoparticles: a review. Sci Rev Chem Commun 2012; 2(1): 80-102.

[49] Rawat M, Singh D, Saraf S, Saraf S. Lipid carriers: a versatile delivery vehicle for proteins and peptides. Yakugaku Zasshi 2008; 128(2): 269-80. [http://dx.doi.org/10.1248/yakushi.128.269] [PMID: 18239375]

[50] Martins S, Sarmento B, Ferreira DC, Souto EB. Lipid-based colloidal carriers for peptide and protein delivery--liposomes versus lipid nanoparticles. Int J Nanomedicine 2007; 2(4): 595-607. [PMID: 18203427]

[51] Shah K, Date A, Joshi M, Patravale V. Solid Lipid Nanoparticles (SLN) of tretinoin: Potential in topical delivery. Int J Pharm 2007; 345(1-2): 163-71. [http://dx.doi.org/10.1016/j.ijpharm.2007.05.061] [PMID: 17644288]

[52] Agrawal Y, Petkar KC, Sawant KK. Development, evaluation and clinical studies of Acitretin loaded

nanostructured lipid carriers for topical treatment of psoriasis. Int J Pharm 2010; 401(1-2): 93-102. [http://dx.doi.org/10.1016/j.ijpharm.2010.09.007] [PMID: 20858539]

[53] Jensen LB, Magnussson E, Gunnarsson L, Vermehren C, Nielsen HM, Petersson K. Corticosteroid solubility and lipid polarity control release from solid lipid nanoparticles. Int J Pharm 2010; 390(1): 53-60. [http://dx.doi.org/10.1016/j.ijpharm.2009.10.022] [PMID: 19836439]

[54] Lapteva M, Mondon K, Möller M, Gurny R, Kalia YN. Polymeric micelle nanocarriers for the cutaneous delivery of tacrolimus: a targeted approach for the treatment of psoriasis. Mol Pharm 2014; 11(9): 2989-3001. [http://dx.doi.org/10.1021/mp400639e] [PMID: 25057896]

[55] Yadav K, Soni A, Singh D, Singh MR. Polymers in topical delivery of anti-psoriatic medications and other topical agents in overcoming the barriers of conventional treatment strategies. Prog Biomater 2021; 10(1): 1-17. [http://dx.doi.org/10.1007/s40204-021-00154-7] [PMID: 33738750]

[56] Pinto MF, Moura CC, Nunes C, Segundo MA, Costa Lima SA, Reis S. A new topical formulation for psoriasis: Development of methotrexate-loaded nanostructured lipid carriers. Int J Pharm 2014; 477(1-2): 519-26. [http://dx.doi.org/10.1016/j.ijpharm.2014.10.067] [PMID: 25445970]

[57] Torchilin VP. Structure and design of polymeric surfactant-based drug delivery systems. J Control Release 2001; 73(2-3): 137-72. [http://dx.doi.org/10.1016/S0168-3659(01)00299-1] [PMID: 11516494]

[58] Deepak P, Nagaich U, Sharma A, Gulati N, Chaudhary A. Polymeric micelles: potential drug delivery devices. Indones J Pharm 2013; Oct 1: 222-37.

[59] Biswasroy P, Pradhan D, Kar B, Ghosh G, Rath G. Recent advancement in topical nanocarriers for the treatment of psoriasis. AAPS PharmSciTech 2021; 22(5): 164. [http://dx.doi.org/10.1208/s12249-021-02057-z] [PMID: 34041632]

[60] Svenson S, Tomalia DA. Dendrimers in biomedical applications—reflections on the field. Adv Drug Deliv Rev 2012; 64: 102-15. [http://dx.doi.org/10.1016/j.addr.2012.09.030] [PMID: 16305813]

[61] Singh D, Singh MR. Development of antibiotic and debriding enzyme-loaded PLGA microspheres entrapped in PVA-gelatin hydrogel for complete wound management. Artif Cells Blood Substit Immobil Biotechnol 2012; 40(5): 345-53. [http://dx.doi.org/10.3109/10731199.2012.675337] [PMID: 22540900]

[62] Amin S, Rajabnezhad S, Kohli K. Hydrogels as potential drug delivery systems. Sci Res Essays 2009; 4(11): 1175-83.

[63] Peppas N, Bures P, Leobandung W, Ichikawa H. Hydrogels in pharmaceutical formulations. Eur J Pharm Biopharm 2000; 50(1): 27-46. [http://dx.doi.org/10.1016/S0939-6411(00)00090-4] [PMID: 10840191]

[64] Limón D, Talló Domínguez K, Garduño-Ramírez ML, Andrade B, Calpena AC, Pérez-García L. Nanostructured supramolecular hydrogels: Towards the topical treatment of Psoriasis and other skin diseases. Colloids Surf B Biointerfaces 2019; 181: 657-70. [http://dx.doi.org/10.1016/j.colsurfb.2019.06.018] [PMID: 31212138]

[65] Kumar S, Prasad M, Rao R. Topical delivery of clobetasol propionate loaded nanosponge hydrogel for effective treatment of psoriasis: Formulation, physicochemical characterization, antipsoriatic potential and biochemical estimation. Mater Sci Eng C 2021; 119: 111605. [http://dx.doi.org/10.1016/j.msec.2020.111605] [PMID: 33321649]

[66] Singh D, Rawat Singh M, Saraf S, Dixit VK, Saraf S. Formulation optimization of metronidazole loaded chitosan microspheres for wound management by 3-factor, 3-level Box–Behnken design.

Micro Nanosyst 2010; 2(2): 70-7.
[http://dx.doi.org/10.2174/1876402911002020070]

[67] Berkland C, Kipper MJ, Narasimhan B, Kim KK, Pack DW. Microsphere size, precipitation kinetics and drug distribution control drug release from biodegradable polyanhydride microspheres. J Control Release 2004; 94(1): 129-41.
[http://dx.doi.org/10.1016/j.jconrel.2003.09.011] [PMID: 14684277]

[68] Sokolova V, Epple M. Inorganic nanoparticles as carriers of nucleic acids into cells. Angew Chem Int Ed Engl. 2008;47(8):1382-95.
[http://dx.doi.org/10.1002/anie.200703039] [PMID: 18175315]

[69] Dinarvand R, Rahmani E, Farbod E. Gelatin microspheres for the controlled release of all-tran--retinoic acid topical formulation and drug delivery evaluation.

[70] Zhang Z, Tsai PC, Ramezanli T, Michniak-Kohn BB. Polymeric nanoparticles-based topical delivery systems for the treatment of dermatological diseases. Wiley Interdiscip Rev Nanomed Nanobiotechnol 2013; 5(3): 205-18.
[http://dx.doi.org/10.1002/wnan.1211] [PMID: 23386536]

[71] Madawi EA, Al Jayoush AR, Rawas-Qalaji M, *et al.* Polymeric nanoparticles as tunable nanocarriers for targeted delivery of drugs to skin tissues for treatment of topical skin diseases. Pharmaceutics 2023; 15(2): 657.
[http://dx.doi.org/10.3390/pharmaceutics15020657] [PMID: 36839979]

[72] Soppimath KS, Aminabhavi TM, Kulkarni AR, Rudzinski WE. Biodegradable polymeric nanoparticles as drug delivery devices. J Control Release 2001; 70(1-2): 1-20.
[http://dx.doi.org/10.1016/S0168-3659(00)00339-4] [PMID: 11166403]

[73] Sahoo SK, Parveen S, Panda JJ. The present and future of nanotechnology in human health care. Nanomedicine. 2007;3(1):20-31.
[http://dx.doi.org/10.1016/j.nano.2006.11.008] [PMID: 17379110]

[74] Letchford K, Burt H. A review of the formation and classification of amphiphilic block copolymer nanoparticulate structures: micelles, nanospheres, nanocapsules and polymersomes. Eur J Pharm Biopharm 2007; 65(3): 259-69.
[http://dx.doi.org/10.1016/j.ejpb.2006.11.009] [PMID: 17196803]

[75] Gungor S, Rezigue M. Nanocarriers mediated topical drug delivery for psoriasis treatment. Curr Drug Metab 2017; 18(5): 454-68.
[http://dx.doi.org/10.2174/1389200218666170222145240] [PMID: 28228078]

[76] Vincent N, D RD, Bn VH. Progress in psoriasis therapy *via* novel drug delivery systems. Dermatol Rep 2014; 6(1): 5451.
[http://dx.doi.org/10.4081/dr.2014.5451] [PMID: 25386329]

[77] Mora-Huertas CE, Fessi H, Elaissari A. Polymer-based nanocapsules for drug delivery. Int J Pharm 2010; 385(1-2): 113-42.
[http://dx.doi.org/10.1016/j.ijpharm.2009.10.018] [PMID: 19825408]

[78] Ourique AF, Pohlmann AR, Guterres SS, Beck RCR. Tretinoin-loaded nanocapsules: Preparation, physicochemical characterization, and photostability study. Int J Pharm 2008; 352(1-2): 1-4.
[http://dx.doi.org/10.1016/j.ijpharm.2007.12.035] [PMID: 18249513]

[79] Erdoğar N, Akkın S, Bilensoy E. Nanocapsules for drug delivery: an updated review of the last decade. Recent Pat Drug Deliv Formul 2019; 12(4): 252-66.
[http://dx.doi.org/10.2174/1872211313666190123153711] [PMID: 30674269]

[80] Gomes GS, Frank LA, Contri RV, Longhi MS, Pohlmann AR, Guterres SS. Nanotechnology-based alternatives for the topical delivery of immunosuppressive agents in psoriasis. Int J Pharm 2023; 631: 122535.
[http://dx.doi.org/10.1016/j.ijpharm.2022.122535] [PMID: 36566826]

CHAPTER 10

Nanosponges as Drug Carriers for the Management of Psoriasis

Rashmi Ghosh[1], Manish Kumar[1,*], Ankit Awasthi[1], Shubham Thakur[1] and **Prabha Singh[2]**

[1] *Department of Pharmaceutics, ISF College of Pharmacy, Moga 142001, Punjab, India*

[2] *Department of Pharmaceutics, Sanjay College of Pharmacy, Mathura-Delhi Road, Mathura 281406, Uttar Pradesh, India*

Abstract: Psoriasis is a chronic skin condition characterized by the hyperproliferation of keratinocytes in the epidermis, resulting in a high turnover rate of the epidermal cells. Apart from its physical manifestations, it also impacts an individual's psychological well-being. Its symptoms, such as pain, itching, and peeling, are more severe than those of other diseases, leading to a higher prevalence of depression and anxiety. Nanosponges are versatile nanoparticle platforms with porous, three-dimensional structures that can effectively encapsulate and deliver a wide range of drugs and bioactive molecules, owing to their distinct capabilities, including controlled release patterns and the ability to target delivery. In this review, the advantages of nanosponges as a drug delivery system for treating the disease will be discussed.

Keywords: Bioactive molecules, Epidermis, Nanosponges, Psoriasis, Targeted delivery.

INTRODUCTION

Delivery systems are continually improving day by day, enabling the controlled release of the drug at the proper place and precise intensity, providing a great mastermind that deserves all honor, simply trying to get the bull's eye goal while both hands and one leg are tied. [1] Nanofabrication, a new and complex development, can be considered akin to the invention of fire during the Stone Age [2].

Nanofabricationinvolve playing around with materials so tiny that you would need a microscope just to see them properly— materials whose properties can be enhanced by manipulating them at the nanoscale. Nanotechnology deals with

* **Corresponding author Manish Kumar:** Department of Pharmaceutics, ISF College of Pharmacy, Moga 142001, Punjab, India; E-mail: manish_singh17@rediffmail.com

Anjali Sharma, Prerna Sharma, Roy Rillera Marzo & Ahmed A. Al Karmalawy (Eds.)

dimensions at the level of nanometers, which is about as small as you can get without talking about individual atoms. Nanomaterials are real physical substances whose sizes fall within 1-100 nm; nanoparticles make up a special class owing to their size-specific features localized around interfaces — think oasis in a desert [3]. Various forms make up these nanoparticles, such as polymeric pearls, phospholipid pebbles, carbon clusters, spongy spheres (to store treasure troves of drugs), micellar marbles, dendrimer diamonds, *etc.* The impact of nanotechnology is profound, as it allows precise control at both spatial and temporal scales. Through a nanofabrication approach, certain designs of individual components can be manufactured and arranged in a way that the desired final substrate is obtained. This nano-synthesis and nanoassembly of engineered substrates make it possible to tailor chemical and physical features both on specific and macroscopic levels. A variety of substances, including antineoplastic agents, proteins, peptides, essential oils, DNA, and others, are organized into colloidal structures, commonly referred to as self-assembled nanostructures (NSs) [1].

Nanosponges are designated for medication delivery because of their distinctive features. Nanoscale drug carriers can do many beneficial things, like targeted medication delivery, controlled release patterns, and storing drugs of various classes in different sizes [1]. They can hold immiscible liquids, offer sustained release for up to 24 hours, reduce pain, improve flexibility, and stabilize the drugs. They can incorporate holes that are designed to serve the medications that are insoluble in water, in which case the nanosponges enhance the solubility and bioavailability of the drugs [2]. Furthermore, nanosponges are useful and flexible in pharmaceutical applications since they are low in toxicity, biodegradable, and may be designed for several delivery routes such as topical, oral, parenteral, and inhalational [2].

They can transport both hydrophilic and hydrophobic pharmaceuticals, which makes them ideal for drug delivery systems that ensure safe and controlled release of drugs over time [4].

Nanosponges represent a type of nanostructured material obtained by crosslinking polymers to build up a three-dimensional porous entity[2]. These nanosponges are able to encapsulate different types of hydrophilic and hydrophobic drug molecules and offer many benefits in comparison with other drug delivery systems (as shown in Fig. (**1**) below) [4].

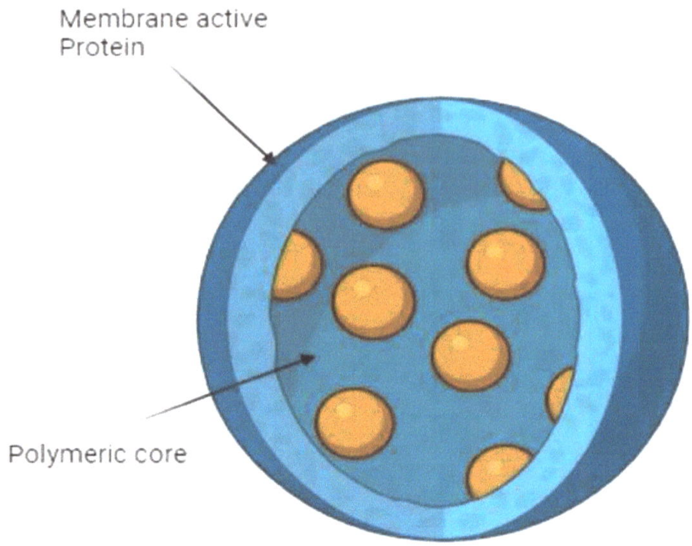

Fig. (1). Nanosponges.

The capacity of nanosponges to encompass the drugs, enhancing their solubility and bioavailability *via* the drug entrapment in their porous nature, results in an additional incredible application. The precise properties of nanosponges, like size, porosity, and surface functionality, can be finely regulated by using different, or tweaking the amount, of crosslinking polymers. It allows quicker disintegration and better control over drug release, which can have a great outcome if more complicated treatment is applied [4].

Not only do the nanosponges play a vital role in drug diffusion, but they also control the onset and duration of the drug's effect. This is because they are 3D-based and capable of holding drugs.

Nanosponges are composed of biodegradable and biocompatible materials, ensuring safety upon usage with a low toxicity level [4]. The efficacy of drug encapsulation relies on the size of the drug molecule and the available void space within the nanosponge structure [4].

Besides being platforms for drug delivery, nanosponges will be investigated for other purposes such as serving as biocatalyst/enzyme carriers and as oxygen delivery vehicles. They will also be used as solubility enhancers and poison sorbents.

Overall, nanosponges form the basis of universal nanoparticle systems that can trap and express a broad spectrum of drugs and biomolecules in a three-dimensional, porous scaffold [2, 3]. Their distinctive features render them viable prospects in relation to medical and pharmaceutical applications.

Psoriasis: A Brief Overview

Psoriasis represents a chronic inflammatory immune-mediated skin disease manifested by dry and raised reddish patches covered with fine silvery scales. It is a multifactorial disorder, which implies that various genetic or environmental factors are responsible for it. Its frequency ranges from 0% to 11.8% worldwide. This illness comes together with cardiovascular, metabolic, and autoimmune comorbidities, so it can also be considered systemic inflammation [4]. Conversely, some researchers argue that psoriasis might not be an autoimmune condition at all but could arise due to abnormal reactions against bacteria living within our epidermis caused by genetic abnormalities affecting innate immunity [5]. Additionally, among other genes involved in the pathogenesis of psoriasis, there is the HLA-Cw6 allele, thus showing a complex genetic background where both innate and adaptive systems fail to work properly [2, 5]. Different omics technologies have helped discover biomarkers that shed light on the molecular mechanisms behind this ailment, thereby facilitating its diagnosis and prognosis [4]. Psoriasis, in brief, is a complicated disease having many faces both outside (cutaneous) and inside (systemic). It represents itself as an immune response gone wrong.

Psoriasis Pathophysiology

Psoriasis is a chronic skin disorder characterized by abnormal, accelerated proliferation of keratinocytes in the epidermis, leading to an increased rate of epidermal cell turnover as compared to normal skin [4]. Although the exact pathogenesis is not completely understood, the disease is thought to result from a complex interaction of genetic, environmental, and immunologic factors. Psoriasis is an immune-mediated disease, defined by complex immune responses leading to increased activation of T cells in the skin that stimulate hyperproliferation of keratinocytes. Thick plaques, acanthosis (epidermal hyperplasia), and parakeratosis lead to the characteristic scaling of the skin in psoriasis [2]. The effects of psoriasis are systemic and not limited to the skin (as shown in Fig. (**2**)). Patients with psoriasis have an increased prevalence of other systemic conditions associated with chronic inflammation, including hyperlipidemia (23-34%), hypertension (in up to 43%), Coronary Artery Disease (CAD), obesity, and type 2 diabetes [5]. Psychosocial burden of disease can be more significant than the physical appearance of the skin. Psoriasis can lead to pruritus, pain, and bleeding from the skin lesions, and increased prevalence of depression and anxiety [5]. Treatment options are vast and range from topicals for mild disease to biologics for moderate to severe plaque psoriasis. Biologics that block TNF-α, IL-12, IL-17, and IL-23 are now in common use, as well as oral systemic treatments like methotrexate and apremilast [6].

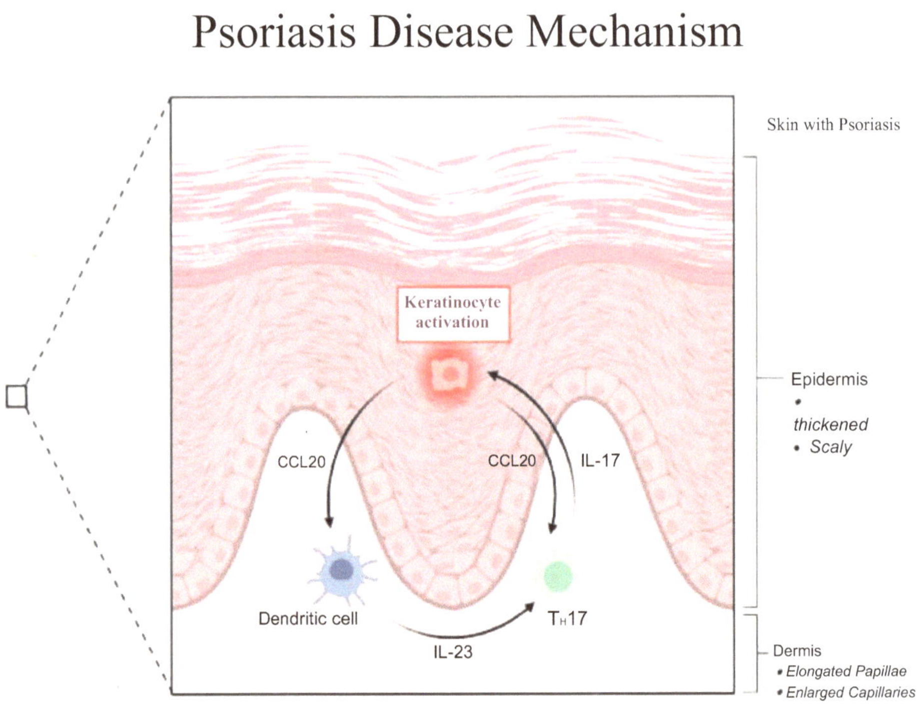

Fig. (2). Pathophysiology of psoriasis.

Current Challenges in Psoriasis Treatment

Psoriasis treatment faces various challenges, including limitations in effectively managing the condition. The main challenges include:

- **Treatment Resistance and Failure**: Despite advancements in psoriasis management, patients may not respond to initial treatments, leading to primary treatment failure. Developing better predictors of treatment response is crucial to identifying patients who are more likely to benefit from a specific biologic agent [5].
- **Adverse Effects and Long-term Safety Concerns**: New treatments like agents have changed how psoriasis is treated, particularly for people with moderate to severe symptoms. However, these treatments come with drawbacks such as treatment not working as expected, safety concerns in the long term, and limitations on how widely they can be used effectively [5, 7].

- **High Costs and Insurance Coverage**: The cost of newer medications, especially biologics, can be a significant barrier to access. Insurance companies may refuse to cover these medications or require patients to try cheaper or older medications, creating an access barrier.
- **Limited Treatment Options for Specific Areas**: Certain areas of the skin, such as the scalp, nails, or genital areas, have limited treatment options. For example, topical creams may not be effective for scalp-only psoriasis, and systemic medications may not be suitable for patients with mild psoriasis.
- **The severity of psoriasis can fluctuate due to various factors**, such as stress, diet, weight changes, and changes in seasons. This variability can make it difficult for patients to find a treatment that consistently works for them.
- **Psoriasis can Present Differently in Patients with Skin of Color**, and there is a lack of representation in medical education materials. This can lead to underdiagnosis and undermanagement of psoriasis in these populations.
- **Addressing Patients' Psychosocial Needs** is a crucial aspect of treating psoriasis, but it is often neglected in the treatment process. This challenge highlights the need for research and innovation in psoriasis treatment to improve patients' outcomes and quality of life [8].

These challenges emphasize the importance of continued research and innovation in psoriasis treatment to improve the outcomes and quality of life of patients affected by this chronic condition.

In psoriasis, there is a need for innovative treatment methods due to the chronic nature of the condition and the challenges associated with existing treatments. Issues like side effects, resistance to treatment, expensive costs, and varying patient responses highlight the need for innovation. While there have been progressions in treatments like innovative biologics and small-molecule inhibitors, challenges such as safety issues and the intricate immunopathogenesis of psoriasis still impede successful therapy outcomes [9]. Interestingly, while the focus on psoriasis has highlighted the potential of personalized medicine and the use of biomarkers for tailored treatments [6], the broader field of dermatology also emphasizes the transformative impact of biologics and targeted therapies for various skin conditions [10]. This suggests a trend towards precision medicine, which is similarly observed in the management of other diseases such as Non-Small Cell Lung Cancer (NSCLC) and cancer in general, where targeted therapies and precision medicine are reshaping treatment paradigms [11]. In summary, the need for innovative treatment approaches in psoriasis is evident, with emerging trends promising to address current challenges through personalized medicine, novel biologics, and small-molecule inhibitors [6, 7]. The advancements in dermatology and other fields reinforce the potential of these approaches to improve patient outcomes and quality of life [10, 11]. Current management strategies for psoriasis focus on symptom relief, enhancing quality of life, and halting disease progression through various methods like topical therapies, phototherapy, systemic medications, and biologic agents targeting specific immune pathways. Recent advancements in psoriasis treatment include new topical products like a JAK inhibitor, combination therapeutic approaches, and the development of fixed-dose combination products that have shown enhanced efficacy compared to individual drugs [12]. Additionally, research is exploring novel techniques such as the use of nanoparticles for topical treatment, indicating a growing intensity in investigating diverse treatment options for psoriasis [13]. The continuous emergence of innovative treatments, including steroid-free topicals, biologics, and oral medications, underscores the importance of ongoing research and development to improve outcomes for individuals with psoriasis [14].

Continued research and collaborations are essential to translate these scientific breakthroughs into clinical practice, thereby optimizing the management of psoriasis and other chronic conditions.

NANOSPONGES IN PSORIASIS MANAGEMENT

The innovative development of these nanosponges is a significant achievement because it has the potential to provide drugs for people with psoriasis, in addition to others. Psoriasis is a skin disease characterized by inflammation of the skin and the formation of silver scales. The local application of corticosteroids, retinoids, or immunosuppressants, which are meant to treat psoriasis, may lead to systemic side effects if they are distributed throughout the body.

The use of nanosponges has emerged as a method for delivering medications to treat psoriasis because of their characteristics and potential benefits. These porous structures in three dimensions can hold substances, such as anti-inflammatory and immunosuppressive drugs, and release them gradually, improving effectiveness while reducing adverse effects. They are very necessary in psoriasis treatment because of their numerous advantages compared to other treatment options. Through their ability to improve both the solubility and skin penetration, they help drug uptake and bioavailability in the process. This is largely true for the psoriasis patients, who may also be subjected to compromised skin barriers, and hence, the drugs will not penetrate the skin adequately.

Secondly, nanosponges exhibit very promising potential for sustained release of therapeutic agents, thereby ensuring a constant therapeutic effect over a longer period. This may therefore improve patient compliance and reduce the frequency of dosing. A few studies have already revealed the efficacy of nanosponges for psoriasis therapy. In a study published on Biomolecules, curcumin-loaded cellulose nanofiber lipid hybrid films have been found to be effective than imiquimod in ameliorating psoriasis-like dermatitis in mice [12]. In this regard, a research paper in the Pharmaceutics journal reported that a nanosponges gel containing curcumin and caffeine demonstrated to be more efficient in treating psoriasis and to shorten the treatment duration [10]. There are extensive possibilities of applying nanosponges in the treatment of psoriasis. They can therefore increase the efficacy of drugs at the skin level, reduce side effects, and extend the drug release time. Besides, nanosponges can be modified to penetrate the particular skin layers or specific cells, and due to this, they become much more accurate and effective in delivering the therapy.

Advantages of Using Nanosponges for Psoriasis Management

Nanosponges as an Aid in Psoriasis Treatment: Nanosponges play a crucial role in psoriasis therapy. Nevertheless, they must be used with caution. They must be proportioned with the right length, width, and a steady surface. These factors influence the nanosponges' behaviour in the skin and the way they work.

Additionally, these cells must be safe for the body and should also break down easily to minimize side effects. In short, nanosponges might be effective in transporting drugs to treat psoriasis. They may spread the medicines more evenly on your skin. They could cut down on side effects and give a continuous release of the drugs over time. However, more research is needed to determine how effectively nanosponges work for psoriasis treatment and to establish the optimal method for their production [14].

Potential Applications and Benefits

Thanks to their unique mode of action, nanosponges offer a promising approach for treating psoriasis in the future. The advantages of using nanosponges to treat psoriasis include:

- Enhanced Skin Penetration: Nanosponges may penetrate deeper into the skin, allowing for better delivery of therapeutic agents directly to the affected areas. Generally, an increase in tissue penetration leads to improved therapeutic efficacy and reduced systemic side effects [10, 14].
- Reduced Stratum Corneum Inflammation: Owing to their nanosize, nanosponges have the potential to mitigate inflammation within the stratum corneum, a skin layer that is highly affected by psoriasis. Diminishing the inflammation might result in better treatment efficiencies.
- Enhanced Keratinocyte Proliferation: It is on record that nanosponges are capable of fostering the proliferation of keratinocytes, an essential step in the

healing of psoriasis. This will lead to faster therapies that are more effective due to an increased number of cells produced for healing purposes.

- Sustained Drug Release: The manner in which drugs are released into the body is controlled by nanosponges to ensure that they are released over time. This makes them remain effective continually over a period of time. It also raises patient compliance while slashing down costs for treatments, among other things [14, 15].
- Potential for Combination Therapy: Because nanosponges may hold several therapeutic chemicals, it is possible to create combination treatments that address various psoriasis symptoms. This pharmacophore modeling may result in better drugs with fewer side effects.
- Better Patient Compliance: Patients are more likely to utilize treatments when using nanosponges because they tend to be more enjoyable and to increase patient compliance and the overall success of a therapy in general [15].
- Decreased adverse Effects: Skin atrophy, oil acne, hypopigmentation, and allergic contact dermatitis are among some of the side effects that traditional treatment could bring. Nanosponge is one of the drugs that has lowered the incidence of toxicity. Such a reduction in negative outcomes may result in both higher and better patient satisfaction, as well as the success of treatment.
- Enhanced Bioavailability: The utilization of nanosponges enables a significant increase in the bioavailability of therapeutic substances, resulting in more effective treatments that require fewer dosage frequencies. Increased absorption leads to improved treatment outcomes and reduced healthcare costs.
- Possibility for Customized Medicine: As nanosponges show a high level of specificity, targeting unique characteristics of psoriasis, they will be able to offer individualized therapies for each patient. The drug development process may become more efficient and drugs may be delivered to the targeted site with higher purity and less or no toxic effects [16].
- Research Advancements: Nanosponges have become a useful tool for research and it is through their use that various inventive and revolutionary solutions for psoriasis have been discovered. Besides this continuous research, it may be expected to come up with more newly-developed therapeutic strategies and promising outcomes.

To summarize, nanosponges are potentially advantageous for managing psoriasis due to the following reasons, enhanced skin permeability, decreased inflammation in the stratum corneum, increased proliferation of keratinocytes, sustained drug release, the possibility of combination therapy, accepted patients' medicine regimen, fewer side effects, increased bioavailability, the potential for personalized medicine, and research leadership. Due to these reasons, nanosponges are a unique and truly attractive research subject in the field of psoriasis treatment [12].

Marketed Topical Corticosteroids Formulation for Psoriasis

Psoriasis has been treated with various topical corticosteroids available on the market. A summary of these products is provided here, including the active ingredient, manufacturer, and risks associated with the dosage form. This summary is displayed in Table **1**.

Table 1. A list of topical corticosteroids and commercial formulations classification by WHO [15].

Potency	BCS class	Topical corticosteroids	Formulations
Ultra-high	I	Clobetasol propionate Cream, 0.05% Diflorasone diacetate	Cream, 0.05% Ointment, 0.05%
High	II	Amcinonide Betamethasone Dipropionate Desoximetasone Fluocinonide Cream,	Ointment, 0.1% Ointment, 0.05% Cream or ointment, 0.025% ointment, or gel, 0.05%
-	II	Halcinonide Betamethasone dipropionate Betamethasone valerate	Cream, ointment, or gel, 0.05% Cream, 0.1% Cream, 0.05%Ointment, 0.1%
Moderate	IV	Desoximetasone Fluocinolone acetonide Fludroxycortide Hydrocortisone valerate Triamcinolone acetonide	Cream0.05% Ointment, 0.025% Ointment, 0.05% Ointment, 0.2% Cream, 0.1%
-	V	Betamethasone Dipropionate Betamethasone valerate Fluocinolone acetonide Fludroxycortide Hydrocortisone butyrate Hydrocortisone valerate Triamcinolone acetonide	Lotion, 0.02% Cream, 0.1% Cream, 0.025% Cream, 0.05% Cream, 0.1% Cream, 0.2% Lotion, 0.1%
Low	VI	Betamethasone valerate Desonide Fluocinolone acetonide	Lotion, 0.05% Cream, 0.05% Solution, 0.01%
-	VII	Dexamethasone sodium phosphate Hydrocortisone acetate Methylprednisolone acetate	Cream, 0.1% Cream, 1% Cream, 0.25%

METHOD OF PREPARATION OF NANOSPONGES

Solvent Method

Proper solvents, *e.g.*, dimethyl sulfoxide (DMSO) and dimethylformamide (DMF), polar aprotic solvents are used. These are suitable for mixing polymers. The methods begin by adding the polymer to the solvent blend, then blending it well until it is uniformly distributed. A ratio of 8:2 is considered the best for this particular application, as it is the crosslinker to polymer ratio. The mixture needs to be reacted for 48 hours at 10°C, up to the solvent reflux temperature. Cooling the solution back down to room temperature happens after the reaction has completed [16]. As shown in Fig. (**3**) below.

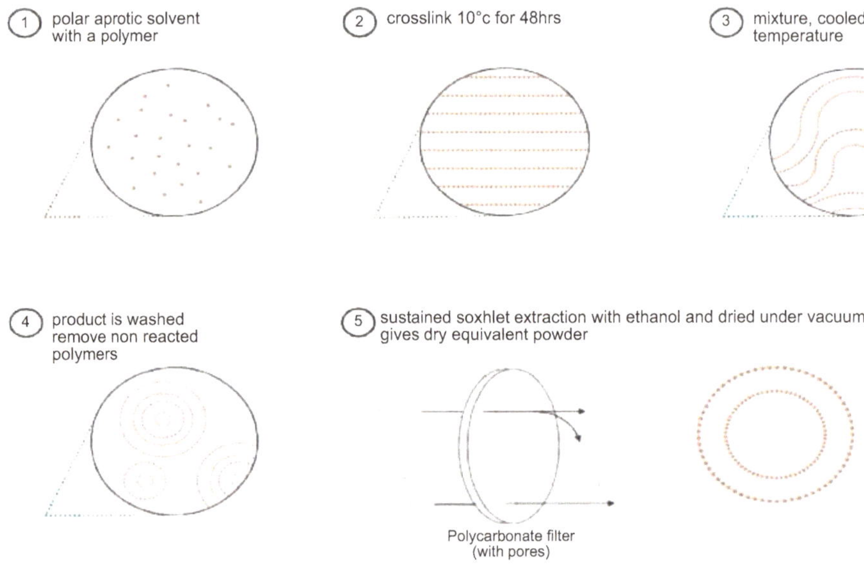

Fig. (3). Solvent evaporation method.

Ultrasound-Assisted Method

Synthesis with the assistance of ultrasound comprises a polymer ultrasonic fusion. This phenomenon is generated without the need for a solvent for cross-linking, as ultrasonic waves penetrate the polymer.

In a test tube, a proper molar ratio of polymer to crosslinker was pre-mixed. Then, the flask was placed in an ultrasound bath, the temperature of which was set at 50°C. The ultrasonication procedure was then carried out for 56 minutes. After sonication, the mixture was cooled to the required temperature, and then it was vigorously agitated and purified. Excess water was added to purify it from unreacted polymer and reagents. The clean, isolated solid was then subjected to

Soxhlet extraction with ethyl alcohol. As a result of the filtration, NSs (nanospheres) were developed and dried under vacuum. The next run was dedicated to drug loading and bonding with the skin, and the mechanism is affected by these factors, as shown in Fig. (**4**) below [17].

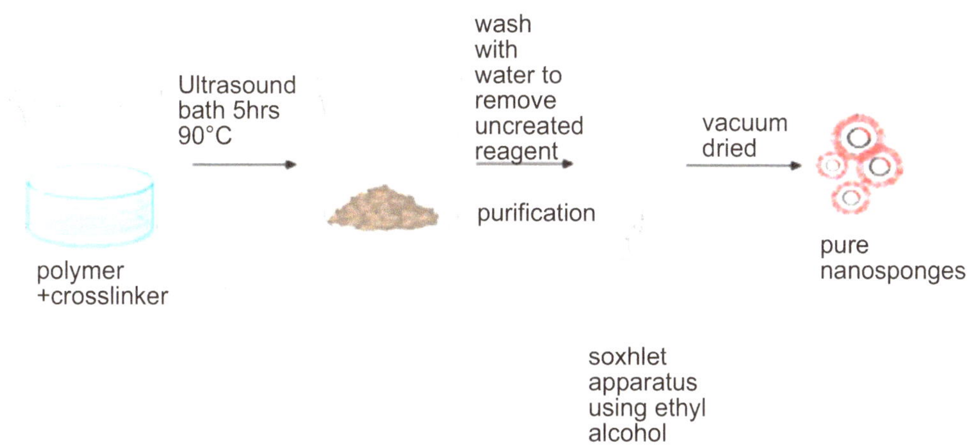

Fig. (4). Ultrasound-assisted method.

Bubble Electrospinning

A common electrospinning system typically consists of a syringe, syringe pump, high-voltage power supply, and a grounded collector, as illustrated in the literature. Nonetheless, a crucial obstacle to their widespread adoption is the limited production output of nanofibers. Polyvinyl alcohol is utilized as the polymer for bubble electrospinning. Homogeneity is guaranteed by adding distilled water to the 10% polymer solution and heating it to 80-90 °C for 2 hours. The solution is then left to cool to room temperature before being used to make nanoporous fibres [18].

Synthesis by the Use of Microwave Radiation

This method utilizes microwave irradiation to fabricate CD NSs, significantly reducing reaction times and enhancing crystallinity. With traditional heating techniques, the reaction duration is reduced fourfold by microwave-assisted synthesis, leading to NSs with a consistent particle size distribution and crystallinity. Are there any experiments performed between microwave-assisted heating and traditional ways of synthesizing CD-based NSs? Can microwave synthesis increase the drug loading capacity of the model drug by four times, as revealed during an investigation where they used HRTEM (High Resolution

Transmission Electron Microscopy), which displayed highly crystalline NSs with narrow size distribution, indicating superior results when microwaves are used for heating reactors? In addition, does irradiating molecules directly with microwaves result in higher efficiency than through whole systems, such as solvent container walls surrounding liquids, which absorb some heat before transferring it to the desired locations, thereby losing a significant amount of energy required for reactions? Consequently, the overall reaction rate increases [19].

Synthesis and Application of Beta-Cyclodextrin Nanosponges as Drug Transporters

Recently, innovative drug delivery systems have attracted attention in the pursuit of more effective drugs. These systems are designed to modify the pharmacokinetics and bioavailability of drugs in a way that increases their efficacy and bioavailability [20], and one promising example is the use of beta-cyclodextrin (β-CD) nanosponges as carriers or transporters. The inner part of such a "nanosponge" consists of a circular assembly with a 3-dimensional (3D) structure that has direct tunnels or passages through which molecules can be engulfed for subsequent release elsewhere within the body while bypassing cells, tissues, and biological membranes that would otherwise have been obstacles. Being carriers for drug conveyance, these nanosponges are 3D structures featuring circles with openings towards them, facilitating drug transportation. This has made them gain interest due to their ability to solubilize and stabilize drugs through the generation of a greater surface area range provided by their unique constructions. Additionally, β-CD nanosponges can be prepared easily by reacting β-CD with cross-linkers such as diisocyanates, diaryl carbonates, and carbonyl diimidazoles, among others. Synthesis of β-CD nanosponges involves β-CD cross-linked by these cross-linkers, hence leading to the formation of nanosponge materials [21].

Preparation of Naproxen Sodium Nanosponges by Solvent Diffusion Method

Let's explore how the Naproxen sodium nanosponges were prepared in the work of Ilyas *et al.* The scientists chose the solvent diffusion technique because it permits unique control over the herbal and aqueous ingredients, specifically ethyl cellulose and polyvinyl alcohol. In this method, the scattered phase was dissolved in a mixture of ethyl cellulose and the drug, using dichloromethane and polyvinyl alcohol. During this process, they thoroughly mixed the blend for 2 hours at 1000 rpm. After this, they collected the resulting nanosponges using filtration and dried them in an oven at 40°C for 24 hours. To ensure the removal of residual dyes, the dried nanosponges were stored in a dryer. This careful process emphasizes the caution with which these miniaturized drug delivery systems are prepared [17].

These little sponges can do a cool job as they deliver drugs well and help the drugs dissolve faster. Wc made one using a technique called "solvent diffusion." It's like mixing things up and letting them stay. The nanosponges we created were particularly effective at soaking up the blue dye from the water. This means that they can help clean up pollutants in the environment. In our study, we employed the solvent dispersion method to prepare Naproxen sodium nanosponges, which is a common method for their development [20].

CHARACTERIZATION OF NANOSPONGES

Preparation of Drug-Loaded Nanosponges

Currently, the development of nano-sized drug delivery systems for various applications, such as wound healing and skin regeneration, is widely explored [18]. One of several novel ways is the application of drug-loaded nanosponges, which are regarded as a new element in targeted drug delivery. Polymeric micelles for drug delivery are constructed through several steps to perform their function. Initially, nanosponges need to avoid aggregation in water due to their presence. To ensure that the dispersed nanoparticles do not achieve peak aggregation, the nanosponges will be sonicated. The centrifugation of the sonicated dispersion will yield the colloidal nanosponges solution. This colloidal dispersion forms an aqueous phase containing sponge nanoparticles (SNPs), which remain in the insoluble microspheres during the freeze-drying process, resulting in the separation of the supernatant and the dehydrated SNPs.

The step of drug loading into nanosponges consists of suspending the nanosponges in water and performing ultrasonication to avoid aggregation. Centrifugation is the technique employed to obtain a colloidal solution, which, after freeze-drying, separates the nanospheres from the other parts.

In the next step, an excess amount of drug is dispersed and constantly stirred for a specified duration of time to allow the process of complexation to occur and form the nanosponges in an aqueous suspension. After complexation, the uncomplexed drug is separated by repeated centrifugation. Finally, the nanosponges are obtained through the use of solvent evaporation or freeze-drying methods [22].

Particle Size Determination

The size of the particles is maintained during polymerization to produce free-flowing powders with fine aesthetic properties. Laser light diffractometry, or the Malvern Zeta Sizer, is used to determine the particle size of loaded and unloaded nanosponges. To investigate the influence of particle size on drug release, a cumulative graph plotting particle size vs time is used. Particles bigger than 30 μm might have a gritty sensation. Particles between 10-25 μm are ideal for topical medication administration due to their appropriate size for effective and pleasant application [23].

Pore Analysis of Nanosponges

Pore investigations are conducted to obtain information on the size of nanochannels and nanocavities generated by the formation of nanosponges. The porosity of nanosponges is typically determined by helium pycnometry, which allows for the permeation of both inter and intraparticle voids within the material. The real volume of the nanosponge material is calculated using the helium displacement technique. This approach determines the volume of the sample by quantifying the quantity of helium gas displaced, thereby providing an accurate representation of the substance's actual volume.

Calculating Percent Porosity

Due to the intrinsic porous nature of nanosponges, these systems often exhibit greater porosity than the parent polymer used in their manufacture. The percentage porosity may be computed. The percentage porosity may be calculated using the following equation: % Porosity = [Bulk volume - True volume] / Bulk volume multiplied by 100 This formula quantifies porosity, a crucial factor in understanding the structural features and prospective uses of nanosponges.

Swelling and Water Uptake

Immersing swellable polymers, such as polyamidoamine nanosponges, in an aqueous solution enables the determination of the degree of water absorption. Swelling and water absorption may be measured using the following formulas:

Percentage of Swelling:

% Swelling = [Marking of cylinder at a specified time point / Initial marking before soaking] × 100.

Percentage of Water Uptake:

% Water Uptake = [Mass of hydrogel after 72 hours / Initial mass of dry polymer] × 100

In vitro Drug Release

The multi-fluidity cell rotation design is combined for the *in vitro* release kinetics research investigation. The configuration holds a 1ml volume-based formulation consisting of nanosponges impregnated with medicine in the donor reservoir. The space for a receptor, divided by a hydrophilic membrane of the dialysis method, is filled by phosphate buffer at pH 7.4 or pH 1.2.

Each experiment lasts 24 hours, with the old buffer being removed at regular intervals and a new buffer fully refilled. The targeted drug is then added to the medium, and its release can be analyzed using an appropriate analytical methodology to assess the release pattern.

Microscopic Study

The use of Electron Microscopy (SEM) and Transmission Electron Microscopy (TEM) in studying the microscopic details of these formulations is a fundamental part of understanding the formation of complexes and their transformation and interaction with the drug itself. Using SEM and TEM allows differentiating these methods and their features which are both advantages and disadvantages. Thus, for certain purposes in electron microscopy they are suitable while others are not.

SEM shows its capacity to examine the surface topologies and structures of the drug, nanosponges, and their complexes of various sizes. It produces high-quality photographs of the sample's exterior at the nanoscale, highlighting features like texture, topography, and chemical elements. The SEM is great for examining the state of the surface in detail, revealing the roughness, contamination, and defects precisely. These data will help researchers build a clearer picture of the mechanisms by which the drug works on nanosponges and further our understanding of possible outcomes related to the drug's stability and bioavailability.

However, TEM is better equipped for identifying the constituent parts and components of the material's internal structure. It can achieve high image resolution, which stems from the fact that its accuracy allows for observing the image of atomic structures and even the way the atoms are located on the sample. TEM study of raw materials and the final product holds crystal state details about the crystal structure and the crystal shapes of the materials. This data may be of great importance in revealing the inner workings of inclusion complex formation and the potential consequences for product properties, serving as an observatory.

In the course of studying the microscopic (nano sponges and the complex formation), SEM and TEM both can be used independently for gaining a wider range of understanding as to how the transformation and interactions deal with the formation of these complexes. SEM leads to a surface survey of materials, whereas TEM results in an internal examination of the structure and composition of the materials. In terms of SEM and TEM, the LE differences are to analyze the objectives of the research and the type of information required. If the properties of the materials are at the heart of the issue, then the SEM is likely the most appropriate method to employ. But if the intention is to study the internal structure and composition of the related materials, TEM can be easily used as a qualitative method. Combining the advantages of both techniques, researchers will be able to gain a more detailed insight into the microscopic nature of the drug and nanosponges, as well as their complexes, which will help build better products and optimize the process [24].

CASE STUDIES

Kumar *et al.* [2021] reveal the efficacy of Clobetasol Propionate (CP) in managing psoriasis. By entrapping CP into nanosponges and integrating them with hydrogel, a safer alternative for improved treatments is proposed. Cyclodextrin-based nanosponges loaded with CP were successfully engineered and characterized, showing good payload and controlled release. *In vitro* evaluation showed its efficacy against THP1 cells, demonstrating anti-inflammatory and immune modulatory effects. The nanosponges also exhibited pseudoplastic behavior, acceptable spreadability, and mechanical properties, making them more effective for topical application. The nanoformulation showed anti-psoriatic activity *in vivo* using a mouse tail model [25].

Kumar *et al.* [2021] developed a dithranol nanosponge integrated Carbopol hydrogel as a new approach for psoriasis management. The nanosponges were synthesized using diphenyl carbonate and β-cyclodextrin and embedded into Carbopol hydrogels. The formulations were evaluated *in vivo* for their antipsoriatic potential and as markers of oxidative stress. The hydrogel showed satisfactory results in spreadability, viscosity, and texture profiles. The findings suggest a new delivery method for dithranol in topical psoriasis treatments [25].

Ravi *et al.* [2019] created and evaluated celecoxib nanosponges, which were freeze-dried. The optimized nanosponge formulation showed maximum drug release at 24 hours, demonstrating sustained celecoxib drug delivery. This formulation was prepared for the treatment of psoriatic arthritis [26].

Iriventi *et al.* [2020] developed a beta-cyclodextrin-based nanosponge of curcumin and caffeine, which was synthesized and characterized, showing superior characteristics and better performance. Incorporating these nanosponges in a topical gel showed better therapeutic effects than conventional formulations. Sustained drug release was achieved for 12 hours, and promising *in vivo* and *ex vivo* permeation studies suggest this gel could be a promising local treatment for psoriasis [27].

Shaikh *et al.* [2023] created psoralen-loaded nanosponges and assessed their antipsoriatic activity. Thc different polymers at various ratios were used to formulate the nanosponges. The prepared formulations were evaluated for different parameters. The nanosponges made using PVA: EC [1:1] were determined to be superior in the *in vitro* testing and were subsequently selected for antipsoriatic potential investigation [28].

CONCLUSION AND FUTURE PROSPECTS

Nanosponges have surfaced as a hopeful system for the delivery of drugs that would help in dealing with psoriasis, owing to their distinct capabilities, including the patterns of the drug release, which are under control, and the capabilities of targeted delivery. Some advantages make nanosponges stand out among other delivery systems. They can encapsulate various substances, both hydrophilic and lipophilic molecules, and elevate solubility for poorly water-soluble molecules, which is not common. Besides, nano sponges are robust, capable of surviving temperatures reaching up to 300°C — hence being fit for diverse applications.

Nanosponges have shown their potential in treating psoriasis through a number of studies. An example would be the use of nanosponge-loaded topical gels containing curcumin and caffeine, which have been shown to significantly enhance anti-psoriatic efficacy. In another case, the formulation of nanosponge-loaded hydrogels with Clobetasol propionate was found to have much more anti-psoriatic effect compared to plain and Clobetasol propionate hydrogels.

In the future, the horizons for nanosponges in psoriasis containment could see the emergence of more advanced formulations that can penetrate specific skin layers with the drug and sustainably release active pharmaceutical ingredients. Moreover, scientists are investigating the capabilities of nanosponges to carry different therapeutic agents simultaneously, which should significantly improve their effectiveness.

Conclusively, the nano sponges have demonstrated themselves highly effective as drug delivery system for psoriasis. Their unique features including controlled drug release patterns and targeted delivery capabilities, make them an ideal choice in treating this chronic autoimmune disease. However, more research should be conducted to fully investigate the potential of nanosponges in managing psoriasis. This calls for more innovative formulations with sustained relief to patients who are affected by the condition; the chronically deprived plight must also be considered during the formulation processes.

REFERENCES

[1] Upadhyay RK. Drug delivery systems, CNS protection, and the blood brain barrier. BioMed research international. 2014; 2014.
[http://dx.doi.org/10.1155/2014/869269] [PMID: 25136634]

[2] Swaminathan S, Vavia PR, Trotta F. Cyclodextrin-based nanosponges: a promising platform for drug delivery. Drug Deliv. 2016;23(3):848-66.
[http://dx.doi.org/10.3109/10717544.2014.962043] [PMID: 25262753]

[3] Pandey P, Purohit D, Dureja H. Nanosponges–A promising novel drug delivery system. Recent Pat Nanotechnol 2018; 12(3): 180-91.
[http://dx.doi.org/10.2174/1872210512666180925102842] [PMID: 30251614]

[4] Ravi SC, Krishnakumar K, Nair SK. Nano sponges: A targeted drug delivery system and its applications. GSC Biological and Pharmaceutical Sciences. 2019; 7(3): 040-7.
[http://dx.doi.org/10.30574/gscbps.2019.7.3.0098]

[5] Gupta R, Debbaneh MG, Liao W. Genetic epidemiology of psoriasis. Curr Dermatol Rep 2014; 3(1): 61-78.
[http://dx.doi.org/10.1007/s13671-013-0066-6] [PMID: 25580373]

[6] Jiang S, Hinchliffe TE, Wu T. Biomarkers of an autoimmune skin disease—psoriasis. Genomics Proteomics Bioinformatics 2015; 13(4): 224-33.
[http://dx.doi.org/10.1016/j.gpb.2015.04.002] [PMID: 26362816]

[7] Ravi SCKK. NSNs A targeted drug delivery system and its applications GSC Biological and Pharmaceutical Sciences. GSC Biological and Pharmaceutical Sciences 2019.

[8] Hoffman MB, Hill D, Feldman SR. Current challenges and emerging drug delivery strategies for the treatment of psoriasis. Expert Opin Drug Deliv 2016; 13(10): 1461-73.
[http://dx.doi.org/10.1080/17425247.2016.1188801] [PMID: 27164301]

[9] Singh D. Challenges in immunomodulation for psoriasis: recent advancements and need of therapies. Curr Drug Ther 2024; 19(3): 275-8.
[http://dx.doi.org/10.2174/0115748855274998231113110529]

[10] Bashir B. Advancements in dermatological therapies. The therapist (Journal of Therapies & Rehabilitation Sciences). 2023: 01.
[http://dx.doi.org/10.54393/tt.v4i03.137]

[11] Rai V, Gupta Y, Srivastava SP, Shukla A, Bano N, Khan S. Targeted therapies in cancer treatment: unveiling the latest breakthroughs and promising approaches. Journal for Research in Applied Sciences and Biotechnology 2024; 2(6): 175-83.
[http://dx.doi.org/10.55544/jrasb.2.6.26]

[12] Lequang JA. Innovations in psoriasis management: Based on selected presentations from the symposium for cosmetic advances & laser education (SCALE) virtual congress-July 24 to 26, 2020. J Clin Aesthet Dermatol 2020; 13(11) (Suppl. 2): S8-S23.
[PMID: 33362902] [PMCID: PMC7733677]

[13] Bodnár K, Fehér P, Ujhelyi Z, Bácskay I, Józsa L. Recent approaches for the topical treatment of psoriasis using nanoparticles. Pharmaceutics 2024; 16(4): 449.
[http://dx.doi.org/10.3390/pharmaceutics16040449] [PMID: 38675110]

[14] Schön MP. Advances in psoriasis treatment. Lancet 2005; 366(9494): 1333-5.
[http://dx.doi.org/10.1016/S0140-6736(05)67542-3] [PMID: 16226595]

[15] Shetty K, Sherje AP. Nano intervention in topical delivery of corticosteroid for psoriasis and atopic dermatitis—a systematic review. J Mater Sci Mater Med 2021; 32(8): 88.
[http://dx.doi.org/10.1007/s10856-021-06558-y] [PMID: 34331599]

[16] Rubin Pedrazzo A, Caldera F, Zanetti M, Appleton SL, Dhakar NK, Trotta F. Mechanochemical green

synthesis of hyper-crosslinked cyclodextrin polymers. Beilstein J Org Chem 2020; 16(1): 1554-63. [http://dx.doi.org/10.3762/bjoc.16.127] [PMID: 32704321]

[17] Asfaram A, Ghaedi M, Dashtian K. Ultrasound assisted combined molecularly imprinted polymer for selective extraction of nicotinamide in human urine and milk samples: Spectrophotometric determination and optimization study. Ultrason Sonochem 2017; 34: 640-50. [http://dx.doi.org/10.1016/j.ultsonch.2016.06.018] [PMID: 27773291]

[18] Yang R, He J, Xu L, Yu J. Bubble-electrospinning for fabricating nanofibers. Polymer (Guildf) 2009; 50(24): 5846-50. [http://dx.doi.org/10.1016/j.polymer.2009.10.021]

[19] Singireddy A, Rani Pedireddi S, Nimmagadda S, Subramanian S. Beneficial effects of microwave assisted heating versus conventional heating in synthesis of cyclodextrin based nanosponges. Mater Today Proc 2016; 3(10): 3951-9. [http://dx.doi.org/10.1016/j.matpr.2016.11.055]

[20] Garcia-Orue I, Gainza G, Villullas S, Pedraz JL, Hernandez RM, Igartua M. Nanotechnology approaches for skin wound regeneration using drug-delivery systems Nanobiomaterials in soft tissue engineering. Elsevier 2016; pp. 31-55. [http://dx.doi.org/10.1016/B978-0-323-42865-1.00002-7]

[21] Moscovici1 M, Hlevca2 C, Casarica1 A, Pavaloiu2 RD. Nanocellulose and nanogels as modern drug delivery systems. Nanocellulose and Nanohydrogel Matrices: Biotechnological and Biomedical Applications. 2017: 209-69. [http://dx.doi.org/10.1002/9783527803835.ch9]

[22] McBain SC, Yiu HH, Dobson J. Magnetic nanoparticles for gene and drug delivery. Int J Nanomedicine 2008; 3(2): 169-80. [PMID: 18686777]

[23] Danaei M, Dehghankhold M, Ataei S, *et al.* Impact of particle size and polydispersity index on the clinical applications of lipidic nanocarrier systems. Pharmaceutics 2018; 10(2): 57. [http://dx.doi.org/10.3390/pharmaceutics10020057] [PMID: 29783687]

[24] Tiwari K, Bhattacharya S. The ascension of nanosponges as a drug delivery carrier: preparation, characterization, and applications. J Mater Sci Mater Med 2022; 33(3): 28. [http://dx.doi.org/10.1007/s10856-022-06652-9] [PMID: 35244808]

[25] Kumar S, Prasad M, Rao R. Topical delivery of clobetasol propionate loaded nanosponge hydrogel for effective treatment of psoriasis: Formulation, physicochemical characterization, antipsoriatic potential and biochemical estimation. Mater Sci Eng C 2021; 119: 111605. [http://dx.doi.org/10.1016/j.msec.2020.111605] [PMID: 33321649]

[26] Ravi G, Bose PSC, Ravi V, Sarita D. Preparation, characterization and evaluation of celecoxib loaded nanosponges for the treatment of psoriatic arthritis. International Journal of Medical and Biomedical Studies 2019; 3(12): 181-5. [http://dx.doi.org/10.32553/ijmbs.v3i12.828]

[27] Iriventi P, Gupta NV, Osmani RAM, Balamuralidhara V. Design & development of nanosponge loaded topical gel of curcumin and caffeine mixture for augmented treatment of psoriasis. Daru 2020; 28(2): 489-506. [http://dx.doi.org/10.1007/s40199-020-00352-x] [PMID: 32472531]

[28] Shaikh AAK, DAQ, UAS, RB, Rajmane. Nanosponges-based hydrogel formulation containing psoralen to enhance topical delivery. european chemical bulletin. 2023;ISSN 2063-5346 (2023).

CHAPTER 11

Polymeric Nanoparticles Based Pharmacotherapy for the Management of Psoriasis

Prachi Saini[1], **Kanika Mangla**[1], **Girish Kumar**[2], **Reshu Virmani**[1] and **Tarun Virmani**[2,*]

[1] *School of Pharmaceutical Sciences, MVN University, Palwal, Haryana, India*

[2] *Amity Institute of Pharmacy, Amity University, Greater Noida, Uttar Pradesh, India*

Abstract: Psoriasis is a chronic inflammatory skin disorder affecting millions worldwide, posing significant therapeutic challenges due to its complex pathophysiology and diverse clinical manifestations. Conventional treatment options often yield suboptimal results and are associated with adverse effects, highlighting the need for innovative therapeutic strategies. Polymeric nanoparticles [PNPs] have emerged as a promising approach, offering enhanced drug bioavailability, sustained release, and reduced systemic toxicity. This chapter provides a comprehensive overview of the application of PNPs in psoriasis management, emphasizing their advantages over conventional therapies. By addressing the limitations of existing treatments, PNPs offer a viable strategy for enhancing therapeutic outcomes and improving patient care in psoriasis management.

Keywords: Bioavailability enhancement, Drug delivery systems, Nanotechnology in dermatology, Psoriasis treatment, Polymeric nanoparticles, Sustained drug release, Targeted therapy.

INTRODUCTION

Psoriasis is an immune-mediated chronic skin condition. It is characterized by hyperproliferation and poor differentiation of keratinocytes, leading to patchy, scaly skin lesions. It can extend from a single location to the entire body, causing severe inflammation and the development of skin plaques. The prevalence of psoriasis varies across different regions, with higher reported incidence rates in Western countries compared to tropical and subtropical regions. Epidemiological studies indicate that genetic predisposition, environmental factors, and lifestyle differences contribute to this variation. An estimated 2-4% of people worldwide suffer from psoriasis; hence, anti-psoriatic drugs are predicted to command a

* **Corresponding author Tarun Virmani:** Amity Institute of Pharmacy, Amity University, Greater Noida, Uttar Pradesh, India; E-mail: tarun2feb@gmail.com

Anjali Sharma, Prerna Sharma, Roy Rillera Marzo & Ahmed A. Al Karmalawy (Eds.)

nearly 18.8 billion USD market in 2021. Since psoriasis is a chronic illness, its effects extend beyond the patient's physical discomfort; they also impair their social and psychological well-being, which lowers their overall quality of life. In addition to affecting the skin, psoriasis exacerbates a number of comorbid conditions, including hyperlipidaemia, diabetes, peptic ulcers, psoriatic arthritis, cardiac problems, metabolic disorders, *etc.* Therefore, a major area of concentration in global public health and dermatology is conducting thorough studies on psoriasis to determine its risk factors, develop efficient therapies and preventive measures, and understand its pathophysiology. Although psoriasis can affect any part of the body, it typically begins in certain areas, such as the scalp, knees, or groin. Although there are other types of psoriasis based on appearance, plaque psoriasis, the most prevalent type, is distinguished by silvery skin scales caused by psoriasis vulgaris.

Plaque psoriasis, the most common variety of psoriasis, is characterized by psoriasis plaques of red, scaly lesions on the skin that are covered in silvery-white scales. Psoriasis has a pathophysiology that is linked to both the immune system and genetics [1]. Psoriasis is currently understood to be caused by the stimulation of dendritic cells in the skin, which activate the defense mechanism, including macrophages and T-cells, along with the facilitation of communication between the immune system and epidermal keratinocytes. These circumstances lead to an increase in cytokine production, which in turn triggers an overabundance of keratinocytes beginning in the basal layer of epidermis and the general inflammation of the skin linked to the development of psoriasis lesions. The pathophysiology of psoriasis is illustrated in Fig. (**1**).

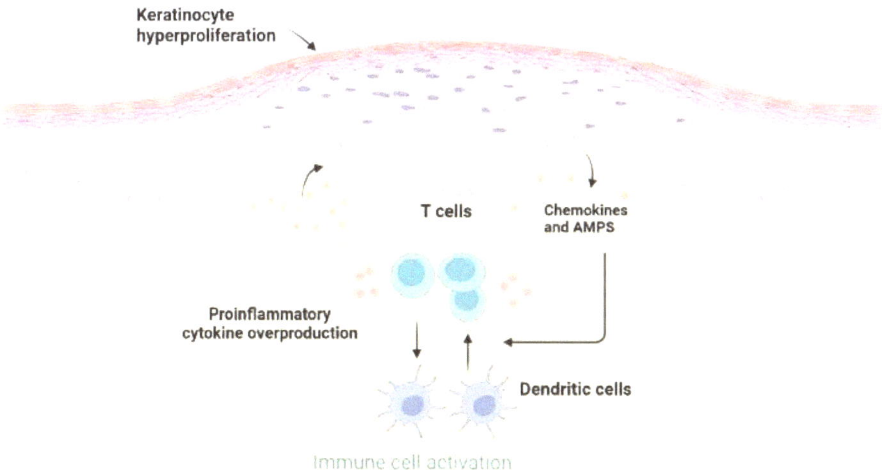

Fig. (1). Regulatory steps in psoriasis development.

This figure illustrates the key regulatory mechanisms involved in the pathophysiology of psoriasis, including immune system activation, inflammatory cytokine release, and keratinocyte proliferation. Understanding these steps is essential for identifying therapeutic targets and developing effective treatment strategies.

Conventional Treatment of Psoriasis

Many traditional psoriasis therapies are now available in the market and have been shown to be effective in alleviating discomfort and symptoms; however, the majority of them have several drawbacks.

Four primary methods are used in the management of conventional psoriasis: topical therapy, systemic therapy, biologic systemic therapy, and phototherapy [2]. Drugs administered systemically are typically needed for moderate-to-severe diseases. These consist of methotrexate [MTX], cyclosporine, fumaric acid esters, and acitretin. DNA synthesis is inhibited by MTX, a folic acid antagonist [3]. Nausea, loss of appetite, hepatotoxicity, and vomiting are the common adverse effects [4]. Cyclosporine is a potent immunosuppressant that can be used to produce remission and as a maintenance treatment for psoriasis [3]. Because of its retinoid side effects, which include teratogenicity, dry skin, conjunctivitis, and hair loss, acitretin is also used in very small dosages to treat psoriasis [5]. Fumaric acid esters are also used to treat psoriasis due to their anti-oxidative, anti-inflammatory, and immunomodulatory effects [6]. Along with a decrease in lymphocyte and leukocyte numbers, they frequently cause gastrointestinal symptoms [7]. Topical distribution is better than systemic dosage due to less immunosuppression and toxicity. The most common therapeutic agents used to treat psoriasis are retinoid analogues, corticosteroids, immunosuppressants, and dithranol; however, inadequate drug absorption *via* the skin continues to be a major barrier to traditional topical treatment [8]. Phototherapy is another fitting alternative to treat psoriasis. Various sources such as light-emitting diodes, strong pulsed light, pulsed dye laser, psoralen UVA, UVB, and photodynamic therapy have been studied [9]. Scholars have created a variety of lipid-based nanoparticles, including solid lipid nanoparticles, ethosomes, transethosomes, liposomes, niosomes, and nanostructured lipid carriers [10].

Psoriasis treatment is categorized into topical therapy, systemic therapy, and phototherapy, depending on the severity of the condition. Phototherapy and systemic treatments are primarily reserved for severe cases due to their potential carcinogenic and toxic effects. In contrast, topical therapies are considered safer as they directly target the basal layer of the epidermis, where psoriasis originates [2 - 4]. Commonly prescribed topical formulations include anti-inflammatory agents such as corticosteroids, along with vitamin A, synthetic vitamin D3, and anthralin. Additionally, over-the-counter treatments containing coal tar and salicylic acid are also available. However, topical therapies may lead to side effects such as skin irritation, thinning, and dilated blood vessels. To enhance psoriasis management, controlled drug delivery systems that facilitate deeper penetration of medications while minimizing adverse effects could serve as an effective alternative [5].

Advantages of Nanotechnology Over Conventional Treatment

Various drug therapies, including calcitriol, tacrolimus, steroids, and calcineurin inhibitors, provide symptomatic relief in psoriasis by modulating the immune system. However, these treatments often lead to serious side effects and increase the risk of other illnesses. Additionally, frequent dosing and inadequate skin penetration pose significant challenges in conventional psoriasis treatment, necessitating the development of advanced drug delivery systems. Nanocarriers have emerged as a promising solution, offering targeted and sustained drug delivery with improved bioavailability, reduced toxicity, extended circulation, lower dosing frequency, and enhanced skin penetration. Among these, lipid-based nanocarriers such as liposomes, nanostructured lipid carriers, nanoemulsions, and solid lipid nanoparticles have demonstrated superior efficacy due to their lipid content, which facilitates drug absorption while minimizing adverse effects. However, lipid-based systems suffer from limitations such as poor encapsulation efficiency and low stability. These challenges can be addressed by incorporating polymers, leading to the development of polymeric nanoparticles [PNPs]. Various polymers have been explored for formulating PNPs of antipsoriatic drugs, as discussed in this chapter.

Nanoparticles for the Pharmacotherapy of Psoriasis

Advancements in drug therapy require more than just the development of new therapeutic agents; overcoming challenges such as low drug solubility, poor bioavailability, first-pass metabolism, rapid elimination, and plasma level fluctuations is essential. An effective strategy to address these limitations is the use of controlled and targeted drug delivery systems [6, 7]. The choice of drug carrier depends on the intended route of administration, with sizes ranging from nanometres [colloidal carriers] to micrometres [microparticles] or even millimetres [implants]. However, microparticles and implants are unsuitable for intravenous delivery and targeted therapy, making colloidal carriers—such as nanoparticles—an increasingly attractive option. Various nanoscale drug delivery systems, including nanoparticles, liposomes, ethosomes, nanoemulsions, nanosuspensions, polymer-drug conjugates, and micelles, are being explored for enhanced treatment of psoriasis [8].

Topical Applications of Polymers

Chitosan and Derivatives

Chitosan is a naturally occurring polysaccharide that has gained a lot of recognition in the pharmaceutical sector because of its distinct qualities of biodegradability, biocompatibility, mucoadhesiveness, and low toxicity [9]. It also has antibacterial and antifungal properties, which help treat various skin conditions. It is produced from chitin through a deacetylation process using various chemical or enzymatic routes. It consists of N-acetyl-d-glucosamine and glucosamine connected by β [1 - 4] glycosidic linkages. The physicochemical characteristics of chitosan can be improved by chemical modification owing to the presence of amino groups in its structure. Chitosan and its derivatives are utilized to develop nanocarriers which have shown great potential as drug delivery system in dermal diseases due to their many positive attributes, including nanosize, enhanced stability, suitable pharmacokinetic and pharmacodynamic profile, non-immunogenicity, and increased drug loading capacity [10]. These also have shown permeation enhancement activity due to their polyatomic nature. Owing to their polyatomic nature, chitosan nanoparticles have greater mucoadhesiveness with the skin surface, having negative charges, resulting in prolonged contact time. Chitosan nanoparticles also provide stimulus-responsive release of the drug, which increases the therapeutic efficiency of the treatment [11]. Numerous investigations have shown that chitosan is a powerful drug carrier due to its diverse physicochemical properties, which include increased skin penetration, pH-related swelling, regulated drug properties, hemocompatibility, and cytocompatibility [12].

Experiments have additionally shown that chitosan is a powerful medication carrier component in psoriasis. Ridolfi and companions investigated the efficacy of chitosan with the anti-psoriatic medication tretinoin by creating chitosan-lipid nanoparticles. They found that the drug's ideal encapsulation had low toxicity, great stability, and permeability. It has been demonstrated that the carrier system works well for topically delivering tretinoin to keratinocytes [13].

Poly-[Lactic-Co-Glycolic Acid] [PLGA]

PLGA is a widely studied biocompatible and biodegradable polymer for regulated and prolonged drug administration in topical ailments like psoriasis. It minimizes the toxicity due to the ability to hydrolyze into glycolic acid and lactic acid within the body [14]. It is possible to control PLGA degradation rates to range from months to years, which presents a powerful opportunity for sustained release of the drug, resulting in enhanced therapeutic efficiency. In addition, PLGA nanoparticles can be made target-specific by employing their functionalization with various ligands and their release can be made stimulus-responsive. These are capable of delivering a large variety of therapeutic molecules, including hydrophilic and lipophilic agents [15]. The potential of PLGA nanoparticles to treat psoriasis can be well explained by a study in which a PLGA nanoparticle-based hydrogel was developed to deliver curcumin. PLGA nanoparticles-based hydrogel was administered topically to animals with psoriasis. The findings demonstrated that PLGA nanoparticles-based hydrogel had superior anti-psoriatic activity in animals with psoriasis compared to blank hydrogel, plain curcumin-loaded hydrogel, and tacrolimus ointment. This enhanced therapeutic potential could be due to sustained release, increased deposition and enhanced penetration of curcumin through skin [16].

Polyethylene Glycol [PEG]

PEG is the preferred polymer for drug delivery in various skin conditions. It has been approved by the FDA for human consumption due to its safety and non-toxicity [17]. PEG serves as an ideal drug carrier in the treatment of psoriasis due to various distinct characteristics of enhanced solubility, chemical stability, biocompatibility, and increased flexibility. It reduces immunogenicity by PEGylating, increases drug permeability, permits regulated release, and localizes drug activity, all of which lessen systemic side effects and increase therapeutic efficacy [18]. It has been utilized to develop various formulations, including emulgels, hydrogels, and nanoparticles. Through a procedure known as PEGylation, these PEG configurations are chemically linked to the preferred product. Numerous PEGylation studies have been documented, including PEG-biomolecule conjugations, PEG-based gels, and PEG-based liposomes, among others. PEGylation has demonstrated clinical efficacy as a versatile polymer for innovative delivery techniques in various diseases, including obesity, neurodegeneration, and rheumatoid arthritis [19]. Although topical administration has great promise, its potential for treating psoriasis remains unexplored. Several PEG studies in the treatment of psoriasis have been the subject of numerous research projects in recent years, with the goal of minimizing the issues that arose in the transdermal delivery section that followed [20].

Dextran

Dextran is an important polysaccharide that is extensively researched as a polymeric drug carrier. Dextran is a bacterial polysaccharide consisting essentially of -1,6-linked glucopyranoside residues with a fraction of -1,3-linked residues [21]. It is an exopolysaccharide having extreme biocompatibility and biodegradability. It is ideal for usage as a nanomedicine, cell imaging system, nanodrug carrier, or nano biosensor due to its simple yet unique biopolymeric nature [22]. Because of its exceptional biocompatibility and distinct physicochemical characteristics, dextran-based nanoparticles with high solid contents could be synthesized in a single step from monomers without the need of organic solvents or surfactants [23]. Chemical modification of dextran is simple, and processes including etherification, esterification, amidation, and oxidation can be used to derive different glycoconjugates.

Dextran, in particular, is highly water soluble, biocompatible, and biodegradable. It also improves the stability of the drug delivery system and keeps the medication from building up in the bloodstream [24]. Dextran-based nanoparticles of acitretin were developed by Lan *et al.* to treat psoriasis. Acitretin-loaded dextran nanoparticles ameliorated psoriasis at lower doses than plain acitretin with reduced adverse effects. In addition, nanoparticles suppressed the proliferation of keratinocytes greater than plain acitretin [25]. These findings revealed the potential of dextran-based nanoparticles to ameliorate skin conditions like psoriasis.

Carbopol

In the different pharmaceutical formulations, Carbopol is of interest as an excipient. It is derived from the cross-linking of acrylic acid with polyalkenyl ether or divinyl glycol [26]. The versatility of Carbopol as a topical polymer is due to its gelling property, thermal stability, viscoelasticity, and compatibility with a large number of drugs. With its cross-linked composition, complex hydrophobic nature, and particle size ranging from 0.2 and 0.6 microns, Carbopol indicates potential as a delivery system for controlled releases of pharmaceutical products. These characteristics render it a viable alternative to conventional drug therapy for specific issues [27]. For example, Mittal *et al.* fabricated carbopol-based nanoemulgel loaded with tacrolimus to treat psoriasis. The results of *ex vivo* studies displayed 1.5-fold improved penetration from the nanoemulgel of tacrolimus compared to the commercial formulation. *In vivo* study demonstrated noteworthy anti-psoriatic activity than the commercial conventional formulation of tacrolimus, revealing the potential of carbopol-based nanoemulgel to ameliorate psoriasis [28]. Navdeep and his team had developed Barbaloin gel using Carbopol polymer for safe and effective treatment of Psoriasis. The results of *in vitro* studies demonstrated favourable results for the amelioration of psoriasis, however, animal studies are still pending to confirm it [29].

Hydroxypropyl Methylcellulose [HPMC]

HPMC is a hydrophilic, biocompatible, and biodegradable polymer gaining popularity in drug delivery [30]. Due to swelling, gelling, and thickening properties, it provides controlled release of the drugs. It possesses Bioadhesive characteristics due to the presence of hydroxyl [OH] in its structure, which enables the formation of hydrogen bonds [31]. The Bioadhesive nature facilitates the prolonged retention of the drugs at local sites. HPMC has minimal interaction with a large group of drugs resulting in good compatibility index [32]. For example, Jain *et al.* developed liposphere gel co-loaded with tacrolimus and curcumin to treat psoriasis. The findings demonstrated increased anti-psoriatic activity of liposphere gel in imiquimod induced psoriatic animals compared to plain drugs [33]. In another study, Kilofoyle *et al.* investigated toward HPMC in the paclitaxel nanosphere based on tyrosine in order to ensure a topical treatment of psoriasis. Tyrosphere development, paclitaxel loading, and distribution through the HPMC gel were the primary objectives of the research in order to increase the drug's solubility [34].

Polymeric Nanocarriers Based Topical Delivery of Anti-Psoriatic Drugs

Polymeric carriers play a key role in nanoparticle formulations. Polymers can be obtained from natural as well as synthetic sources. Polymeric nanoparticles are developed using a variety of biodegradable and biocompatible polymers having a size range of 10-1000 nm [35]. These are categorised into two categories, namely nanocapsules and nanospheres. In nanocapsules, the drug is restricted to a cavity enclosed by a distinctive polymeric membrane, while in nanospheres, the drug is dispersed like a matrix system [36]. Polymers are incredibly useful materials for creating a wide variety of molecular designs that can be combined to create distinctive nanoparticle structures with a wide range of possible medical uses [37]. Polymeric nanoparticles offer several favourable advantages, for example, enhancing the stability of medications and proteins, allowing for the simple control of molecule size and surface properties, increasing drug release, and the capacity to target a specific organ [38]. Over the past few years, considerable research has been conducted on nanosized carriers for various biomedical applications, including vaccination, drug delivery, gene therapy, and disease diagnosis. These carriers offer several advantages: regulated and prolonged drug release, stabilization of substances through both physical and chemical protection, higher accumulation in tumors due to the enhanced permeation and retention (EPR) effect, surface modification with peptides and antibodies for cell- and tissue-specific targeting, and gene delivery through the formation of internalizable drug–vehicle complexes. A significant amount of work has been invested in making nanomedicine technology commercially available. The FDA has already approved a number of nanoparticle-based therapies, including Abraxane [albumin-bounded paclitaxel nanoparticles] for the treatment of breast cancer and Estrasorb [micellar nanoparticles] for topical menopausal therapy. Various nanoparticles are examined in Fig. (**2**).

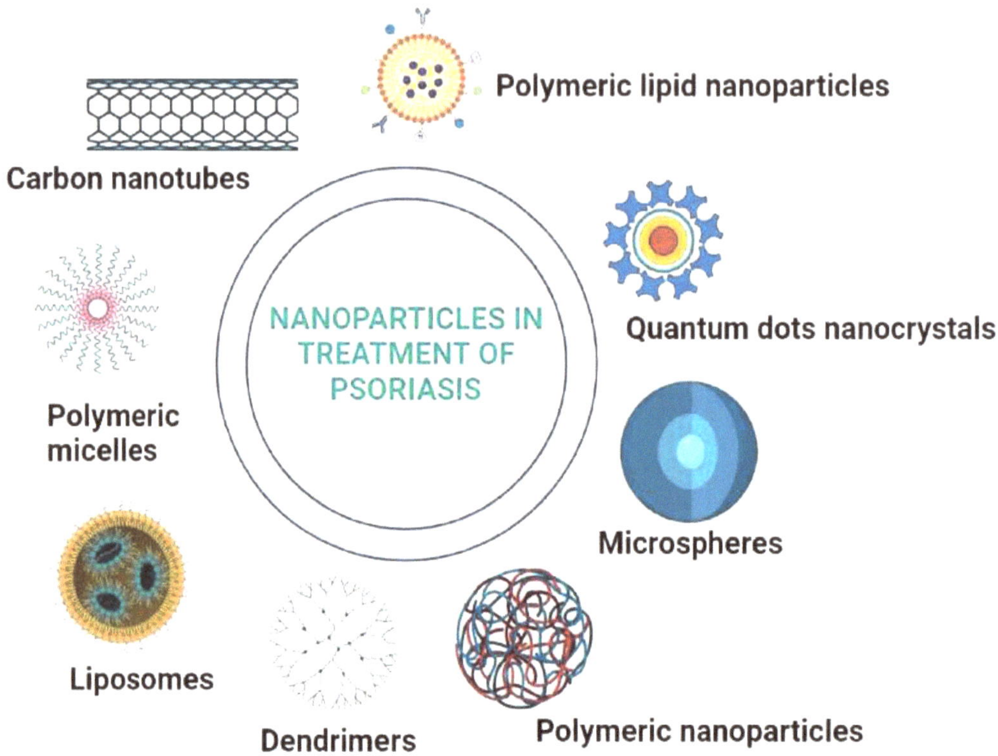

Fig. (2). Nanoparticles for the treatment of psoriasis.

This figure provides an overview of different nanoparticle-based drug delivery systems utilized for psoriasis treatment. It highlights the advantages of nanocarriers, such as enhanced drug bioavailability, targeted delivery, prolonged circulation, and improved skin penetration, thereby addressing the limitations of conventional therapies.

Advantages of Polymeric Nanoparticles

- They increase the stability of the drugs.
- They facilitate improved efficiency and effectiveness over conventional delivery systems.
- They provide the required concentration of drugs at the desired site.
- They can be utilized to treat a large number of diseases.

- They can be easily fabricated and modified to elicit desired action [39].

In order to optimise dermatological distribution, topical formulations containing nanosized carriers like liposomes, lipid nanoparticles, polymeric nanoparticles, and nanoemulsions are extensively utilized [40]. Some of these nanotechnology carriers, nanoparticles of polymeric material with easily adjustable physical and chemical characteristics may mitigate the side effects of toxic drugs with their controlled release, boost the cutaneous penetration of the drugs through the skin barrier by enhancing the concentration gradient, and efficiently safeguard the drugs from degradation. Here, we concentrate on polymeric nanoparticle-based topical delivery. Most current advancements in the transdermal distribution of polymers and polymeric nanocarriers to ameliorate psoriasis are mentioned in Table **1**.

Table 1. Recent research on polymeric nanoparticles-based treatment for psoriasis.

Type of Polymeric Nanoparticle	Therapeutic Agent	Key Findings	Reference
PLGA nanoparticles	Tazarotene	Tazarotene-loaded nanoparticles displayed greater skin and follicular delivery of the drug than its solution.	[41]
Chitosan nanoparticles	Tacrolimus	Provided increased skin deposition of the drug as compared to the commercial conventional ointment	[42]
Polymeric nanoparticles based hydrogel	Methotrexate	Provided improved bioavailability of the drug.	[43]
Chitosan/hyaluronic acid nanoparticles	Alantolactone	Alantolactone-loaded nanoparticles successfully reduced keratinocyte STAT3 hyperactivation and lessened psoriasis symptoms.	[44]
Lecithin/chitosan hybrid nanoparticles	Tacrolimus	Demonstrated enhanced anti-psoriatic potential compared to the conventional commercial formulation.	[45]
Lipid polymer hybrid nanoparticles	Clobetasol	Revealed markedly higher PASI score, less skin injury, and decreased proliferation than the commercial product.	[46]
PLGA nanoparticles based hydrogel	Curcumin	Curcumin-loaded PLGA nanoparticles exhibited superior anti-psoriatic activity compared to plain curcumin hydrogel.	[47]
Chitosan nanoparticles	Epigallocatechin-3-gallate	Demonstrated improved anti-psoriatic activity compared to the free drug.	[48]

(Table 1) cont.....

Type of Polymeric Nanoparticle	Therapeutic Agent	Key Findings	Reference
Hybrid polymer-lipid nanoparticles	TNFα siRNA	Codelivery of TNFα and siRNA in the form of nanoparticles exhibited improved anti-psoriasis activity.	[49]
Poly[ε-caprolactone] based hydrogel	Hydrocortisone	Demonstrated increased anti-psoriasis activity along with safety.	[50]
PLGA-PEG-PLGA Triblock nanoparticles	Cyclosporin A	Drug-loaded nanoparticles showed decreased levels of TNF-α, IL-22, and IL-17A as compared to the cyclosporin A solution.	[51]

This table presents an overview of recent studies exploring the use of polymeric nanoparticles [PNPs] in psoriasis treatment. It summarizes key findings on various polymeric nanocarrier formulations, the therapeutic agents encapsulated, their mechanisms of action, and the observed benefits over conventional therapies. The table highlights advancements in drug delivery, such as improved bioavailability, enhanced skin penetration, prolonged drug release, and reduced systemic toxicity. By providing insights into the latest research, this table emphasizes the growing potential of PNPs as a promising approach for more effective and safer psoriasis management.

Marketed Formulation

Table **2** summarises the many market items used in the treatment of psoriasis, including the active medication and the manufacturer of the dose type. This table provides a comprehensive summary of commercially available formulations used in psoriasis treatment. It includes details on the active pharmaceutical ingredients [APIs], their respective dosage forms, and the manufacturers. By outlining these marketed products, the table offers insights into the therapeutic options currently available, ranging from topical treatments and systemic therapies to biologics. It also highlights the role of different drug delivery systems in improving treatment efficacy, patient compliance, and minimizing adverse effects.

Table 2. Marketed formulation for the treatment of psoriasis.

Company	Drug	Brand Name	References
Valeant	Methoxalen	Oxsoralen [1%]	[52]
Valeant Astellas	Pimecrolimus and tacrolimus	Elidelprograf [1.5mg]	[53]
LEO pharma	Calcipotriol	Dovonex[0.005%]	[54]
Allergan	Tazarotene	Tazorac[0.1%]	[55]
Biorga	Dithranol	Psoriatec[1%]	[56]

(Table 2) cont.....

Company	Drug	Brand Name	References
Medimetrics	Fluocinolone	Synalar[0.025mg]	[57]
Person and covey	Coal tar	DHS tar [0.5%]	[58]
Merk	Betamethasone	Diprolene[0.05%]	[59]
Allergan indiapvt.Ltd. Cipla Ltd.	Cyclosporine	Restasis[0.4ml] Imusporin[25mg]	[60]
Ranbaxy Laboratories Ltd.	Aciterin	Acrotac[10mg] SandimmunNeoral[50mg/ml]	[61]

CONCLUSION

This chapter underscores the promising potential of nanoparticle-based approaches in revolutionizing the treatment landscape of psoriasis. Through meticulous research and innovative formulations, scientists have harnessed the unique properties of polymeric nanoparticles to enhance drug delivery, prolong therapeutic effects, and mitigate the adverse effects associated with conventional treatments. As we navigate the complexities of psoriasis management, the advent of polymeric nanoparticle technology offers a beacon of hope, promising improved efficacy, patient compliance, and ultimately, a better quality of life for individuals afflicted by this chronic inflammatory condition. Moving forward, continued research will be paramount in these exciting advancements into tangible therapeutic options, thereby reshaping the paradigm of psoriasis treatment for years to come.

REFERENCES

[1] Bowcock AM, Krueger JG. Getting under the skin: the immunogenetics of psoriasis. Nat Rev Immunol 2005; 5(9): 699-711. [http://dx.doi.org/10.1038/nri1689] [PMID: 16138103]

[2] Virmani T, Kumar G, Pathak K. Non-aqueous nanoemulsions: An innovative lipid-based drug carrier. In: Advancements in Controlled Drug Delivery Systems [Internet]. IGI Global; 2022 [cited 2023 Oct 29]. p. 134–58. Available from: https://www.igi-global.com/chapter/non-aqueo-s-nanoemulsions/300404

[3] Virmani R, Virmani T, Singh C, Sorout G, Gupta J. Hidden potential of natural herb *Carissa carandas* (Karonda). Res Pharm Health Sci 2017; 3: 294-302.

[4] van de Kerkhof P, Vissers W. Established treatments of psoriasis. Curr Drug Targets Inflamm Allergy 2004; 3(2): 145-56. [http://dx.doi.org/10.2174/1568010043343967] [PMID: 15180467]

[5] Naldi L, Griffiths CEM. Traditional therapies in the management of moderate to severe chronic plaque psoriasis: an assessment of the benefits and risks. Br J Dermatol 2005; 152(4): 597-615. [http://dx.doi.org/10.1111/j.1365-2133.2005.06563.x] [PMID: 15840088]

[6] Virmani T, Gupta J. Pharmaceutical application of microspheres: an approach for the treatment of various diseases. Int J Pharm Sci Res 2017; 8(8): 3253-60.

[7] Mehnert W, Mäder K. Solid lipid nanoparticles production, characterization and applications. Adv

Drug Deliv Rev 2001; 47(2-3): 165-96.
[http://dx.doi.org/10.1016/S0169-409X(01)00105-3] [PMID: 11311991]

[8] Nanjwade BK, Patel DJ, Udhani RA, Manvi FV. Functions of lipids for enhancement of oral bioavailability of poorly water-soluble drugs. Sci Pharm 2011; 79(4): 705-27.
[http://dx.doi.org/10.3797/scipharm.1105-09] [PMID: 22145101]

[9] Virmani T, Kumar G, Sharma A, *et al.* Amelioration of cancer employing chitosan, its derivatives, and chitosan-based nanoparticles: recent updates. Polymers (Basel) 2023; 15(13): 2928.
[http://dx.doi.org/10.3390/polym15132928] [PMID: 37447573]

[10] Gupta S, Bansal R, Gupta S, Jindal N, Jindal A. Nanocarriers and nanoparticles for skin care and dermatological treatments. Indian Dermatol Online J 2013; 4(4): 267-72.
[http://dx.doi.org/10.4103/2229-5178.120635] [PMID: 24350003]

[11] Virmani T, Kumar G, Virmani R, Sharma A, Pathak K. Nanocarrier-based approaches to combat chronic obstructive pulmonary disease. Nanomedicine (Lond) 2022; 17(24): 1833-54.
[http://dx.doi.org/10.2217/nnm-2021-0403] [PMID: 35856251]

[12] Goy RC, Assis OBG. Antimicrobial analysis of films processed from chitosan and N,N,N-trimethylchitosan. Braz J Chem Eng 2014; 31(3): 643-8.
[http://dx.doi.org/10.1590/0104-6632.20140313s00003014]

[13] Ridolfi F, Renzulli A. Calcic amphiboles in calc-alkaline and alkaline magmas: thermobarometric and chemometric empirical equations valid up to 1,130°C and 2.2 GPa. Contrib Mineral Petrol 2012; 163(5): 877-95.
[http://dx.doi.org/10.1007/s00410-011-0704-6]

[14] Kapoor N, Tran A, Kang J, Zhang R, Philipson KD, Goldhaber JI. Regulation of calcium clock-mediated pacemaking by inositol-1,4,5-trisphosphate receptors in mouse sinoatrial nodal cells. J Physiol 2015; 593(12): 2649-63.
[http://dx.doi.org/10.1113/JP270082] [PMID: 25903031]

[15] Roberts R, Smyth JW, Will J, *et al.* Development of PLGA nanoparticles for sustained release of a connexin43 mimetic peptide to target glioblastoma cells. Mater Sci Eng C 2020; 108: 110191.
[http://dx.doi.org/10.1016/j.msec.2019.110191] [PMID: 31923988]

[16] Li J, Zhuang Y, Zhang Y, Zhang Y, Shen H, Zhang H. Curcumin-loaded polymeric nanomicelles for enhanced treatment of psoriasis. J Biomater Appl. 2021;36(4):707-18.
[http://dx.doi.org/10.1177/08853282211043299] [PMID: 34542884]

[17] Harris JM, Martin NE, Modi M. PEGylation. Clin Pharmacokinet 2001; 40(7): 539-51.
[http://dx.doi.org/10.2165/00003088-200140070-00005] [PMID: 11510630]

[18] Santhanakrishnan KR, Koilpillai J, Narayanasamy D. PEGylation in pharmaceutical development: current status and emerging trends in macromolecular and immunotherapeutic drugs. Cureus 2024; 16(8): e66669.
[http://dx.doi.org/10.7759/cureus.66669] [PMID: 39262507]

[19] Kumar G, Virmani T, Sharma A, Pathak K. Codelivery of phytochemicals with conventional anticancer drugs in form of nanocarriers. Pharmaceutics 2023; 15(3): 889.
[http://dx.doi.org/10.3390/pharmaceutics15030889] [PMID: 36986748]

[20] Veronese FM, Pasut G. PEGylation, successful approach to drug delivery. Drug Discov Today 2005; 10(21): 1451-8.
[http://dx.doi.org/10.1016/S1359-6446(05)03575-0] [PMID: 16243265]

[21] Ukkund S, Alke B, Taqui S, Syed U. Dextran nanoparticles: Preparation and applications. In 2022. p. 1–31.

[22] Banerjee A, Bandopadhyay R. Use of dextran nanoparticle: A paradigm shift in bacterial exopolysaccharide based biomedical applications. Int J Biol Macromol 2016; 87: 295-301.
[http://dx.doi.org/10.1016/j.ijbiomac.2016.02.059] [PMID: 26927936]

[23] Dou H, Xu B, Tao K, Tang M, Sun K. The one-pot synthesis of dextran-based nanoparticles and their application in *in-situ* fabrication of dextran-magnetite nanocomposites. J Mater Sci Mater Med 2008; 19(7): 2575-80.
[http://dx.doi.org/10.1007/s10856-007-3202-7] [PMID: 17665106]

[24] Varshosaz J. Dextran conjugates in drug delivery. Expert Opin Drug Deliv 2012; 9(5): 509-23.
[http://dx.doi.org/10.1517/17425247.2012.673580] [PMID: 22432550]

[25] Lan J, Li Y, Wen J, *et al.* Acitretin-conjugated dextran nanoparticles ameliorate psoriasis-like skin disease at low dosages. Front Bioeng Biotechnol 2022; 9: 816757. Available from: https://www.frontiersin.org/journals/bioengineering-an--biotechnology/articles/10.3389/fbioe.2021.816757/full
[http://dx.doi.org/10.3389/fbioe.2021.816757] [PMID: 35071218]

[26] Panzade P, Puranik PK. Carbopol polymers: a versatile polymer for pharmaceutical applications. Research Journal of Pharmacy and Technology 2010; 3(3): 672-5.

[27] Gaikwad DrV, Yadav V, Dhavale R, Choudhari P, Jadhav S. Effect of carbopol 934 and 940 on fluconazole release from topical gel formulation: a factorial approach. Current Pharma Research 2012; 1(2): 487-93.
[http://dx.doi.org/10.33786/JCPR.2012.v02i02.004]

[28] Mittal S, Ali J, Baboota S. Enhanced anti-psoriatic activity of tacrolimus loaded nanoemulsion gel *via* omega 3 - Fatty acid (EPA and DHA) rich oils-fish oil and linseed oil. J Drug Deliv Sci Technol 2021; 63: 102458.
[http://dx.doi.org/10.1016/j.jddst.2021.102458]

[29] Singh N, Goyal K, Sondhi S, Jindal S. Development and characterization of barbaloin gel for the safe and effective treatment of psoriasis. J Drug Deliv Ther 2020; 10(5): 188-97.
[http://dx.doi.org/10.22270/jddt.v10i5.4299]

[30] Deshmukh K, Ahamed B, Deshmukh R, Pasha SK, Bhagat P, Chidambaram K. Biopolymer composites with high dielectric performance: interface engineering. In: Biopolymer Composites in Electronics. 2017. p. 27–128.

[31] Pan P, Svirskis D, Waterhouse GIN, Wu Z. Hydroxypropyl methylcellulose bioadhesive hydrogels for topical application and sustained drug release: the effect of polyvinylpyrrolidone on the physicomechanical properties of hydrogel. Pharmaceutics 2023; 15(9): 2360.
[http://dx.doi.org/10.3390/pharmaceutics15092360] [PMID: 37765328]

[32] Siepmann J, Peppas NA. Modeling of drug release from delivery systems based on hydroxypropyl methylcellulose (HPMC). Adv Drug Deliv Rev 2001; 48(2-3): 139-57.
[http://dx.doi.org/10.1016/S0169-409X(01)00112-0] [PMID: 11369079]

[33] Jain A, Doppalapudi S, Domb AJ, Khan W. Tacrolimus and curcumin co-loaded liposphere gel: Synergistic combination towards management of psoriasis. J Control Release 2016; 243: 132-45.
[http://dx.doi.org/10.1016/j.jconrel.2016.10.004] [PMID: 27725194]

[34] Kilfoyle BE, Sheihet L, Zhang Z, Laohoo M, Kohn J, Michniak-Kohn BB. Development of paclitaxel-TyroSpheres for topical skin treatment. J Control Release 2012; 163(1): 18-24.
[http://dx.doi.org/10.1016/j.jconrel.2012.06.021] [PMID: 22732474]

[35] Virmani T, Parvez N, Yadav S, Pathak K. Solid inclusion complexes of class II imidazole derivative with β–cyclodextrin. Continental Journal of Pharmaceutical Sciences 2007; 1: 1-8.

[36] Kumari A, Yadav SK, Yadav SC. Biodegradable polymeric nanoparticles based drug delivery systems. Colloids Surf B Biointerfaces 2010; 75(1): 1-18.
[http://dx.doi.org/10.1016/j.colsurfb.2009.09.001] [PMID: 19782542]

[37] Peer D, Karp JM, Hong S, Farokhzad OC, Margalit R, Langer R. Nanocarriers as an emerging platform for cancer therapy. Nat Nanotechnol 2007; 2(12): 751-60.
[http://dx.doi.org/10.1038/nnano.2007.387] [PMID: 18654426]

[38] Kumar A, Garg T, Sarma GS, Rath G, Goyal AK. Optimization of combinational intranasal drug delivery system for the management of migraine by using statistical design. Eur J Pharm Sci 2015; 70: 140-51.
[http://dx.doi.org/10.1016/j.ejps.2015.01.012] [PMID: 25676136]

[39] Abhilash M. Potential applications of nanoparticles. 2010 Jan 1; 1.

[40] Kayser O, Lemke A, Hernández-Trejo N. The impact of nanobiotechnology on the development of new drug delivery systems. Curr Pharm Biotechnol 2005; 6(1): 3-5.
[http://dx.doi.org/10.2174/1389201053167158] [PMID: 15727551]

[41] Kshirsagar SM, Shrestha N, Kipping T, Banga AK. Formulation development of tazarotene-loaded PLGA nanoparticles for follicular delivery in the treatment of inflammatory skin diseases. Eur J Pharm Biopharm 2024; 200: 114346.
[http://dx.doi.org/10.1016/j.ejpb.2024.114346] [PMID: 38823541]

[42] Fereig SA, El-Zaafarany GM, Arafa MG, Abdel-Mottaleb MMA. Tacrolimus-loaded chitosan nanoparticles for enhanced skin deposition and management of plaque psoriasis. Carbohydr Polym 2021; 268: 118238.
[http://dx.doi.org/10.1016/j.carbpol.2021.118238] [PMID: 34127220]

[43] Asad MI, Khan D, Rehman A, Elaissari A, Ahmed N. Development and in *vitro/in vivo* evaluation of ph-sensitive polymeric nanoparticles loaded hydrogel for the management of psoriasis. Nanomaterials (Basel) 2021; 11(12): 3433.
[http://dx.doi.org/10.3390/nano11123433] [PMID: 34947782]

[44] Chen R, Zhai YY, Sun L, *et al.* Alantolactone-loaded chitosan/hyaluronic acid nanoparticles suppress psoriasis by deactivating STAT3 pathway and restricting immune cell recruitment. Asian Journal of Pharmaceutical Sciences 2022; 17(2): 268-83.
[http://dx.doi.org/10.1016/j.ajps.2022.02.003] [PMID: 35582636]

[45] Fereig SA, El-Zaafarany GM, Arafa MG, Abdel-Mottaleb MMA. Self-assembled tacrolimus-loaded lecithin-chitosan hybrid nanoparticles for *in vivo* management of psoriasis. Int J Pharm 2021; 608: 121114.
[http://dx.doi.org/10.1016/j.ijpharm.2021.121114] [PMID: 34543618]

[46] Pukale SS, Sharma S, Dalela M, *et al.* Multi-component clobetasol-loaded monolithic lipid-polymer hybrid nanoparticles ameliorate imiquimod-induced psoriasis-like skin inflammation in *Swiss albino* mice. Acta Biomater 2020; 115: 393-409.
[http://dx.doi.org/10.1016/j.actbio.2020.08.020] [PMID: 32846238]

[47] Sun L, Liu Z, Wang L, *et al.* Enhanced topical penetration, system exposure and anti-psoriasis activity of two particle-sized, curcumin-loaded PLGA nanoparticles in hydrogel. J Control Release 2017; 254: 44-54.
[http://dx.doi.org/10.1016/j.jconrel.2017.03.385] [PMID: 28344018]

[48] Chamcheu JC, Siddiqui IA, Adhami VM, *et al.* Chitosan-based nanoformulated (–)-epigallocatechi--3-gallate (EGCG) modulates human keratinocyte-induced responses and alleviates imiquimod-induced murine psoriasiform dermatitis. Int J Nanomedicine 2018; 13: 4189-206.
[http://dx.doi.org/10.2147/IJN.S165966] [PMID: 30057446]

[49] Suzuki IL, de Araujo MM, Bagnato VS, Bentley MVLB. TNFα siRNA delivery by nanoparticles and photochemical internalization for psoriasis topical therapy. J Control Release 2021; 338: 316-29.
[http://dx.doi.org/10.1016/j.jconrel.2021.08.039] [PMID: 34437914]

[50] Kondiah PPD, Rants'o TA, Mdanda S, Mohlomi LM, Choonara YE. A poly (caprolactone)-cellulose nanocomposite hydrogel for transdermal delivery of hydrocortisone in treating psoriasis vulgaris. Polymers (Basel) 2022; 14(13): 2633.
[http://dx.doi.org/10.3390/polym14132633] [PMID: 35808678]

[51] Kagawa A, Sato A, Makino K, Takeuchi I. Therapeutic effects of 30 nm cyclosporin a-loaded

nanoparticles using PLGA-PEG-PLGA triblock copolymer for transdermal delivery in mouse models of psoriasis. Appl Sci (Basel) 2024; 14(9): 3791.
[http://dx.doi.org/10.3390/app14093791]

[52] Rishi P, Maitray A. Methoxsalen-induced macular toxicity. Indian J Ophthalmol 2017; 65(11): 1243-5.
[http://dx.doi.org/10.4103/ijo.IJO_413_17] [PMID: 29133667]

[53] Yin Z, Xu J, Luo D. Efficacy and tolerance of tacrolimus and pimecrolimus for atopic dermatitis: a meta-analysis. J Biomed Res 2011; 25(6): 385-91.
[http://dx.doi.org/10.1016/S1674-8301(11)60051-1] [PMID: 23554715]

[54] Meth MJ, Weinberg JM. Cyclopamine: inhibiting hedgehog in the treatment of psoriasis. Cutis 2006; 78(3): 185-8.
[PMID: 17036662]

[55] Tas S, Avci O. Use of cyclopamine in the treatment of psoriasis [Internet]. US7605167B2, 2009 [cited 2024 Apr 20]. Available from: https://patents.google.com/patent/US7605167B2/en

[56] Benezeder T, Painsi C, Patra V, *et al.* Dithranol targets keratinocytes, their crosstalk with neutrophils and inhibits the IL-36 inflammatory loop in psoriasis. eLife 2020; 9: e56991.
[http://dx.doi.org/10.7554/eLife.56991] [PMID: 32484435]

[57] Kanee B. Clinical studies with topical fluocinolone acetonide in the treatment of various dermatoses. Can Med Assoc J 1963; 88(20): 999-1003.
[PMID: 13962197]

[58] Sekhon S, Jeon C, Nakamura M, *et al.* Review of the mechanism of action of coal tar in psoriasis. J Dermatolog Treat 2018; 29(3): 230-2.
[http://dx.doi.org/10.1080/09546634.2017.1369494] [PMID: 28814117]

[59] Sidgiddi S, Pakunlu RI, Allenby K. Efficacy, safety, and potency of betamethasone dipropionate spray 0.05%: A treatment for adults with mild-to-moderate plaque psoriasis. J Clin Aesthet Dermatol 2018; 11(4): 14-22.
[PMID: 29657667]

[60] Rajagopalan M, Saraswat A, Chandrashekar B, *et al.* Role of cyclosporine (CsA) in immuno-dermatological conditions. Indian Dermatol Online J 2022; 13(5): 585-99.
[http://dx.doi.org/10.4103/idoj.idoj_189_22] [PMID: 36304637]

[61] Pai V, Phadke D, Shukla P, Naik K. Fixed tapering dosage of acitretin in patients with psoriasis: A short-term analysis of clinical efficacy and its effects on biochemical parameters. Indian J Dermatol 2019; 64(3): 213-6.
[http://dx.doi.org/10.4103/ijd.IJD_300_18] [PMID: 31148860]

CHAPTER 12

Metallic Nanoparticles-Based Pharmacotherapy for the Management of Psoriasis

Anjali Mishra[1], **Manisha Bhatia**[1], **Manish Kumar**[2,*] and **G.T. Kulkarni**[3]

[1] *M.M. College of Pharmacy, Maharishi Markandeshwar (Deemed to be University), Mullana, Ambala 133207, Haryana, India*

[2] *Department of Pharmaceutics, ISF College of Pharmacy, Moga 142001, Punjab, India*

[3] *Faculty of Pharmacy, DIT University, Dehradun, Uttarakhand, India*

Abstract: Psoriasis, a chronic inflammatory skin disease, presents a significant therapeutic challenge. Conventional treatments often exhibit limited efficacy and adverse effects. This chapter examines the potential of metallic nanoparticles as a promising approach for managing psoriasis. By harnessing the unique properties of these nanoparticle-based pharmacotherapies, researchers have developed innovative drug delivery systems and therapeutic strategies. These nanoparticles offer advantages such as enhanced drug bioavailability, targeted delivery, and sustained release, leading to improved clinical outcomes. This chapter discusses the current state-of-the-art in metallic nanoparticle-based therapies for psoriasis, highlighting their mechanisms of action, potential benefits, and challenges. Furthermore, this chapter emphasizes the importance of addressing safety and toxicity concerns associated with metallic nanoparticles. While preclinical studies have demonstrated promising results, rigorous evaluation of their long-term effects and biocompatibility is crucial before widespread clinical application. Future research should focus on optimizing nanoparticle formulations, exploring combination therapies, and conducting well-designed clinical trials to establish the efficacy and safety of these nanomaterials in psoriasis management.

Keywords: Drug delivery, Metallic nanoparticles, Psoriasis, Psoriasis management, Skin disease.

INTRODUCTION

Psoriasis, a chronic autoimmune skin disease characterized by excessive inflammation and rapid skin cell turnover, presents significant challenges in long-term management. While current therapies offer relief, limitations exist, including

* **Corresponding author Manish Kumar:** Department of Pharmaceutics, ISF College of Pharmacy, Moga 142001, Punjab, India; E-mail: manish_singh17@rediffmail.com

side effects, lack of sustained efficacy, and difficulty in targeting specific cell types. Metallic nanoparticles (NPs) are emerging as a promising approach for treating psoriasis. This chapter explores the potential of AuNPs, AgNPs, and other metallic NPs for enhanced drug delivery, targeted therapy, and modulation of the inflammatory response in psoriatic lesions. We will discuss the mechanisms of action, recent clinical studies, remaining challenges, and future directions of metallic NP-based pharmacotherapy for improved psoriasis management.

Psoriasis: Overview and Burden

Psoriasis is a chronic, immune-mediated inflammatory skin condition that affects around 2% of the worldwide population [1]. It manifests as raised, red, scaly plaques typically on the elbows, knees, scalp, and lower back [2]. Psoriasis goes beyond a skin condition, significantly impacting patients' quality of life. Itching, burning, and pain associated with the lesions can cause significant discomfort and sleep disturbances [3]. The psychological burden is substantial, with increased rates of depression, anxiety, and social isolation due to the visible nature of the disease [4]. Furthermore, psoriasis is linked to an increased risk of developing comorbidities like cardiovascular disease, metabolic syndrome, and depression, highlighting its systemic impact [5]. Psoriasis represents a significant healthcare burden, with high costs associated with treatment and lost productivity. With no cure currently available, the focus lies on effective management strategies to improve patients' quality of life and well-being.

Current Psoriasis Treatments: Limitations and Challenges

Current treatment options for psoriasis offer varying degrees of success, but all have limitations. Topical corticosteroids are often the first line of defence, effective for mild to moderate cases but with potential for side effects like skin thinning with long-term use [6]. Systemic medications like methotrexate and cyclosporine can be highly effective but come with a risk of serious side effects requiring close monitoring [7]. Biologic therapies, a newer class of drugs targeting specific inflammatory pathways, have revolutionized treatment for moderate to severe psoriasis. However, these medications can be expensive, require injection or infusion, and may lose effectiveness over time, necessitating a switch to a different biologic [8]. Additionally, some patients with psoriasis do not respond well to any of the currently available treatments, highlighting the need for novel therapeutic approaches.

Promise of Nanomedicine in Psoriasis Management

Psoriasis, a chronic inflammatory skin disease, presents a significant challenge in achieving long-term control. Current therapies, while effective in some cases, have limitations including side effects, lack of sustained efficacy, and difficulty targeting specific cell types. Nanomedicine, utilizing nanoparticles (NPs) in the 1-100 nanometre range, offers a promising avenue for overcoming these limitations [9]. NPs possess unique properties that make them ideal for psoriasis treatment. Their small size allows for deeper penetration into psoriatic lesions, enhancing drug delivery and potentially reducing systemic side effects [10]. Additionally, NPs can be functionalized to target specific cell types within the lesion, such as activated immune cells, for a more localized therapeutic effect [11].

Metallic nanoparticles, like gold and silver nanoparticles (AuNPs and AgNPs), are particularly promising due to their inherent anti-inflammatory and anti-proliferative properties, potentially offering therapeutic benefits beyond simple drug delivery [12]. Studies suggest these NPs can modulate the immune response, reduce inflammation, and inhibit the excessive growth of keratinocytes, key factors in psoriatic plaques [13]. Nanomedicine holds immense potential for revolutionizing the treatment of psoriasis. By combining targeted drug delivery, enhanced therapeutic efficacy, and potentially reduced side effects, metallic NPs offer a novel approach for improved patient outcomes and disease management.

METALLIC NANOPARTICLES FOR PSORIASIS TREATMENT

Metallic nanoparticles (NPs), like gold and silver nanoparticles (Fig. **1**), are emerging as a potential game-changer in psoriasis treatment. Their small size allows for deeper penetration into psoriatic lesions, potentially delivering drugs more effectively and reducing side effects. Beyond drug delivery, these NPs possess inherent anti-inflammatory and anti-proliferative properties. Studies suggest they can modulate the immune response, decrease inflammation, and inhibit excessive skin cell growth, all key contributors to psoriatic plaques. This unique combination of targeted delivery and therapeutic benefits makes metallic NPs a promising avenue for improved psoriasis management.

Types of Metallic Nanoparticles for Psoriasis

Gold Nanoparticles (AuNPs)

Gold nanoparticles (AuNPs) have become a star player in the field of nanomedicine due to their unique properties and potential applications in various diseases. These nanoparticles are essentially gold particles sized between 1-100 nanometres, offering a fascinating combination of physical, chemical, and biological characteristics [14]. One of the key advantages of AuNPs is their biocompatibility. Unlike some other nanoparticles, AuNPs exhibit minimal toxicity in human cells, making them a promising candidate for drug delivery systems [15]. Additionally, AuNPs possess a tunable surface chemistry, allowing them to be customized with various molecules for targeted therapy [16]. AuNPs hold immense potential for diagnostics and therapeutics. Their ability to interact with light makes them useful for imaging techniques like photothermal therapy, where they can be used to target and destroy diseased cells upon exposure to light [17]. Furthermore, AuNPs can be conjugated with drugs or biomolecules for targeted drug delivery, potentially reducing systemic side effects and enhancing therapeutic efficacy [18].

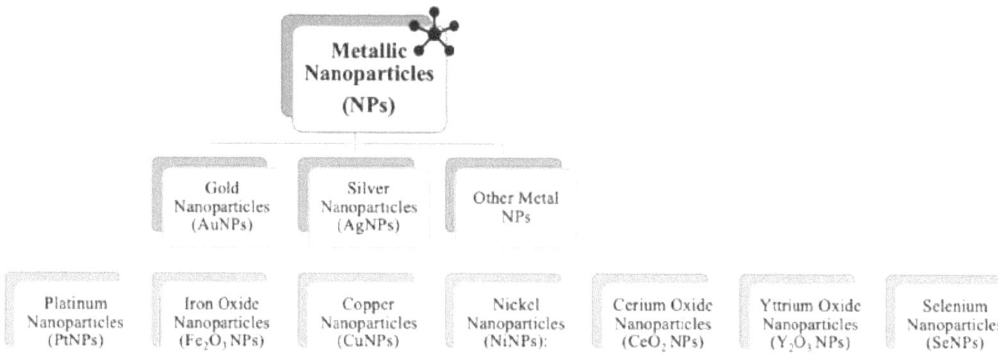

Fig. (1). Types of metallic nanoparticles.

Research on AuNPs is rapidly expanding, with ongoing exploration for applications in cancer treatment, infectious diseases, and gene therapy [19]. However, challenges remain. Long-term safety and biodistribution of AuNPs require further investigation [20]. Additionally, optimizing large-scale production and ensuring cost-effectiveness are crucial for widespread clinical use. Despite these challenges, AuNPs offer a bright future for nanomedicine. Their unique properties and versatility hold immense potential for revolutionizing disease diagnosis and treatment.

Silver Nanoparticles (AgNPs)

Silver nanoparticles (AgNPs) have garnered significant interest in the realm of nanomedicine due to their potent antimicrobial properties. These nanoparticles, typically ranging from 1-100 nanometres in size, exhibit a broad spectrum of activity against bacteria, viruses, and fungi [21]. This makes them attractive candidates for various applications, including wound healing, disinfection, and combating infectious diseases [22].

The antimicrobial efficacy of AgNPs stems from their ability to interact with microbial membranes, disrupt their function, and ultimately lead to cell death [23]. Additionally, AgNPs possess anti-inflammatory properties, potentially offering benefits in wound healing and inflammatory skin conditions [24]. However, the very properties that make AgNPs attractive also raise concerns. Silver ions released from these nanoparticles can be cytotoxic, potentially harming healthy human cells alongside microbes [25]. This cytotoxicity necessitates careful consideration of dosage and potential side effects when exploring AgNPs for therapeutic applications [26]. Furthermore, concerns exist regarding the environmental impact of AgNPs. Their release into the environment could disrupt ecosystems and potentially contribute to the development of antibiotic-resistant bacteria [27]. Strict regulations and responsible production practices are crucial to ensure the safe use of AgNPs. In conclusion, AgNPs offer a promising avenue for combating infections and potentially managing inflammatory conditions. However, their cytotoxicity and environmental impact require careful consideration. Continued research is needed to optimize their therapeutic benefits while mitigating potential risks.

Other Metallic Nanoparticles

While gold and silver nanoparticles (AuNPs and AgNPs) have garnered significant attention in nanomedicine, other metallic nanoparticles are emerging as promising candidates for various therapeutic applications. Here, we explore some of these possibilities, highlighting their potential benefits and ongoing research.

- Platinum Nanoparticles (PtNPs):

Platinum nanoparticles (PtNPs) hold particular interest in cancer treatment due to their unique catalytic properties. They can be used in a process called "tumour catalytic therapy" where PtNPs are delivered to tumours and activated with light or ultrasound. This activation triggers the production of Reactive Oxygen Species (ROS) that can destroy cancer cells [28]. Additionally, PtNPs are being explored for drug delivery applications due to their ability to be conjugated with therapeutic molecules and released in a controlled manner. Recent studies explore the potential of platinum nanoparticles as topical drug delivery systems for improved management of psoriasis [29].

- Iron Oxide Nanoparticles (Fe_2O_3NPs):

Iron oxide nanoparticles (Fe_2O_3NPs) offer unique advantages in diagnostics and therapeutics. Their magnetic properties allow them to be manipulated using external magnetic fields, enabling targeted drug delivery to specific sites within the body [30]. Additionally, IONPs can be used for Magnetic Resonance Imaging (MRI), providing a tool for disease diagnosis and monitoring treatment progress.

Studies suggest iron oxide nanoparticles may possess inherent anti-inflammatory properties, potentially aiding in reducing psoriasis symptoms [31].

• Copper Nanoparticles (CuNPs):

Copper nanoparticles (CuNPs) exhibit potent antimicrobial properties similar to AgNPs but may offer advantages in terms of biocompatibility [32]. Research suggests CuNPs can be effective against a broad spectrum of bacteria, including antibiotic-resistant strains. Additionally, CuNPs possess anti-inflammatory properties, making them potentially useful for treating inflammatory skin conditions like psoriasis.

• Nickel Nanoparticles (NiNPs):

Research on NiNPs for psoriasis management is limited. However, some studies suggest their potential for antimicrobial activity, which could be beneficial in managing secondary infections associated with psoriasis [33]. However, safety concerns regarding nickel cytotoxicity and potential allergic reactions necessitate further investigation before clinical applications can be considered [34].

• Cerium Oxide Nanoparticles (CeO_2 NPs):

CeO_2 NPs possess antioxidant and anti-inflammatory properties, potentially offering benefits in psoriasis treatment [35]. Studies suggest CeO_2 NPs can scavenge free radicals and modulate inflammatory pathways, potentially reducing psoriatic plaque formation [36]. However, further research is needed to determine optimal dosages and delivery methods for safe and effective use in psoriasis patients [37].

• Yttrium Oxide Nanoparticles (Y_2O_3 NPs):

Y_2O_3 NPs are being explored for their potential wound healing properties. Psoriasis can lead to impaired skin barrier function and chronic wounds. Studies suggest Y_2O_3 NPs may promote wound healing by stimulating collagen synthesis and cell proliferation. However, more research is required to understand the specific effects of Y_2O_3 NPs on psoriatic lesions and their safety profile in this context [38].

- Selenium Nanoparticles (SeNPs):

SeNPs exhibit antioxidant and anti-inflammatory properties similar to CeO_2 NPs. Studies suggest SeNPs may improve skin health and reduce inflammation. However, the specific effects of SeNPs on psoriasis require further investigation. Additionally, the potential for selenium toxicity necessitates careful consideration of dosage and administration routes.

Advantages of Metallic Nanoparticles for Psoriasis Therapy

Psoriasis, a chronic inflammatory skin condition, poses a significant challenge due to limitations of current treatments. Metallic nanoparticles (NPs) emerge as a promising avenue to overcome these limitations, offering several advantages:

- Enhanced Drug Delivery: Metallic NPs, typically sized 1-100 nanometres, can penetrate deeper into psoriatic lesions compared to traditional medications [39]. This targeted delivery allows for lower drug doses, potentially reducing systemic side effects associated with oral or topical medications [40]. Studies suggest NPs can be loaded with corticosteroids or other anti-psoriatic drugs, improving drug efficacy at the site of inflammation [41].
- Inherent Therapeutic Properties: Certain metallic NPs, like gold (AuNPs) and silver (AgNPs), possess inherent anti-inflammatory and anti-proliferative properties [42]. AuNPs have been shown to modulate the immune response, potentially reducing inflammation in psoriatic plaques [43]. AgNPs exhibit antimicrobial activity, potentially providing additional benefits in managing secondary infections associated with psoriasis.
- Targeted Therapy: Metallic NPs can be functionalized with specific molecules that target activated immune cells within psoriatic lesions. This targeted approach allows for a localized therapeutic effect, minimizing damage to healthy tissues compared to traditional broad-spectrum medications.
- Combination Therapy: Metallic NPs can be combined with existing psoriasis treatments, potentially improving overall efficacy. For example, NPs loaded with corticosteroids could be used alongside phototherapy, potentially offering a more potent therapeutic approach with reduced reliance on high drug doses.

MECHANISMS OF ACTION OF METALLIC NANOPARTICLES IN PSORIASIS

Psoriasis, a chronic autoimmune inflammatory skin disease, is characterized by excessive inflammation and rapid skin cell turnover. Current therapies offer varying degrees of success but have limitations. Metallic nanoparticles (NPs) present a promising approach due to their unique properties and potential mechanisms of action (Fig. **2**) in psoriasis. Here, we delve into the key mechanisms by which metallic NPs might influence psoriatic lesions:

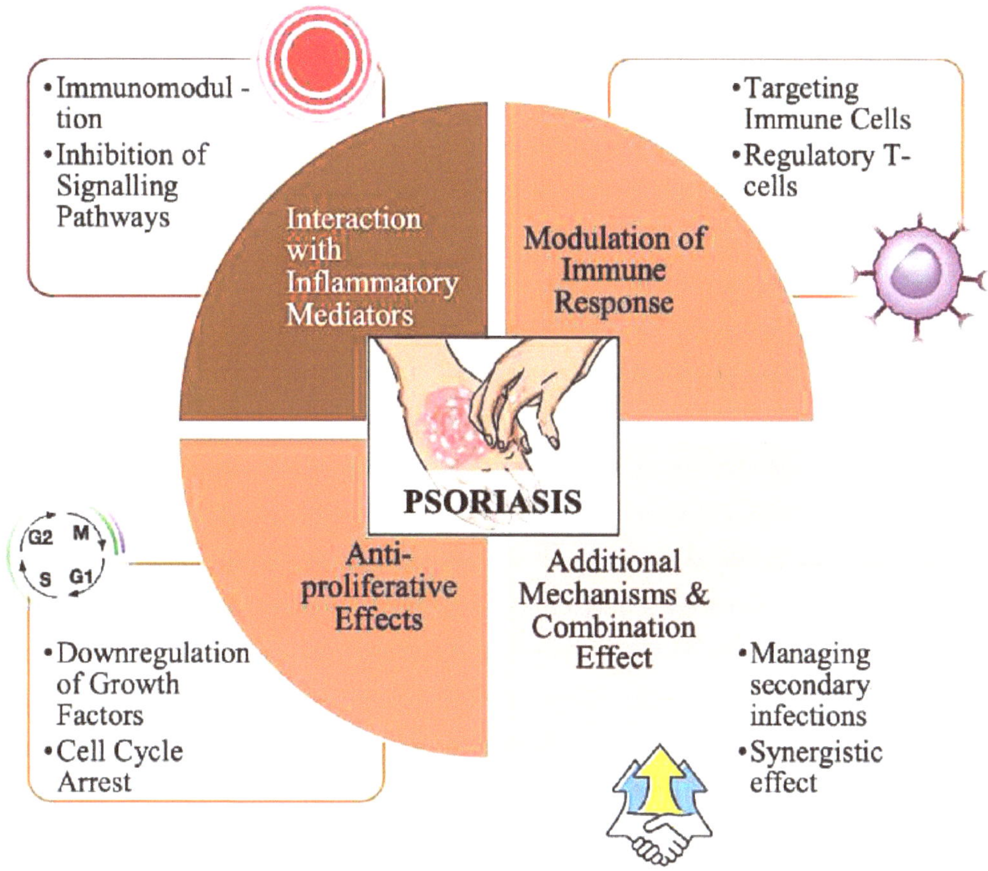

Fig. (2). Mechanism of Action of Metallic NPs for Psoriasis.

Interaction with Inflammatory Mediators

Psoriasis is driven by an overactive immune response, with the release of pro-inflammatory cytokines and infiltration of immune cells into the skin. Metallic NPs can interact with these inflammatory mediators in several ways:

- Immunomodulation: Certain NPs, like AuNPs, have been shown to downregulate the production of pro-inflammatory cytokines such as TNF-alpha and IL-17. This can help to dampen the inflammatory response and reduce psoriatic plaque formation [44].
- Inhibition of Signalling Pathways: NPs can interfere with specific signalling pathways involved in inflammation. For example, studies suggest AgNPs might

inhibit the NF-κB pathway, a key regulator of inflammatory gene expression [45].

Modulation of Immune Response

Psoriatic lesions are heavily infiltrated by immune cells like T-lymphocytes. Metallic NPs can modulate the immune response by:

- Targeting Immune Cells: NPs can be functionalized with antibodies or other targeting moieties to specifically interact with activated immune cells within the psoriatic plaque [46]. This targeted approach can suppress the activity of these pro-inflammatory cells.
- Regulatory T-cells: Some NPs may promote the activity of regulatory T-cells, which play a crucial role in dampening the immune response. This can help to restore immune balance and alleviate psoriatic inflammation [47].

Anti-proliferative Effects

Psoriasis is characterized by excessive keratinocyte proliferation in the skin. Metallic NPs can exert anti-proliferative effects through various mechanisms:

- Downregulation of Growth Factors: NPs may inhibit the expression or activity of growth factors like keratinocyte growth factor (KGF), which stimulate keratinocyte proliferation [48].
- Cell Cycle Arrest: Studies suggest some NPs can induce cell cycle arrest in keratinocytes, preventing their uncontrolled proliferation.

Additional Mechanisms

Metallic NPs like AgNPs possess inherent antimicrobial properties, potentially beneficial in managing secondary infections associated with psoriasis. Furthermore, certain NPs may enhance skin barrier function, potentially improving overall skin health in patients with psoriasis.

Combination Effects

It is important to consider the potential for combined effects of metallic NPs. For instance, NPs loaded with anti-inflammatory drugs might not only deliver the drug but also exert their own immunomodulatory effects, leading to a synergistic therapeutic outcome.

PRE-CLINICAL AND CLINICAL STUDIES

Pre-Clinical Studies

Psoriasis, a chronic inflammatory skin condition, seeks novel therapeutic approaches. Metallic nanoparticles (NPs) with their unique properties hold promise for improved psoriasis management (Table **1**). Pre-clinical studies play a vital role in evaluating the potential of a drug before human trials.

Table 1. Pre-clinical studies of metallic nps for psoriasis management.

S. No.	Metallic Nanoparticle (NPs)	Findings	Refs.
1.	Gold, Silver, Titanium Dioxide, Selenium, and Zinc Oxide NPs	Psoriasis is a serious inflammatory disease with limited treatment options due to side effects. Nanoparticles offer promise for targeted drug delivery, reducing side effects and improving treatment efficacy. Metal-based nanoparticles with anti-inflammatory properties are being explored for psoriasis treatment, with research focusing on delivery methods and mechanisms of action.	[49]
2.	Nanoparticles	Psoriasis is a common autoimmune skin condition affecting millions globally. Current treatments offer some relief, but a complete cure remains elusive. This review explores the potential of nanoparticles for targeted drug delivery in psoriasis treatment. Nanoparticles offer advantages like improved drug delivery and reduced side effects compared to conventional methods. Research suggests that nanoparticles could significantly enhance the effectiveness of existing psoriasis treatments.	[50]
3.	Cerium Oxide NPs	This research investigates the potential protective effects of cerium oxide nanoparticles (CeO_2NPs) against chemically induced damage in mice and rats. The study explores CeO_2NPs' ability to: - Reduce liver and testicular damage caused by specific chemicals. - Protect against mammary gland issues. - Offer antioxidant and anti-inflammatory benefits in these tissues. The findings suggest CeO_2NPs might hold promise for mitigating some types of organ damage, but further research is needed to fully understand their safety and efficacy.	[51]
4.	Gold, Copper Oxide, Platinum, Ceria, and Zinc Oxide NPs	Metallic nanoparticles offer a promising alternative to the limited treatments currently available. These nanoparticles are small enough to deliver anti-inflammatory properties directly to the affected area and can be tracked to monitor their effectiveness. While research is ongoing, metal-based nanoparticles show potential for future treatment of inflammatory diseases like psoriasis.	[52]

(Table 1) cont.....

S. No.	Metallic Nanoparticle (NPs)	Findings	Refs.
5.	Lecithin–Chitosan Nanoparticles *via* Hybridization with Gold Nanoparticles	Researchers investigated using gold nanoparticles to improve the delivery of existing anti-psoriasis medications. They attached gold nanoparticles to existing successful formulations like tacrolimus-loaded nanoparticles. Animal studies showed that gold nanoparticle conjugates improved the anti-inflammatory effects of the medications in a psoriasis model, suggesting promise for this approach in future psoriasis treatments.	[53]
6.	Selenium NPs	This study explores using selenium nanoparticles (SeNPs) as a potential treatment. SeNPs were shown to reduce inflammation and cell proliferation in a psoriasis model, suggesting they might be a promising candidate for future psoriasis therapies with fewer side effects.	[54]
7.	Gold, Silver and Platinum NPs	This review highlighted that these nanoparticles target immune cells in psoriatic lesions without harming healthy skin cells. Studies suggest they can decrease inflammatory molecules and suppress pathways involved in psoriasis. Early research shows promise for their effectiveness and reduced side effects compared to current treatments.	[55]
8.	Silver NPs	Silver nanoparticles (AgNPs) hold promise for treating psoriasis due to their anti-inflammatory effects. Studies show AgNPs can reduce inflammatory molecules like TNF-α and IL-1β in skin cells, potentially mimicking the effects of anti-inflammatory drugs. Research suggests AgNPs might specifically target immune cells in psoriatic lesions, further reducing inflammation without harming healthy skin. Early findings from cell and animal studies, as well as a clinical trial, indicate AgNPs could be a future psoriasis treatment with fewer side effects.	[56]
9.	Titanium Dioxide NPs	Titanium dioxide nanoparticles (TiO_2 NPs) are being explored for use in photodynamic therapy (PDT), a treatment that uses light to kill cells. When exposed to ultraviolet light, TiO_2 NPs generate Reactive Oxygen Species (ROS) that can damage and kill cells. This approach shows promise for treating various skin conditions like psoriasis and even cancer cells. Researchers are exploring ways to improve TiO_2 NPs for targeted therapy in medicine.	[57]
10.	Cyclodextrin-Modified CeO_2 NPs	This study explores cerium oxide nanoparticles (β-CDs/CeO_2 NPs) as a potential treatment for psoriasis. These nanoparticles act as antioxidants, mimicking enzymes that clear harmful molecules in the skin. They can also carry anti-psoriasis drugs (like dithranol) and release them slowly. Early research in mice suggests these nanoparticles may be effective in reducing inflammation and improving psoriasis symptoms.	[58]

(Table 1) cont.....

S. No.	Metallic Nanoparticle (NPs)	Findings	Refs.
11.	Silver NPs	Silver nanoparticles show promise for various medical applications, including treating psoriasis. However, more research is needed before they can be safely used in humans. While studies suggest silver nanoparticles have potential benefits, large-scale production methods and potential side effects need to be addressed. Toxicity is a major concern, and researchers need to thoroughly investigate how these nanoparticles interact with the body and how they are eliminated. Only a few studies have explored the safety of bio-synthesized silver nanoparticles, which are seen as a promising option for future psoriasis treatment.	[59]
12.	Silver, Gold, Zinc Oxide, Titanium Dioxide, and Selenium NPs	Metallic nanoparticles are being explored as a new approach to treat inflammation, including psoriasis because of the fact that traditional treatments for inflammation have limitations. These metallic nanoparticles are being studied for their potential due to their small size and ability to enter cells. This review study focuses on how these nanoparticles are made from natural sources (green synthesis) and how they reduce inflammation in different ways.	[60]
13.	silver and gold nanoparticles complexed with *Cornus mas*	Researchers investigated how nanoparticles made from silver and gold, combined with an extract from the Cornelian cherry (*Cornus mas*), reduced inflammation in psoriasis. These nanoparticles were applied topically and targeted at inflammatory cells in the skin. Lab studies and analysis of skin from psoriasis patients showed that the nanoparticles significantly reduced inflammatory molecules and markers. This suggests these "green" nanoparticles could be a new psoriasis treatment that avoids side effects associated with some current medications.	[61]
14.	Silver and Gold Nanoparticles Complexed with Polyphenolic Compounds	Psoriasis is an inflammatory skin disease where immune cells called macrophages release inflammatory molecules that worsen the condition. Current medications that target these molecules can cause serious side effects. This study explores nanoparticles made from silver and gold combined with a natural extract. The researchers applied these nanoparticles topically to patients with psoriasis. The nanoparticles significantly reduced inflammation in the skin by targeting and reducing the number of macrophages. Lab studies support these findings and suggest the nanoparticles work by blocking the pathway that activates macrophages and reducing their production of inflammatory molecules. This new approach offers promise for a safe and effective psoriasis treatment with fewer side effects than current medications.	[62]

(Table 1) cont.....

S. No.	Metallic Nanoparticle (NPs)	Findings	Refs.
15.	Silver NPs	This study discusses the potential negative effects of silver nanoparticles (Ag-NP) on the immune system, highlighting the following: - Silver nanoparticles are widely used, but concerns exist about their safety. - A previous study showed Ag-NP exposure harms immune system function in rats. - This study focused on how Ag-NP exposure affects the body's ability to produce antibodies in response to a vaccine. - The results confirm that Ag-NP exposure weakens the immune response, suggesting potential health risks. - The study highlights the importance of thorough testing to assess the safety of nanoparticles.	[63]
16.	Silver NPs	Researchers investigated the safety of AgNPs by injecting them into rats. The results showed liver damage and chromosomal abnormalities in the bone marrow at higher doses, suggesting that AgNPs might be toxic at high levels. This study highlights the importance of safety assessments when considering using nanoparticles in medicine.	[64]
17.	Silver NPs	This study explored the safety of silver nanoparticles (AgNPs) for potential medical uses. They injected AgNPs at various doses into rats. While the lower doses (less than 10mg/kg) didn't cause harm, higher doses (more than 20mg/kg) resulted in negative effects like liver damage, blood cell abnormalities, and DNA damage. This suggests that AgNPs might be safe for medical applications, but only at very low doses. The study highlights the importance of finding the right dosage to avoid negative side effects when considering AgNPs for treatments like psoriasis.	[65]
18.	Cerium Oxide NPs	This study explores cerium oxide nanoparticles as a potential treatment for inflammation, including psoriasis. Nanoceria can act like antioxidants, potentially reducing harmful free radicals involved in inflammation. Lab studies in mouse cells showed they were non-toxic and reduced inflammatory molecules. Animal studies suggest they are well tolerated and may offer a new approach to treating chronic inflammatory diseases like psoriasis.	[66]

Exploring the Potential of Metallic NPs

Pre-clinical studies investigate the therapeutic potential of various metallic NPs in psoriasis. Here are some key areas of exploration:

- Anti-inflammatory effects: Studies assess the ability of NPs to modulate the immune response, potentially reducing inflammation within psoriatic lesions.
- Targeted drug delivery: Researchers explore using NPs as carriers for existing

psoriasis medications. This could enhance drug delivery to the affected area, minimizing side effects associated with systemic treatments.

- Antimicrobial properties: Certain metallic NPs possess inherent antimicrobial activity. Pre-clinical studies investigate whether these NPs can target bacteria associated with psoriasis, potentially contributing to symptom improvement.
- Safety evaluation: A crucial aspect of pre-clinical studies is assessing the safety profile of metallic NPs. This includes investigating potential cytotoxicity, immune reactions, and long-term toxicity concerns.

Methods of Exploration

- Cellular models: Skin cells and immune cells are cultured in a lab setting to analyze the interactions of NPs with these cells and their impact on relevant cellular pathways in psoriasis.
- Animal models: Mice with induced psoriatic symptoms are used to test the therapeutic efficacy and safety of NPs in a whole organism. These models allow researchers to observe the effects of NPs on disease progression and potential side effects.

Benefits of Pre-clinical Studies

- Optimize NP design: Pre-clinical studies help identify the optimal size, shape, surface properties, and composition of NPs to maximize their therapeutic effects and minimize potential risks.
- Inform clinical trial design: The data collected from pre-clinical studies informs the design of future clinical trials, establishing safe dosages, delivery methods, and potential outcomes to be measured in human studies.
- Reduce risk in human trials: By identifying potential safety concerns early on, pre-clinical studies ensure a more ethical and safer approach to testing these novel therapies in humans.

Clinical Trials: Current Status and Future Directions

Clinical trials are the cornerstone of medical advancement, rigorously evaluating the safety and efficacy of new drugs, treatments, and medical devices in humans. Understanding the current landscape and future directions of clinical trials is crucial for progress in healthcare.

Current Status

- Growth and Efficiency: The number of registered clinical trials globally has been steadily increasing, indicating a robust pipeline of potential new therapies. More research on humans with psoriasis is needed. Most studies so far have only used animals or cells to mimic the condition.

- Standardization and Transparency: Efforts are underway to standardize clinical trial protocols and reporting, aiming for greater transparency and generalizability of results.
- Diversity and Inclusion: A growing emphasis is placed on including more diverse patient populations in clinical trials to ensure generalizability and address the specific needs of underrepresented groups.
- Technology Integration: Advancements in digital technologies like Electronic Health Records (EHRs) and telemedicine are facilitating remote data collection and patient monitoring within trials, improving efficiency and accessibility.

Researchers investigated nanoparticles loaded with an extract from Cornelian cherry (*Cornus mas*) for treating psoriasis. They tested these nanoparticles in several stages: first in the lab using cells that mimic inflamed psoriatic skin, then on actual skin biopsies from psoriasis patients, and finally in a clinical trial with people who have psoriasis. Both silver and gold nanoparticles significantly reduced inflammatory molecules in all stages of testing. The nanoparticles appear to target immune cells in the skin (macrophages) and prevent them from releasing harmful molecules that worsen psoriasis. This approach, using nanoparticles and a natural extract, shows promise as a new psoriasis treatment [62].

Researchers explored gold nanoparticles loaded with a natural anti-inflammatory berry extract for treating psoriasis. Lab studies using skin cells showed that these nanoparticles significantly reduced inflammatory molecules compared to the extract alone. A clinical study involving patients with psoriasis also found that creams containing these nanoparticles were more effective than a common steroid cream (hydrocortisone). The longer-lasting presence of the nanoparticles on the skin may explain their superior effectiveness. This suggests that gold nanoparticles loaded with natural extracts hold promise as a new treatment for psoriasis [67].

Another study explored using silver nanoparticles loaded with the same berry extract for psoriasis. While these nanoparticles reduced inflammatory molecules, like other studies, they also harmed the skin cells. This suggests that silver nanoparticles might not be a good option for psoriasis treatment because they can damage the skin, even though other natural materials combined with nanoparticles may avoid this side effect [68].

Challenges and Limitations

- High Costs: Clinical trials can be expensive to conduct, limiting the number and variety of therapies investigated.
- Recruitment Difficulties: Enrolling a sufficient number of qualified participants can be challenging, delaying trials and potentially hindering the generalizability

of results.

- Regulatory Burden: The complex regulatory processes for clinical trial approval can lengthen timelines and hinder innovation.
- Data Sharing and Open Science: Concerns persist regarding data sharing between pharmaceutical companies, academic institutions, and independent researchers, potentially hampering scientific collaboration and progress.

Future Directions

- Precision Medicine: Clinical trials are increasingly incorporating biomarkers and genetic testing to identify patients who are most likely to benefit from a specific treatment, leading to a more personalized approach to medicine.
- Adaptive Designs: The use of adaptive trial designs allows for ongoing modification based on accumulating data, potentially improving efficiency and allowing for faster evaluation of promising therapies.
- Patient Engagement: There is a growing focus on patient engagement throughout the clinical trial process, from design to dissemination of results, empowering patients and fostering trust in research.
- Decentralized Trials: The use of telemedicine and remote monitoring technologies holds promise for decentralized clinical trials, allowing participation from a wider range of patients and potentially reducing costs.

CHALLENGES AND FUTURE CONSIDERATIONS

Nanoparticle-based therapeutics hold immense promise for revolutionizing medicine. However, significant challenges need to be addressed before widespread clinical application becomes a reality. Here, we delve into key concerns and future considerations:

Biocompatibility and Long-Term Toxicity

- Cytotoxicity: Nanoparticles can potentially interact with healthy cells, leading to unintended cytotoxicity. Careful evaluation of potential cellular interactions and long-term effects is crucial [69].
- Immune Response: Nanoparticles can trigger immune responses, including inflammation or allergic reactions. Understanding the specific immune response elicited by different nanoparticles and their surface modifications is essential [70].
- Biodistribution and Clearance: Understanding the fate of nanoparticles after administration is vital. Their biodistribution patterns and clearance mechanisms need to be thoroughly investigated to minimize potential accumulation and long-term toxicity in organs [71].

Scalability and Manufacturing Costs

- Reproducibility: Scaling up production of nanoparticles with consistent size, shape, and surface properties remains a challenge. Reproducible manufacturing is essential for maintaining safety and efficacy.
- Cost-Effectiveness: Current manufacturing processes for nanoparticles can be expensive, hindering their widespread use. Developing cost-effective and scalable production methods is crucial for making these therapies accessible.

Regulatory Landscape

- Regulatory Uncertainty: Regulatory frameworks for nanoparticle-based therapeutics are still evolving. Clear guidelines for pre-clinical and clinical testing are needed to ensure safety and efficacy while fostering innovation.
- Environmental Impact: The potential environmental impact of nanoparticle production and disposal needs careful consideration. Regulations may be necessary to mitigate potential environmental risks.

Future Directions

- Advanced Characterization Techniques: Developing sophisticated techniques to characterize and monitor the behavior of nanoparticles *in vivo* will be crucial for assessing their safety and efficacy.
- Computational Modeling: Utilizing computational modeling can aid in predicting the behavior of nanoparticles and designing them for optimal biocompatibility and targeted delivery.
- Nanoparticle Design and Engineering: Tailoring the size, shape, surface chemistry, and functionality of nanoparticles can optimize their therapeutic properties and minimize potential toxicity.
- Collaboration between Researchers, Industry, and Regulatory Agencies: Stronger collaboration among researchers, industry, and regulatory agencies will be essential to efficiently translate promising nanoparticle-based therapeutics into clinical practice.

CONCLUSION

Psoriasis, a chronic inflammatory skin condition, poses a significant challenge due to limitations of current treatments. Metallic nanoparticles (NPs) emerge as a promising avenue to address these limitations. Their small size and unique properties offer exciting possibilities for improved psoriasis management. Metallic NPs can revolutionize drug delivery for psoriasis. By penetrating deeper into psoriatic lesions, they can deliver medications directly to the site of inflammation, potentially reducing the need for high drug doses and minimizing systemic side effects. Additionally, certain metallic NPs possess inherent anti-inflammatory and anti-proliferative properties, offering additional therapeutic benefits beyond simple drug delivery. They can modulate the immune response, suppress excessive skin cell growth, and potentially contribute to alleviating psoriatic symptoms. Furthermore, metallic NPs can be functionalized for targeted therapy. By attaching specific molecules to their surface, they can be directed to interact with activated immune cells within psoriatic plaques. This targeted approach allows for a localized therapeutic effect, minimizing damage to healthy tissues compared to traditional broad-spectrum medications. Metallic NPs can also be combined with existing psoriasis treatments, potentially leading to improved overall efficacy and reduced reliance on high drug doses. Despite these exciting possibilities, challenges remain before metallic NPs can be widely used for psoriasis treatment. Ensuring biocompatibility and addressing long-term safety concerns are paramount. Additionally, developing cost-effective and scalable production methods is crucial for making these therapies accessible. The regulatory landscape for nanoparticle-based therapeutics is still evolving, and clear guidelines for pre-clinical and clinical testing are needed. Future Directions and the Road to Clinical Translation: Future research directions hold the key to unlocking the full potential of metallic NPs for psoriasis management. Advanced characterization techniques will allow for a deeper understanding of how these nanoparticles interact with the body. Computational modelling can play a vital role in optimizing their design for targeted delivery and minimizing potential toxicity. Additionally, continued research on nanoparticle engineering will enable the tailoring of size, shape, and surface functionalities to achieve optimal therapeutic effects. The successful translation of these promising findings into clinical practice hinges on strong collaboration between researchers, industry, and regulatory agencies. By working together, these stakeholders can navigate the challenges, design and test safe and effective nanoparticle-based therapies, and ultimately bring relief to patients suffering from psoriasis. Metallic nanoparticles hold immense promise for revolutionizing psoriasis management, offering a future filled with hope for improved patient outcomes and a better quality of life.

REFERENCES

[1] Bodemer AA. Psoriasis. 2nd ed. Integrative Medicine 2007; pp. 757-69.
[http://dx.doi.org/10.1016/B978-1-4160-2954-0.50073-9]

[2] Griffiths CEM, Armstrong AW, Gudjonsson JE, Barker JNWN. Psoriasis. Lancet 2021; 397(10281): 1301-15.
[http://dx.doi.org/10.1016/S0140-6736(20)32549-6] [PMID: 33812489]

[3] Bhosle MJ, Kulkarni A, Feldman SR, Balkrishnan R. Quality of life in patients with psoriasis. Health Qual Life Outcomes 2006; 4(1): 35.
[http://dx.doi.org/10.1186/1477-7525-4-35] [PMID: 16756666]

[4] Lee HJ, Kim M. Challenges and future trends in the treatment of psoriasis. Int J Mol Sci 2023; 24(17): 13313.
[http://dx.doi.org/10.3390/ijms241713313] [PMID: 37686119]

[5] Nestle FO, Kaplan DH, Barker J. Psoriasis. N Engl J Med 2009; 361(5): 496-509. [http://dx.doi.org/10.1056/NEJMra0804595] [PMID: 19641206]

[6] Castela E, Archier E, Devaux S, *et al.* Topical corticosteroids in plaque psoriasis: a systematic review of efficacy and treatment modalities. J Eur Acad Dermatol Venereol 2012; 26(s3) (Suppl. 3): 36-46. [http://dx.doi.org/10.1111/j.1468-3083.2012.04522.x] [PMID: 22512679]

[7] Wilsmann-Theis D, Funk R, Mössner R, Bieber T, Wenzel J. Efficacy and safety of methotrexate in psoriasis vulgaris long-term treatment: a real-world observation study. Indian J Dermatol 2023; 68(6): 669-73. [http://dx.doi.org/10.4103/ijd.ijd_551_23] [PMID: 38371546]

[8] Gordon K, Papp K, Poulin Y, Gu Y, Rozzo S, Sasso EH. Long-term efficacy and safety of adalimumab in patients with moderate to severe psoriasis treated continuously over 3 years: Results from an open-label extension study for patients from REVEAL. J Am Acad Dermatol 2012; 66(2): 241-51. [http://dx.doi.org/10.1016/j.jaad.2010.12.005] [PMID: 21752491]

[9] Zhao Q, Cheng N, Sun X, Yan L, Li W. The application of nanomedicine in clinical settings. Front Bioeng Biotechnol 2023; 11: 1219054. [http://dx.doi.org/10.3389/fbioe.2023.1219054] [PMID: 37441195]

[10] Bodnár K, Fehér P, Ujhelyi Z, Bácskay I, Józsa L. Recent approaches for the topical treatment of psoriasis using nanoparticles. Pharmaceutics 2024; 16(4): 449. [http://dx.doi.org/10.3390/pharmaceutics16040449] [PMID: 38675110]

[11] Afzal O, Altamimi ASA, Nadeem MS, *et al.* Nanoparticles in drug delivery: from history to therapeutic applications. Nanomaterials (Basel) 2022; 12(24): 4494. [http://dx.doi.org/10.3390/nano12244494] [PMID: 36558344]

[12] Dreaden EC, Alkilany AM, Huang X, Murphy CJ, El-Sayed MA. The golden age: gold nanoparticles for biomedicine. Chem Soc Rev 2012; 41(7): 2740-79. [http://dx.doi.org/10.1039/C1CS15237H] [PMID: 22109657]

[13] Chen R, Zhai YY, Sun L, *et al.* Alantolactone-loaded chitosan/hyaluronic acid nanoparticles suppress psoriasis by deactivating STAT3 pathway and restricting immune cell recruitment. Asian Journal of Pharmaceutical Sciences 2022; 17(2): 268-83. [http://dx.doi.org/10.1016/j.ajps.2022.02.003] [PMID: 35582636]

[14] Mieszawska AJ, Mulder WJM, Fayad ZA, Cormode DP. Multifunctional gold nanoparticles for diagnosis and therapy of disease. Mol Pharm 2013; 10(3): 831-47. [http://dx.doi.org/10.1021/mp3005885] [PMID: 23360440]

[15] Ghosh P, Han G, De M, Kim C, Rotello V. Gold nanoparticles in delivery applications. Adv Drug Deliv Rev 2008; 60(11): 1307-15. [http://dx.doi.org/10.1016/j.addr.2008.03.016] [PMID: 18555555]

[16] Mahato K, Nagpal S, Shah MA, *et al.*; Gold nanoparticle surface engineering strategies and their applications in biomedicine and diagnostics; 3 Biotech; 2019; 9(2): 57. [http://dx.doi.org/10.1007/s13205-019-1577-z]

[17] Kong FY, Zhang JW, Li RF, Wang ZX, Wang WJ, Wang W. Unique roles of gold nanoparticles in drug delivery, targeting and imaging applications. Molecules 2017; 22(9): 1445. [http://dx.doi.org/10.3390/molecules22091445] [PMID: 28858253]

[18] Huang H, Liu R, Yang J, *et al.* Gold nanoparticles: construction for drug delivery and application in cancer immunotherapy. Pharmaceutics 2023; 15(7): 1868. [http://dx.doi.org/10.3390/pharmaceutics15071868] [PMID: 37514054]

[19] Roma-Rodrigues C, Rivas-García L, Baptista PV, Fernandes AR. Gene therapy in cancer treatment: why go nano? Pharmaceutics 2020; 12(3): 233. [http://dx.doi.org/10.3390/pharmaceutics12030233] [PMID: 32151052]

[20] Alkilany AM, Murphy CJ. Toxicity and cellular uptake of gold nanoparticles: what we have learned so far? J Nanopart Res 2010; 12(7): 2313-33.
[http://dx.doi.org/10.1007/s11051-010-9911-8] [PMID: 21170131]

[21] Bruna T, Maldonado-Bravo F, Jara P, Caro N. Silver nanoparticles and their antibacterial applications. Int J Mol Sci 2021; 22(13): 7202.
[http://dx.doi.org/10.3390/ijms22137202] [PMID: 34281254]

[22] Paladini F, Pollini M. Antimicrobial silver nanoparticles for wound healing application: progress and future trends. Materials (Basel) 2019; 12(16): 2540.
[http://dx.doi.org/10.3390/ma12162540] [PMID: 31404974]

[23] Akter M, Sikder MT, Rahman MM, *et al.* A systematic review on silver nanoparticles-induced cytotoxicity: Physicochemical properties and perspectives. J Adv Res 2018; 9: 1-16.
[http://dx.doi.org/10.1016/j.jare.2017.10.008] [PMID: 30046482]

[24] Burduşel AC, Gherasim O, Grumezescu AM, Mogoantă L, Ficai A, Andronescu E. Biomedical applications of silver nanoparticles: an up-to-date overview. Nanomaterials (Basel) 2018; 8(9): 681.
[http://dx.doi.org/10.3390/nano8090681] [PMID: 30200373]

[25] Gherasim O, Puiu RA, Bîrcă AC, Burduşel AC, Grumezescu AM. An updated review on silver nanoparticles in biomedicine. Nanomaterials (Basel) 2020; 10(11): 2318.
[http://dx.doi.org/10.3390/nano10112318] [PMID: 33238486]

[26] Xu L, Wang YY, Huang J, Chen CY, Wang ZX, Xie H. Silver nanoparticles: Synthesis, medical applications and biosafety. Theranostics 2020; 10(20): 8996-9031.
[http://dx.doi.org/10.7150/thno.45413] [PMID: 32802176]

[27] Kampe S, Kaegi R, Schlich K, Wasmuth C, Hollert H, Schlechtriem C. Silver nanoparticles in sewage sludge: Bioavailability of sulfidized silver to the terrestrial isopod *Porcellio scaber*. Environ Toxicol Chem 2018; 37(6): 1606-13.
[http://dx.doi.org/10.1002/etc.4102] [PMID: 29363840]

[28] Abed A, Derakhshan M, Karimi M, *et al.* Platinum nanoparticles in biomedicine: preparation, anti-cancer activity, and drug delivery vehicles. Front Pharmacol 2022; 13: 797804.
[http://dx.doi.org/10.3389/fphar.2022.797804] [PMID: 35281900]

[29] Fereig SA, El-Zaafarany GM, Arafa MG, Abdel-Mottaleb MMA. Tackling the various classes of nano-therapeutics employed in topical therapy of psoriasis. Drug Deliv 2020; 27(1): 662-80.
[http://dx.doi.org/10.1080/10717544.2020.1754527] [PMID: 32393082]

[30] Pankhurst QA, Connolly J, Jones SK, Dobson J. Applications of magnetic nanoparticles in biomedicine. J Phys D Appl Phys 2003; 36(13): R167-81. [DOI:10.1088/0022-3727/36/13/201].
[http://dx.doi.org/10.1088/0022-3727/36/13/201]

[31] Nandhini J, Karthikeyan E, Rajeshkumar S. Nanomaterials for wound healing: Current status and futuristic frontier. Biomedical Technology 2024; 6: 26-45. [DOI:10.1016/j.bmt.2023.10.001.].
[http://dx.doi.org/10.1016/j.bmt.2023.10.001]

[32] Longano D, Ditaranto N, Sabbatini L, *et al.*; Synthesis and antimicrobial activity of copper nanomaterials; nano-antimicrobials; 2011: 85–117.
[http://dx.doi.org/10.1007/978-3-642-24428-5_3]

[33] Berhe MG, Gebreslassie YT. Biomedical applications of biosynthesized nickel oxide nanoparticles. Int J Nanomedicine 2023; 18: 4229-51.
[http://dx.doi.org/10.2147/IJN.S410668] [PMID: 37534055]

[34] Sunderman FW, Range CL, Sunderman FW Jr, Donnelly AJ, Lucyszvn GW. Nickel poisoning. XII. Metabolic and pathologic changes in acute pneumonitis from nickel carbonyl. Am J Clin Pathol 1961; 36(6): 477-91.
[http://dx.doi.org/10.1093/ajcp/36.6.477] [PMID: 13918426]

[35] Das S, Dowding JM, Klump KE, McGinnis JF, Self W, Seal S. Cerium oxide nanoparticles: applications and prospects in nanomedicine. Nanomedicine (Lond) 2013; 8(9): 1483-508. [http://dx.doi.org/10.2217/nnm.13.133] [PMID: 23987111]

[36] Hirst SM, Karakoti AS, Tyler RD, Sriranganathan N, Seal S, Reilly CM. Anti-inflammatory properties of cerium oxide nanoparticles. Small. 2009;5(24):2848–56. [http://dx.doi.org/10.1002/smll.200901048] [PMID: 19802857]

[37] Lee HJ, Kim M. Challenges and future trends in the treatment of psoriasis. Int J Mol Sci 2023; 24(17): 13313. [http://dx.doi.org/10.3390/ijms241713313] [PMID: 37686119]

[38] Chawla V, Sharma S, Singh Y. Yttrium oxide nanoparticle-loaded, self-assembled peptide gel with antibacterial, anti-inflammatory, and proangiogenic properties for wound healing. ACS Biomater Sci Eng 2023; 9(5): 2647-62. [http://dx.doi.org/10.1021/acsbiomaterials.3c00134] [PMID: 37097124]

[39] Thirumal D, Sindhu RK, Goyal S, *et al.* Pathology and treatment of psoriasis using nanoformulations. Biomedicines 2023; 11(6): 1589. [http://dx.doi.org/10.3390/biomedicines11061589] [PMID: 37371684]

[40] Rahman M, Akhter S, Ahmad J, Ahmad MZ, Beg S, Ahmad FJ. Nanomedicine-based drug targeting for psoriasis: potentials and emerging trends in nanoscale pharmacotherapy. Expert Opin Drug Deliv 2015; 12(4): 635-52. [http://dx.doi.org/10.1517/17425247.2015.982088] [PMID: 25439967]

[41] Faraji AH, Wipf P. Nanoparticles in cellular drug delivery. Bioorg Med Chem 2009; 17(8): 2950-62. [http://dx.doi.org/10.1016/j.bmc.2009.02.043] [PMID: 19299149]

[42] Mendes C, Thirupathi A, Corrêa MEAB, Gu Y, Silveira PCL. The use of metallic nanoparticles in wound healing: new perspectives. Int J Mol Sci 2022; 23(23): 15376. [http://dx.doi.org/10.3390/ijms232315376] [PMID: 36499707]

[43] Koushki K, Keshavarz Shahbaz S, Keshavarz M, Bezsonov EE, Sathyapalan T, Sahebkar A. Gold nanoparticles: multifaceted roles in the management of autoimmune disorders. Biomolecules 2021; 11(9): 1289. [http://dx.doi.org/10.3390/biom11091289] [PMID: 34572503]

[44] Koushki K, Keshavarz Shahbaz S, Keshavarz M, Bezsonov EE, Sathyapalan T, Sahebkar A. Gold nanoparticles: multifaceted roles in the management of autoimmune disorders. Biomolecules 2021; 11(9): 1289. [http://dx.doi.org/10.3390/biom11091289] [PMID: 34572503]

[45] Dhayalan M, Karikalan P, Umar RS, *et al.*; Biomedical applications of silver nanoparticles; Intech Open; 2021. [http://dx.doi.org/10.5772/intechopen.99367]

[46] Brusini R, Varna M, Couvreur P. Advanced nanomedicines for the treatment of inflammatory diseases. Adv Drug Deliv Rev 2020; 157: 161-78. [http://dx.doi.org/10.1016/j.addr.2020.07.010] [PMID: 32697950]

[47] Nussbaum L, Chen YL, Ogg GS. Role of regulatory T cells in psoriasis pathogenesis and treatment. Br J Dermatol 2021; 184(1): 14-24. [http://dx.doi.org/10.1111/bjd.19380] [PMID: 32628773]

[48] Li Y, Xu C, Lei C. The delivery and activation of growth factors using nanomaterials for bone repair. Pharmaceutics 2023; 15(3): 1017. [http://dx.doi.org/10.3390/pharmaceutics15031017] [PMID: 36986877]

[49] Singh S, Sharma K, Sharma H; Green extracts with metal-based nanoparticles for treating inflammatory diseases: a review; Current Drug Delivery; 2024; 21(4); 544-570 (27). [http://dx.doi.org/10.2174/1567201820666230602164325]

[50] Dadwal N, Kurmi BD, Singh D, *et al.*; Recent advancements in novel formulations of anti-psoriatic agents for effective delivery: clinical importance and patent survey; Recent Patents on Nanotechnology; 2024; 18(3); 259-277(19).
[http://dx.doi.org/10.2174/1872210517666230601124620]

[51] Adebayo OA; Biochemical evaluation of peptide-based cerium oxide nanoparticles on structure and function of vital organs in adult rodent; PhD dissertation; University of Ibadan; 2023.

[52] Han R, Xiao Y, Bai Q, Choi CHJ. Self-therapeutic metal-based nanoparticles for treating inflammatory diseases. Acta Pharm Sin B 2023; 13(5): 1847-65.
[http://dx.doi.org/10.1016/j.apsb.2022.07.009] [PMID: 37250153]

[53] Fereig SA, El-Zaafarany GM, Arafa MG, Abdel-Mottaleb MMA. Boosting the anti-inflammatory effect of self-assembled hybrid lecithin–chitosan nanoparticles *via* hybridization with gold nanoparticles for the treatment of psoriasis: elemental mapping and *in vivo* modeling. Drug Deliv 2022; 29(1): 1726-42.
[http://dx.doi.org/10.1080/10717544.2022.2081383] [PMID: 35635314]

[54] Gangadevi V, Thatikonda S, Pooladanda V, *et al.*; Selenium nanoparticles produce a beneficial effect in psoriasis by reducing epidermal hyperproliferation and inflammation; J Nanobiotechnol; 2021; 19, 101 (2021).
[http://dx.doi.org/10.1186/s12951-021-00842-3]

[55] Fereig SA, El-Zaafarany GM, Arafa MG, Abdel-Mottaleb MMA. Tackling the various classes of nano-therapeutics employed in topical therapy of psoriasis. Drug Deliv 2020; 27(1): 662-80.
[http://dx.doi.org/10.1080/10717544.2020.1754527] [PMID: 32393082]

[56] Mikhailova EO. Silver nanoparticles: mechanism of action and probable bio-application. J Funct Biomater 2020; 11(4): 84.
[http://dx.doi.org/10.3390/jfb11040084] [PMID: 33255874]

[57] Ziental D, Czarczynska-Goslinska B, Mlynarczyk DT, *et al.* Titanium dioxide nanoparticles: prospects and applications in medicine. Nanomaterials (Basel) 2020; 10(2): 387.
[http://dx.doi.org/10.3390/nano10020387] [PMID: 32102185]

[58] Wu L, Liu G, Wang W, *et al.* Cyclodextrin-modified CeO_2 nanoparticles as a multifunctional nanozyme for combinational therapy of psoriasis. Int J Nanomedicine 2020; 15(15): 2515-27.
[http://dx.doi.org/10.2147/IJN.S246783] [PMID: 32368038]

[59] Kotcherlakota R, Das S, Patra CR; Therapeutic applications of green-synthesized silver nanoparticles, Chapter 16- Green Synthesis, Characterization and Applications of Nanoparticles; 2019; 389-427.
[http://dx.doi.org/10.1016/B978-0-08-102579-6.00017-4]

[60] Agarwal H, Nakara A, Shanmugam VK. Anti-inflammatory mechanism of various metal and metal oxide nanoparticles synthesized using plant extracts: A review. Biomed Pharmacother 2019; 109: 2561-72.
[http://dx.doi.org/10.1016/j.biopha.2018.11.116] [PMID: 30551516]

[61] Crisan D, Scharffetter-Kochanek K, Crisan M, *et al.* Topical silver and gold nanoparticles complexed with *Cornus mas* suppress inflammation in human psoriasis plaques by inhibiting NF-κB activity. Exp Dermatol 2018; 27(10): 1166-9.
[http://dx.doi.org/10.1111/exd.13707] [PMID: 29906306]

[62] Crisan D; Anti-inflammatory effect of metallic silver and gold nanoparticles complexed with polyphenolic compounds in human chronic stationary plaque psoriasis; PhD dissertation; University of Ulm; 2016.

[63] Vandebriel RJ, Tonk ECM, de la Fonteyne-Blankestijn LJ, *et al.* Immunotoxicity of silver nanoparticles in an intravenous 28-day repeated-dose toxicity study in rats. Part Fibre Toxicol 2014; 11(1): 21.
[http://dx.doi.org/10.1186/1743-8977-11-21] [PMID: 24885556]

[64] El Mahdy MM, Eldin TAS, Aly HS, Mohammed FF, Shaalan MI. Evaluation of hepatotoxic and genotoxic potential of silver nanoparticles in albino rats. Exp Toxicol Pathol 2015; 67(1): 21-9. [http://dx.doi.org/10.1016/j.etp.2014.09.005] [PMID: 25446800]

[65] Tiwari DK, Jin T, Behari J. Dose-dependent in-vivo toxicity assessment of silver nanoparticle in wistar rats. Toxicol Mech Methods 2011; 21(1): 13-24. [http://dx.doi.org/10.3109/15376516.2010.529184] [PMID: 21080782]

[66] Hirst SM, Karakoti AS, Tyler RD, Sriranganathan N, Seal S, Reilly CM. Anti-inflammatory properties of cerium oxide nanoparticles. Small 2009; 5(24): 2848-56. [http://dx.doi.org/10.1002/smll.200901048] [PMID: 19802857]

[67] Crisan M, David L, Moldovan B, *et al.* New nanomaterials for the improvement of psoriatic lesions. J Mater Chem B Mater Biol Med 2013; 1(25): 3152-8. [http://dx.doi.org/10.1039/c3tb20476f] [PMID: 32260915]

[68] David L, Moldovan B, Vulcu A, *et al.* Green synthesis, characterization and anti-inflammatory activity of silver nanoparticles using European black elderberry fruits extract. Colloids Surf B Biointerfaces 2014; 122: 767-77. [http://dx.doi.org/10.1016/j.colsurfb.2014.08.018] [PMID: 25174985]

[69] Gupta R, Xie H. Nanoparticles in daily life: applications, toxicity and regulations. J Environ Pathol Toxicol Oncol 2018; 37(3): 209-30. [http://dx.doi.org/10.1615/JEnvironPatholToxicolOncol.2018026009] [PMID: 30317972]

[70] Liu Y, Hardie J, Zhang X, Rotello VM. Effects of engineered nanoparticles on the innate immune system. Semin Immunol 2017; 34: 25-32. [http://dx.doi.org/10.1016/j.smim.2017.09.011] [PMID: 28985993]

[71] Xuan L, Ju Z, Skonieczna M, *et al.*; Nanoparticles-induced potential toxicity on human health: Applications, toxicity mechanisms, and evaluation models;MedComm (2020); 2023; 4(4). [http://dx.doi.org/10.1002/mco2.327]

CHAPTER 13

Ethosomes – Based Pharmacotherapy for the Management of Psoriasis

Ritika Saini[1], **Jasmine Chaudhary**[1,*], **Akash Jain**[1] and **Bhawna Chopra**[2]

[1] *M.M. College of Pharmacy, Maharishi Markandeshwar (Deemed to be University), Mullana, Ambala, Haryana, India*

[2] *Department of Pharmaceutical Chemistry, Guru Gobind Singh College of Pharmacy, Yamuna Nagar 135001, Haryana, India*

Abstract: Psoriasis is a chronic inflammatory skin disease in which over-activation of the immune system (T-cells, keratinocytes) leads to dilation of dermal capillaries of the epidermis and dermis due to excessive production of cytokines. It is primarily characterized by erythematous, itchy, and scaly patches on the exposed surfaces of the body, mainly the scalp, elbows, and knees. Environmental factors, genetics, bacterial infections, *etc*., also play a significant role in its occurrence. Numerous therapies like acupuncture, water therapy, phototherapy, meditation, herbal treatment, moisturizing treatment, use of nutritional supplements, and different drug formulations for topical (salicylic acid, dithranol, vitamin D, corticosteroids, tacrolimus) and systemic (methotrexate, cyclosporine, acitretin) use are beneficial in its management. Topical therapies, due to the skin's barrier effect, have poor penetration and absorption; therefore, to provide more controlled, targeted, nontoxic, secure drug delivery, nanoformulations are used nowadays. Local administration of drug-loaded nanocarriers, *viz*. liposomes, niosomes, ethosomes, nanoemulsions, transferosomes, *etc*. demonstrated improved penetrability and effectiveness at lesser doses while causing little systemic side effects. Ethosomes are emerging lipid vesicular nanocarriers containing phospholipids along with relatively high amounts of alcohol (mainly ethanol), which are responsible for the penetration of entrapped drugs (having diverse physicochemical parameters) deep into the skin. Because of their high safety, efficacy, stability, patient compliance, and simple manufacturing procedures, ethosomes act as one of the effective carriers for transdermal drug delivery. Various drug-containing ethosomes have been successfully designed and evaluated for the pharmacotherapy of psoriasis. Therefore, in this chapter, the main focus is to collate all the ethosomes-based drug formulations designed for the management of psoriasis.

Keywords: Ethosomes, Liposomes, Nanoemulsions, Niosomes, Pharmacotherapy, Transferosomes.

* **Corresponding author Jasmine Chaudhary:** M.M. College of Pharmacy, Maharishi Markandeshwar (Deemed to be University), Mullana, Ambala, Haryana, India; E-mail: jasmine.jain@mmumullana.org

Anjali Sharma, Prerna Sharma, Roy Rillera Marzo & Ahmed A. Al Karmalawy (Eds.)

INTRODUCTION

The skin is the human body's largest organ, with a complex structure comprising the epidermis and the underlying dermis, the two skin layers playing a substantial role in percutaneous absorption [1, 2].

Transdermal drug delivery is one of the frequently employed techniques for the administration of drugs having less stability in the gastrointestinal tract, high first-pass metabolism, or significant undesirable effects when taken orally. High patient compliance, non-invasive nature, ease of administration, controlled drug distribution, and less dose frequency are other major benefits [3]. Initially, the transdermal drug delivery approach (first generation) involves the usage of topical formulations in the form of gel or liquid spray to deliver the medication directly to the skin without using any complicated apparatus [4, 5]. Later, drug administration was made more effective with the use of vehicles and their analogs (second generation).

Nanovesicles, including liposomes, transfersomes, ethosomes, niosomes, and phytosomes, are some methods for transdermal drug delivery. These are nano-sized spherical bilayer vesicles composed of lipids or similar products like surfactants [6]. The ethosomes are among the innovative, novel lipid-based vesicular systems that provide superior drug delivery compared to other nanoparticles, particularly for transdermal applications. A phospholipid bilayer and an inner aqueous core containing the medication make up ethosomal vesicles [3]. The combination of lipid content and high ethanol concentration enhances their affinity towards lipophilic and hydrophilic (high molecular weight) compounds and significantly augments flexibility and deformability, enabling passing across the spaces between cells with negligible medication loss [6, 7].

The large ethanolic content also moves the vesicle's surface charge toward strong negative values, causing electrostatic repulsions and thereby preventing vesicle aggregation. It alters the structure of the cell membrane and outer lipid layers of the skin, allowing vesicles to penetrate the skin layers. Thus, ethosomes can be regarded as soft, elastic vesicles with dimensions varying from 30 nm to several microns, which can transport the drug in both occlusive and non-occlusive conditions across the skin [3]. Considering all of these qualities, ethosomes can be regarded as an efficient method (lipid-based) for active drug distribution into or across the skin, and thus have numerous applications in various biological fields [7].

The Transdermal Drug Delivery System (TDDS) is preferred over conventional drug administration methods nowadays, as drugs can be administered accurately and safely using various delivery techniques across different types of skin, with no first-pass metabolism [5], *i.e.*, they do not undergo any metabolic changes until they arrive at their target location. TDDS is non-invasive and non-allergenic if administered properly within the scheduled period and mechanism [8]. This enables the uniform delivery of medications at predetermined and regulated rates. Because of this, administering drugs *via* the transdermal route has gained wide popularity in the pharmaceutical sector. The incorporation of chemical enhancers, however, has shown no remarkable effect in improving the transdermal transport of small molecules [9].

Ethosomes are also preferred over liposomes because classic liposomes only reach the top layer of the stratum corneum and do not profoundly enter the skin. Transdermal delivery is established to be possible only with specialized vesicles like ethosomes containing good ethanolic content. Ethanol is a widely recognized effective permeability enhancer [10]. However, the ethanol content in liposome formulations is very low. Lipid vesicular systems *i.e.*, ethosomes, contain ethanol in quite high concentrations and thus are highly effective in increasing the penetration of various drugs through the skin.

Mechanism of Action of Ethosomes

Ethosomes work efficiently when vesicles, ethanol, and skin lipids work together. Due to better dispersion of active components, a more competent interaction is observed between ethosomes and skin lipids rather than with liposomes [3]. The ethanol-lipid interaction in the polar head group area lowers its transition temperature in the stratum corneum. This reduces the density of the lipid multilayer and increases fluidity, permitting the easy pervasion of the drug into deep skin layers [11]. Moreover, ethanol gives vesicles a smoother, more flexible texture, which allows them to penetrate the epidermal layer more deeply [12, 13].

Ethosomal Delivery Systems

The first ethosomes were discovered by Touitou and his students at the Hebrew University School of Pharmacy in 1995 [14] to transport active substances into deep layers of the skin and systemic circulation. The vesicular structure and the transition temperature of the lipids in ethosomes were studied using TEM and DSC, and it was concluded that, depending on the composition of the system, ethosomes may have one or many lamellar layers. Ethosomes were found to possess a higher degree of fluidity because of their low lipid levels [15].

Ethosomes are vesicular carriers composed of hydro/alcoholic/glycolic phospholipid, with a comparatively high amount of alcohol [11]. Ethosome-based drug delivery is gaining popularity in the present era [7]. Based on the components utilized in the formulations, there are three varieties of ethosomes [3]

- Classical ethosomes
- Transethosomes
- Invasomes

Classic Ethosomes

Introduction of hydrophilic *i.e.*, water or buffer solutions to the lipophilic portion *i.e.* dissolvable lipids/organic components using “rotary film evaporation method” under consistent velocity and temperature (between 40°C and room temperature) leads to the development of organic film on the classical ethosomes [16]. The film is then moisturized with a hydrophilic solution, which causes the lipids to swell and create bilayer vesicles.

The hydrophilic solution is combined with the organic solution at a consistent volume and stirred at a high temperature and constant velocity in the “ethanol injection” technique leading to precipitation of lipid molecules forming bilayer structure. By adjusting the ratio of the organic and hydrophilic solvents in each of these techniques, the physicochemical characteristics of the nanostructures may be altered. The produced ethosomes may optionally be homogenized or subjected to sonication following the stirring procedure to decrease their size and distribution [7].

Transethosomes

The presence of penetration enhancers and edge activators in transethosomes makes their structure extremely deformable. They can permeate *via* small pores (around 5-10 times smaller). The charged head group of amphiphilic compounds (edge activators) provides the ionic characteristics of the surfactant and lipophilic alkyl groups [17]. They aid the destabilization of lipid bilayers inside the vesicles, leading to changes in their flexibility and deformability.

Transethosomes, in contrast to classic ethosomes, lack a regular shape and size. The kind and number of agents that increase penetration (edge activators) govern their morphological variability. Furthermore, transethosomes have comparatively better encapsulation effectiveness than ethosomes, and this efficiency is often unaffected by the molecular weight, charge, and polarity [7].

Invasomes

Invasomes are compounds characterized by hydrocarbon chains and a lipid bilayer vesicle containing terpenes, the main component of essential oils. Terpenes perturb the compact order of lipid bilayers, increasing the vesicles' deformability and flexibility, and improving their capacity to reach the underlying layers of the skin. Utilizing several terpenes in combination has synergistic effects and increases the vesicles' flexibility. For example, when compared to structures having only citral, invasomes can be manufactured by adding three distinct types of terpenes—cineol, limonene, and citral—which provides a greater concentration of the active compound in the stratum corneum. Furthermore, the concentration of terpenes in the vesicle structure is co-related to the amount of active chemicals deposited in the stratum corneum [7].

Preparation of Ethosomes

Ethosomes can be formulated using either the cold method or the hot method.

Cold Method (Cold Approach)

In the cold approach, the active component (drug), phospholipids, or other lipid components are dissolved in ethanol with vigorous stirring and heated at 30°C, which are then added with continuous stirring into water heated at 30°C. After five minutes of churning, the vesicles begin to emerge. The dimensions of the vesicles can be adjusted to the required extent by sonication or extrusion. Lastly, the mixture is refrigerated for storage [11]. Cold storage of generated vesicles is crucial [12].

Hot Method

This process involves heating phospholipids at 400°C till a colloidal solution is produced. Similarly, ethanol mixed with propylene glycol is heated up to 400°C in another vessel. After both phases have achieved 400°C, the organic phase is added to the aqueous phase [12]. After heating this final mixture to 30°C, size reduction is accomplished by extrusion or sonication.

Some other methods have also found utility in the preparation of ethosomes and are discussed briefly:

Classic Method

This method involves dissolution of the drug and phospholipid in ethanol by heating to 30°C ± 1°C. In a closed vessel, the mixture of lipids and double-distilled water is continuously stirred at 700 rpm [13]. A hand extruder is used to homogenize the resultant vesicle suspension.

Mechanical Dispersion Method

Soya phosphatidylcholine is dissolved in a mixture of methanol and chloroform. A rotary vacuum evaporator is then used to remove the organic solvents, leaving behind a thin lipid coating on the flask walls. The lipid film deposited is subjected to an overnight vacuum to eliminate any remaining traces of the solvent. By rotating the flask at the required temperature, hydration is accomplished with different amounts of the hydroethanolic-drug combination [18].

Vortex/sonication Method

Because of ease and efficiency, this method is widely used for preparing ethosomes. Edge activators and phospholipids are combined with phosphate buffer and vigorously shaken and vortexed to ensure uniform dispersion of the components. Sonication is then done using a sonicator/vortex to form vesicles. The duration and intensity of sonication can be adjusted to regulate the vesicle size. The suspension is then forced through different-sized membranes to form vesicles of the desired size [19].

Rotary Film Evaporation

In this method, phospholipids are dispersed in a spherical bottom flask with an organic solvent. Similar to the mechanical dispersion method, the organic solvent is evaporated, leaving behind a thin lipid layer on the inner wall of the flask. The drug-containing aqueous medium is then used to hydrate the lipid film, resulting in the production of lipid bilayer vesicles containing the target drug [19].

Ethanol injection-prepared NBD-PC labelled ethosomes and RhB-labelled ethosomes are examples of fluorescence labelling ethosomes [20].

Additives used in the Formulation of Ethosomes

Phospholipids, a significant amount of ethanol, and water form the major part of ethosomes. The high ethanol level of the ethosomes makes them unique. The hydro/alcoholic/glycolic phospholipid ethosomes are vesicular carriers with a relatively high concentration of alcohols or their combination. A wide range of phospholipids (for the formation of vesicles), *viz* phosphatidylcholine, distearoyl phosphatidylcholine, phosphatidic acid, and soya phosphatidylcholine. Phosphatidylserine, phosphatidylethanolamine, phosphatidylglycerol, phosphatidylinositol, and hydrogenated PC are typically found in ethosomes [21]. Various alcohols, including ethanol, isopropyl alcohol, propylene glycol, *etc*. are added to provide softness and easy penetration of vesicles through the membrane. Carbopol as a vehicle, cholesterol as a stabilizer, and certain dyes like Rhodamine 123 for characterization study are also added [22].

Stability of Ethosomes

Ethosomes, due to the presence of colloidal particles, exhibit optical properties and, on long storage, may exhibit issues of cracking and creaming. They are also susceptible to oxidation and hydrolysis due to their phospholipid content. Determination of the colloid's optical characteristics can help predict the shelf life of ethosomes. This approach can help study the process of destabilization caused by different factors like coalescence, sedimentation, or creaming. Turbiscan Lab® Expert, a novel optical analyzer, is used to evaluate the optical characteristics of ethosomes containing linoleic acid to predict its shelf life [23, 3].

Characterisation of Ethosomes

The ethosomes can be characterized by different parameters as discussed below:

Vesicle Shape

The morphological characteristics of ethosomal vesicles can be examined using electron microscopy (TEM and SEM). This involves applying an aqueous solution, such as phosphotungstic acid, to the formulation. Ethosomes have been found to exhibit malleable and vesicular (spherical) structures [24].

Particle size and Zeta Potential

TEM and SEM can be used for particle size determination, while a zeta meter can be used for zeta potential determination.

Entrapment Efficiency

The ultracentrifugation technique is used to determine the ethosomes' entrapment efficiency. Using a high ultracentrifugal speed (20,000 rpm) and a constant temperature maintained at 4°C for 90 minutes, the vesicles are centrifuged, leading to the separation of sediment from supernatant liquid. The quantity of drugs in the sediment is estimated by lysing the vesicles with methanol [21]. The entrapment efficiency is then calculated using the formula:

Entrapment Efficiency = De/Dt* 100

Where De is the drug concentration in the ethosomal sediment and Dt is the theoretical drug concentration used for preparation.

Transition Temperature

It can be determined using differential scanning calorimetry. The aluminium crucibles containing ethosomes are heated at a rate of 10°C per minute at varying temperatures (20-300°C) [25].

Drug Content

Different analytical techniques like UV spectrophotometer, HPLC, *etc*., can be employed to measure the drug content of the ethosomes [21].

Surface Tension Measurement

It can be measured by the ring method using the Du Nouy ring tensiometer.

Skin Permeation Studies

The penetration of ethosomes into the epidermal layer can be estimated by confocal laser scanning microscopy. The results of *in vitro* studies are then used to correlate the rate of drug release using several kinetic models, such as zero-order, first-order, Higuchi's, Hixson-Crowell cube root, and Korsmeyer-Peppas models.

EVALUATION OF ETHOSOMES [26, 27]

Filter Membrane-Vesicle Interaction Study

It includes the application of vesicle suspension (0.2ml) on a filtration membrane having pores (50 nm), which is then placed in diffusion cells. The lower side of the filter should be in touch with the phosphate buffer (pH 6.5), whereas the top side should be exposed to air. After an hour, the filters are taken out for SEM study by fixing them for the whole night at 4°C in Karnovsky's fixative and then dehydrating them with ethanol solutions varying in volume 30%, 50%, 70%, 90%, 95%, and 100% v/v in water.

Skin Permeation

For skin permeation studies, the rat hair was trimmed (less than 2 mm), and then the abdominal skin was separated from the underlying connective tissue using a scalpel. It was then placed on aluminium foil, and the skin's surface was carefully peeled off to remove any remaining fat or subcutaneous tissue. The excised skin was positioned between the receptor and the donor compartment containing phosphate buffer saline solution (pH 6.5) maintained at a constant temperature of 32°C ± 1°C. 1.0 mL of the ethosomal formulation was applied on the skin's surface and samples (0.5mL) were withdrawn from diffusion cells at different intervals (1, 2, 4, 8, 12, 16, 20, and 24 hours) and analyzed using HPLC.

Stability Study

The stability in terms of drug retention capacity of ethosomal formulations can be evaluated by exposing them to varying temperatures, namely 37 ± 2°C, 45 ± 2°C, and 25 ± 2°C. The vehicle's dimensions (size and shape) are then measured using DLS and TEM to assess the stability of ethosomes quantitatively [21].

The vesicles stored at 4°C ± 0.5°C were tested for stability after 180 days and their size, zeta potential, and entrapment efficiency were assessed to ascertain their efficacy.

Vesicle-Skin Interaction Study

The vesicle-skin interaction can be analyzed using TEM (Transmission electron microscope), SEM (Scanning electron microscope), Eosin-hematoxylin staining, or Fluorescence microscopy of the ultrathin sections of separated skin pieces as per the standard procedures [22, 28].

Drug Uptake Studies

The drug uptake is measured using HPLC and it will be a measure of drug absorption.

HPLC Assay

The quantity of drugs penetrating the receptor compartment during skin penetration *in vitro* and in MT-2 cells can be determined using an HPLC assay [29].

APPLICATION OF ETHOSOMES

Therapeutic Applications

Ethosomes are efficient drug delivery systems for different pharmacological compounds *via* skin and thus can help manage various disorders [3]. For instance:

- With transdermal drug delivery *via* ethosomes, various skin diseases can be cured as ethosomes offer more than 65% of the drug to penetrate the affected area of skin efficaciously [30]. Numerous studies have demonstrated the efficacy of ethosomes (ethosomal antibiotics) as a therapy for microbial and viral skin infections. Erythromycin and bacitracin ethosomal systems have already been tested using animal models of deep skin infections [31].

- The improved skin penetration ability and efficacy of the ethosomal-THP formulation in Parkinson's disease have been reported.
- Ethosomes are found capable of delivering genes to the specific site where they can be expressed to become immunologically active [24]. Studies have shown that ethosomes may transfer DNA molecules topically to make certain genes express in skin cells.
- The anti-inflammatory potential of ammonium glycyrrhizinate ethosomes has also been discovered in the affected skin of human patients.
- Hormones administered orally can cause several dose-dependent adverse effects, high first-pass metabolism, and limited oral bioavailability. In comparison, ethosomal formulation containing testosterone had almost 30 times greater skin penetration [25].
- Ethosomal patches gave beneficial results in rabbits and thus may be useful to treat menopausal symptoms in women and androgen deficiency in males.

Cosmeceutical Applications

Ethosomes as cosmeceuticals offer numerous advantages, which include better transdermal penetration (especially in elastic forms), enhanced stability, but less skin irritation from certain dangerous cosmetic chemicals. For instance:

- Ethosomes can be used to treat skin hyperpigmentation as they can easily penetrate the skin and administer the desired drug directly to the impacted region, thus reducing the appearance of uneven skin tone and dark patches [19]. Oxidative damage can be reduced in the skin by topical application of many antioxidants [30]. Ethosomes are also reported to be a possible treatment for acne by administering medications like benzoyl peroxide and retinoids to the affected region.
- Ethosomes can cure hair loss by directly administering medications like finasteride and minoxidil to the hair follicles [32]. These medications may work better and encourage hair growth since ethosomes have a greater ability to penetrate the epidermis [19].

ETHOSOMES FOR THE MANAGEMENT OF PSORIASIS

Psoriasis is an inflammatory skin condition mainly caused by aging and a hereditary predisposition [33]. The exact etiology of the disease is unknown, but several environmental risk factors, including trauma (Koebner phenomenon), physical and mental stress, infection, and certain drugs, are believed to be associated with the development of psoriasis. Although the incidence and prevalence of psoriasis are not well studied, it has been estimated that around 4% of people experience psoriasis worldwide (Rahman *et al.*, 2015).

Based on causes, signs, and symptoms, psoriasis can be plaque, flexural, guttate, nail, psoriatic arthritis, erythrodermic, and pustular psoriasis (Garg *et al.*, 2016).

PATHOPHYSIOLOGY AND PHARMACOTHERAPY OF PSORIASIS

The primary mechanism in the pathophysiology of psoriasis is T-lymphocyte activation. A major histocompatibility complex (MHC) is formed when the surface of antigen-presenting cells in the dermis and epidermis is attacked by antigens. This MHC was carried into the lymph nodes where it binds to T-lymphocyte receptors, activating T cells and forming synapses which include lymphocyte functional antigen 3, cluster differentiation 2 (CD2), etc [34]. An activated cloned T cell quickly enters the bloodstream, moves to different skin layers, and produces a variety of chemokines, growth factors, and cytokines. In psoriatic skin, they accelerate the process of hyperkeratosis and neovascularization.

The pathophysiology of psoriasis is believed to involve other pathways such as abnormal alterations in the metabolism of eicosanoids and polyunsaturated fatty acids, gene expression, lymphokine secretion, and free-radical generation.

ROLE OF MOLECULAR FACTORS RESPONSIBLE FOR PSORIASIS

T-Lymphocytes

T-lymphocytes are the main mediators of the multifaceted processes throughout the illnesses. Inherited immunity, mediated by keratinocytes, neutrophils, mast cells, and antigen-presenting cells (APCs), and acquired immunity, mediated by T-cells, have demonstrated significant roles in the disease [35]. Interaction between the APCs and T-lymphocytes initiates an immune response, leading to the formation of a complex [36]. This complex recognizes an antigen and triggers the formation of cytokines, such as TNF-α and IFN-γ, which are found in greater concentrations in psoriatic lesions and mediate psoriasis.

NKT Cells

The natural killer T cell has a limited capacity to identify a small number of antigens. However, after being activated by certain glycolipids, NKT cells secrete cytokines including IL-4 and IFN, which promote the growth of inflammation and induce cytotoxicity.

Other Leukocytes

Three main categories of dendritic cell (DC)- dermal plasmacytoid DCs (pDCs), dermal myeloid DCs (CD11c+), and epidermal Langerhans cells (iDCs) populations are present in normal human skin. Psoriatic lesions increase DC levels, which mainly comprise mature and immature myeloid DCs (CD11c+) as well as pDCs in small amounts [36].

Chemokines and Cytokines

Psoriatic lesions have elevated levels of many cytokines, including IFN-α, IFN-γ, TNF-α, and Interleukins (IL-1,-6, -17, -22 and -23). Th-17 cell-induced cytokine release (IL-17A, IL-17F, and IL-22) is predominant in the early stages of the disease. Th-1 cells emit cytokines like IFN-α, IFN-γ, and TNF-α, which control the latter stages of the disease.

Approaches for Treatment of Psoriasis

Although the disease cannot be cured, a few strategies may help in the management.

STRATEGIES BASED ON THE SOURCE

Phytotherapeutics

As they are considered to be safer and free of adverse effects as compared to the synthetic treatments available, these are widely accepted. Various natural drugs have been utilized as phytotherapeutics and are discussed below [37].

Aloe vera

It helps to clear psoriatic lesions and possesses keratolytic action, which causes lesions to become desquamated.

Capsicum annum

Substance P stimulates inflammatory cells, inducing keratinocyte proliferation, vasodilation, and angiogenesis in psoriatic lesions [38]. Capsaicin is the principal active component, which releases substance P by binding to the vanilloid receptor and depleting it [39]. It manages psoriasis by reducing the activity of substance P [40].

Curcuma longa

Phosphorylase kinase (PhK), an enzyme present in the epidermal layers of the skin, causes activation of NF-κB, leading to enormous and uncontrolled proliferation of keratinocytes and the development of psoriatic plaque [41].

Curcuminoids and volatile oils in *Curcuma longa* selectively inhibit the enzyme PhK and thus exhibit anti-inflammatory potential in curing psoriatic lesions.

Nigella sativa (Thymoquinone)

The ethanolic extract of *Nigella sativa* seeds has demonstrated anti-psoriatic activity in HaCaT human keratinocyte cell lines. The extract increased the thickness of the epidermal layer, produced considerable epidermal differentiation, and had good anti-proliferative action [42].

Jawad *et al.*, 2014 evaluated the safety and efficacy of *Nigella sativa* (NS) when applied topically and orally in 60 psoriatic patients. Serum levels of malondialdehyde (MDA) and a PASI score were used to evaluate the study's results. Twenty patients received ointment containing 10% w/w Nigella, another 20 patients received an oral capsule containing 500 mg of pure drug powder and the rest of the patients received a combination of the ointment and capsule. After calculating the PASI score, better results were observed in patients getting the ointment formulation [43].

Punica granatum L

Punica granatum L, a member of the Lythraceae family, has certain active compounds, including Punicalagin; 2, 3(S)-hexahydroxydiphenoyl-D-glucose and punicalin. Using the thymidine phosphorylase inhibition assay, Jacob *et al.*, 2019 assessed the aqueous acetone extract of *Punica granatum* fruit for *in vitro* anti-psoriatic activity and discovered that the extract exhibited thymidine phosphorylase-inhibiting action *in-vitro*, but still *in-vivo* testing is required to validate the activity [44].

Wrightia tinctoria (Roxb)

Wrightia tinctoria, family Apocynaceae, has been used for the treatment of skin diseases like psoriasis since traditional times, which may be possibly due to the presence of certain anti-oxidant constituents like flavonoids and glycoflavones—iso orientin and phenolic acids in their leaves.

The antipsoriatic activity of *Wrightia tinctoria* hydroalcoholic leaf extract has also been assessed using the mouse tail technique. Antioxidant activity and orthokeratosis have been reported as a possible mode of action for their anti-psoriatic activity [45].

Reseda luteola

The natural flavonoid luteolin, derived from the leaves of the *Reseda luteola* plant, family Resedaceae, has also been found to exhibit potential benefits in the management of psoriasis. Luteolin has been observed to cause suppression of IL-6, IL-8, and vascular endothelial growth factor levels along with reduced NFkB activation at both transcriptional and translational levels *in vitro* experiments on the HaCaT cell line [46].

Scutellaria lateriflora

Baicalin, a flavonoid isolated from *Scutellaria lateriflora* and *S. baicalensis* roots, family Lamiaceae, has demonstrated anti-inflammatory effects when applied topically to an IMQ-induced psoriasis model. The protective effect against psoriasis is proposed to be due to the inhibition of TNF-α, IL-17A, IL-22, and IL-23 activity, leading to reduced acanthosis, neutrophil infiltration, hyperkeratosis, and epidermal hyperplasia [47].

Genistein

A flavonoid called genistein, derived from soybeans and Prunus trees, family Leguminosae, has been found to suppress inflammatory mediators (TNF-α, IL-1beta, IL-6, IL-17, IL-23), and chemokine ligand 2 (CCL2) *via* NF-kB pathway in IMQ-induced psoriasis in mouse [48].

Synthetic Drugs

Several synthetic compounds are also used to treat psoriasis in addition to herbal remedies; these are included here:

Infliximab, Adalimumab, and Etanercept (TNF-α Inhibitors)

These drugs suppress the activation of immune cells and keratinocytes *via* TNF α inhibition, resulting in less cytokine release, which reduces the severity of psoriasis.

Apilimod and Uztekinumab (IL-12/IL-23 p40 Inhibitors)

These drugs, *via* inhibition of IL-12/IL-23, block cytokine release and thus can actively participate in the pathogenesis of psoriasis.

Alefacept (T-cell Inhibitors)

The only medication in this class to treat psoriasis is Alefacept, injected intramuscularly or intravenously.

Adapalene, Tazarotene, Tazorac, and Zorac (Vitamin A Analogs)

The first-generation retinoic acid analogs were considered unacceptable because of their toxicity and poor effectiveness. However, the second and third generations proved ineffectual when applied topically but worked well when taken orally. However, unfortunately, because of the toxicity problems, they also showed restricted use. Only some fourth-generation analogs like adapalene, tazarotene, tazorac, and zorac have been discovered to be effective in the treatment of psoriasis.

Vitamin D3 Analogues

Because Vitamin D3 Nuclear Receptors (VDR) are present in dermal fibroblasts and keratinocytes, vitamin D3 analogs are used to treat psoriasis.

Strategies based on the mode of Administration

Depending on the kind of psoriasis, there are generally three ways to administer the medicament: topical, systemic, and phototherapy. Patients with mild to severe psoriasis may benefit from a recommendation for milder topical therapies [49]. Conversely, those with moderate to severe psoriasis might benefit from systemic therapy, which includes oral and biologic medications. After topical and systemic therapies fail, phototherapy is frequently recommended for people with moderate to severe psoriasis [50].

Topical Treatment

Psoriasis can be treated with a variety of topical medications having various modes of action [51] like Coal tar, Dithranol, Retinoids, Calcineurin inhibitors, Salicylic acid, Vitamin D analogs, and Corticosteroids [52].

Systemic Treatment

Systemic therapy (in which medication circulates throughout the entire body) can be further separated into two categories *i.e.*, oral agents (including methotrexate and cyclosporine) and biological agents (generally given intravenously) [50, 53].

Phototherapy Treatment

Phototherapy has been used to treat psoriasis since the 1920s and is currently the standard method to treat moderate to severe psoriasis [49]. Compared to systemic therapy, phototherapy treatment has comparatively fewer adverse effects, including immunosuppression. International guidelines offer three different forms of phototherapy treatments to treat psoriasis: psoralen with ultraviolet A (PUVA), excimer laser/lamp (targeted phototherapy), and narrowband ultraviolet B (NB-UVB).

Limitations of the traditional (conventional) drug delivery method for psoriasis Treatment

Both topical and systemic administration of therapeutic drugs for psoriasis are associated with certain limitations including poor oral bioavailability (as a result of hepatic first-pass metabolism), fast clearance, poor skin deposition, incompatibility or adverse interaction with other drugs, poor skin penetration (due to large particle size), *etc.* which makes their usage difficult and necessitate careful monitoring. In addition, these conventional methods cannot achieve targeted delivery to specific tissues or cells, intracellular sites of action, as well as epithelial and endothelial barriers [36]. The low drug penetration through the thick, scaly plaques (psoriatic skin) leads to low ceramide levels and high cholesterol, leading to "stiff" skin in psoriasis [50, 54].

Therefore, many innovative nanotechnology-based psoriasis treatment techniques have been created using nanotechnology to deliver therapeutic compounds for the treatment of psoriasis. Various nanocarriers, viz. lipid-based (solid lipid nanoparticles, polymeric nanoparticles, nanostructured lipid carriers, liposomes, nanoemulsions, ethosomes, transferosomes, and niosomes), polymer-based (microspheres, micelles, nanocapsule), metallic nanaocarriers, *etc.* have been successfully discovered for their role in the treatment of psoriasis.

NANOTECHNOLOGY-BASED DRUG DELIVERY SYSTEMS

Lipid-Based Nanocarriers [55]

Polymeric Nanoparticles

These are drug-containing solid particles or particulate dispersions that have been dispersed, adsorbed, or enclosed in an appropriate polymer matrix [56]. Particles typically have sizes between 10 and 1000 nm. Being able to contain hydrophilic medications, these polymeric nanoparticles may find application as transdermal carriers for the treatment of psoriasis.

Solid Lipid Nanoparticles (SLN)

These lipid-based vesicular systems have become more significant because of their capacity to release medication at a precise location and at a regulated rate. The lipid-based vesicles have the capacity to produce a lipid film on the skin and their tiny size allows deeper penetration into the stratum corneum [57].

Nanostructured Lipid Carriers (NLC)

These are second-generation lipid nanoparticles having sizes in the nanometer range, thus allowing deeper drug penetration into the skin's layers. Using NLCs, the drug molecule can be protected from external environment-dependent degradation processes such as oxidative, chemical, or physical degradation [55, 58].

Liposomes

These are phospholipid-based spherical vesicles (50 nm to several micrometers) used topically to treat a variety of dermatological conditions, including psoriasis and dermatitis. They are able to encapsulate both lipophilic and hydrophilic drugs [59]. Their small size and lipid nature make them efficient for specific drug delivery to certain skin regions.

Nanoemulsions

A nanoemulsion's globule size varies from 50 to 200 nm. High entrapment efficiency, fewer side effects, improved skin permeability, decreased skin irritation, and prolonged drug release make nanoemulsions significant tool for administering drugs into the dermal layers in the management of psoriasis [56].

Transferosomes

Introduced in the early 1990s, transferosomes represent the second generation of elastic, deformable lipid vesicle carriers. Phospholipids and edge activators are coupled to generate these extremely flexible unilamellar vesicles, with a diameter of less than 100 nm [60]. Transferosomes efficiently transport drugs across various layers of the skin without adhering to stratum corneum lipids [61], and this penetration is unaffected by the partition coefficient and concentration gradient.

Niosomes

Niosomes are tiny lamellar structures produced by hydrating cholesterol with non-ionic surfactants. They shield the drug from the environment, increasing its therapeutic efficacy. Their enhanced features over traditional formulations include biodegradable, biocompatible, and non-immunogenic nature [57].

Ethosomes

The third-generation elastic deformable lipid vesicles include ethosomes (etherosomes). These are vesicles consisting of water, phospholipids, and a significant amount of ethanol (around 20-45%), which serves as an enhancer of penetration and improves their fluidity [62].

POLYMER-BASED NANOCARRIER

Microspheres

These occur as solid polymeric spherical particles ranging from 1 to 1000 mm in diameter and contain the drug evenly distributed throughout the polymer matrix. Other significant components include biodegradable proteins or artificial polymers, which are generally free-flowing powders. Their main advantage is the efficient delivery of therapeutic drugs to the target site in a sustained and regulated manner [63]. Other benefits include protection of unstable drugs both before and after delivery, increasing bioavailability, lowering the frequency or severity of side effects, prolonging the therapeutic effects, and enhancing patient compliance.

Micelles

Micelles are spherical structures with a diameter of less than 100 nm formed by the self-aggregation of amphiphilic molecules in an aqueous solution as a result of the hydrophobic effect [64]. The hydrophobic core contains the lipophilic drug, whereas the hydrophilic drug is mainly found in the hydrophilic core of the micelle structure.

Nanocapsule

It is a kind of nanoparticle composed of a protective matrix (shell) with one or more active components (core). The polymer shell makes up the shell, while the core is made up of a liquid suspension containing the medication.

METALLIC NANOCARRIERS (MNPS)

MNPs often have a broad range of uses in biomedical applications, such as controlled release of therapeutic agents, and strong biocompatibility in a variety of diseased conditions. They offer significant benefits not only for anti-aging and anti-acne therapies but also in the management of a variety of skin conditions, including psoriasis.

Gold nanoparticles (GNPs) emerged as the preferred choice for the topical delivery method of several drugs [65]. Recently, alkyl-terminated GNPs to treat psoriasis have been designed [66].

Silver-containing nanoparticles (AgNPs) using European black elderberry fruit extracts have also been designed and their anti-psoriatic effect on UVB-exposed HaCaT cells in an acute inflammatory model has been discovered [65] due to their potential to reduce the production of inflammatory cytokines.

Management of Psoriasis Using Ethosomes

Psoralen-Based Ethosomes

Zhang *et al.* produced ethosomes containing psoralen for the management of psoriasis. A particle size between 56.71-159.07 nm, with the highest entrapment efficiency at 150 nm, was observed. A significant improvement (around 7 times) in penetration of the drug in rat skin has been found when compared with psoralen ethanolic tincture [67]. It was concluded that effective penetration and permeation of ethosomes might reduce toxicity and boost therapeutic results when used in long-term psoriasis treatment [68].

Acitretin-loaded nanoethosomal gel

Nanoethosomal gel containing acitretin, a second-generation systemic drug for the treatment of psoriasis, has been designed using thin-film hydration and evaluated for its effect in psoriasis, cancer, and skin irritation. The vesicle size and zeta potential were observed to be 147 ± 2.15 nm and −11.5 ± 0.25mV respectively with 90.70 ± 0.89%, entrapment efficiency [69]. The discovered nanoethosomal gel was better with greater skin penetration, reduced skin irritation, and reduced cytotoxicity against normal L-929 cells when compared with simple acitretin gel. The *in-vitro* studies also proved the efficacy of ethosomal gel in psoriasis.

Nigella sativa Linn loaded ethosomes and transethosomes gel

Nigella sativa Linn extract loaded ethosomes using thin layer hydration and transethosomes gel using cold method has also been formulated and evaluated for their potential in imiquimod-induced psoriasis and DNCB-induced dermatitis. The particle size was observed to be 172 ± 11 nm and 188 ± 11 nm and the drug content was 74.1 ± 1.9 and 70.5 ± 2.1 for transethosomes and ethosomes, respectively with favourable zeta potential providing better stability to both the formulations. Both ethosomal formulations showed substantial drug entrapment (71.7 ± 2.7% for transethosomes and 78.6 ± 3.1% for ethosomes) and *in vitro* drug release (98.23% for transethosomes and 95.65% for ethosomes) [70]. The better results might be due to the assimilation of phytoconstituents into vesicular systems like ethosomes providing improved absorption, easy permeation, enhanced bioavailability, and prolonged action.

Curcumin and glycyrrhetinic acid-loaded ethosomes

Ethososomes, having exceptional transdermal properties, are ideally suited as skin carriers for hyperplastic diseases. Curcumin-loaded glycyrrhetinic acid-D-α-tocopherol acid polyethylene glycol succinate (GA-TPGS) ethosomes were also discovered to be effective against psoriasis in an IL-6-induced cell model due to their efficacy in reducing oxidative stress, preventing inflammation [71]. These curcumin-loaded ethosomes were found to have enhanced percutaneous absorption upon topical administration in imiquimod-induced psoriatic mice. The synthesized ethosomes ameliorated lipid peroxidation and showed glucocorticoid-like effects, reducing inflammation and exhibiting antipsoriatic activity.

Mangiferin-loaded glycethosomes

Glycethosomes loaded with mangiferin, a naturally occurring phytoconstituent isolated from *Mangifera indica L.,* were also found to be effective in TPA-induced psoriasis as well as hydrogen peroxide-induced damage, confirming their potential use in the management of psoriasis and other skin conditions. The vesicle mean diameter increased to about 288 nm with better biocompatibility and protective action. Entrapment efficiency was inversely related to the amount of loaded mangiferin [72].

Diclofenac potassium-loaded ethosomes

Diclofenac potassium-loaded ethosomal formulation containing 14% phospholipon 90 and 10–40% ethanol was prepared using the conventional mechanical dispersion method. The drug concentration was maintained at 10 mg/ml or 1% w/v [73]. The formulation was also found effective against psoriasis.

Curcumin-Loaded Hyaluronan-Modified Ethosomes

Zhang *et al.* also investigated the advantages of adding hyaluronic acid to curcumin-loaded propylene glycol-based ethosomes for the treatment of psoriasis. Curcumin was loaded into hyaluronic acid-linked propylene glycol-based ethosomes (by covalent binding) to evaluate their efficacy in an imiquimod-induced psoriasis mouse model [74]. Overexpression of CD44 protein in imiquimod-induced psoriasis was about 2.7 times that of normal skin. It was discovered that linking curcumin to hyaluronic acid enhanced drug accumulation and exhibited anti-inflammatory potential by lowering CD44 and CCR6 protein expression, as well as TNF-α, interleukins, *etc.*

Methotrexate-loaded ethosomal topical gel containing salicylic acid

Ethosomal gel prepared by incorporating methotrexate, soy lecithin, and ethanol was found to be very effective as an anti-psoriatic agent in IMQ-induced psoriasis. Smaller vesicle size, good spreadability, and high entrapment efficiency and penetration rate of formulated ethosomes were observed [75]. A drop in PASI score, reduction in epidermal thickness, and 69.14% drug release have been observed, indicating their effectiveness in psoriasis.

Thymoquinone-loaded lipid vesicles

Ethosomal vesicles loaded with thymoquinone, a volatile, lipid-soluble benzoquinone isolated from *Nigella sativa,* along with Phospholipon 90G and ethanol, were also formulated using the cold approach to evaluate their potency in the mouse-tail model. The prepared ethosomal gel was found to have high anti-psoriatic action [76].

Anthralin-loaded ethosomes

To augment anthralin efficacy against psoriasis, it was incorporated into ethosomal preparations using the cold method. Drug encapsulation greater than 77% with particle size between 146 and 381 nm was observed. The clinical efficacy in psoriatic patients was investigated, and an improvement in the PASI score indicated their potential in managing psoriasis [77].

Clobetasol-loaded ethosomal gel

Korade *et al.* reported the efficiency of clobetasol-loaded ethosomal gel for the treatment of psoriasis due to their improved drug release pattern and entrapment efficiency [78].

Tacrolimus-loaded ethosomes

Tacrolimus-loaded ethosomes were also found to exhibit better accumulation and penetration in the skin epidermal layer for treating psoriasis [79].

Resveratrol-loaded ethosomes

The penetration of resveratrol-loaded ethosomal hydrogel in the skin was observed to be 3.5 times more than liposomes with a high permeability coefficient and penetration rate [80].

Advantages of Ethosomal Drug Delivery [81, 12]

Ethosomal drug delivery offers various advantages, which include:

- Good patient adherence rate as the ethosomal drug is supplied in a semisolid form for optimal patient compliance.
- Safe, simple, non-invasive, and passive method to deliver any kind of drug molecule, including hydrophilic, lipophilic, or amphiphilic compounds, peptides, protein molecules, *etc.*
- Enhanced and better permeation and penetration through the skin.
- When coupled with site-specific ligands, ethosomes can be easily coupled to accomplish active targeting.

Despite its various advantages, some drawbacks are also associated with ethosomes, such as:

- Only potent drugs that do not exceed 10 mg/day are permitted.
- The medication must have a suitable size and be sufficiently soluble to permeate the skin's microcirculation and reach the bloodstream in both wet and lipophilic environments.
- It is frequently intended to be a means of obtaining rapid bolus-type drug intake rather than providing gradual, continuous medication administration.
- Enhancers and excipients used in drug delivery systems might induce dermatitis or skin irritation.
- For the drug to reach systemic circulation, it needs to be adequately soluble in both lipophilic and aqueous environments.

CONCLUSION AND FUTURE PROSPECTS

Ethosome-based pharmacotherapy shows promising potential for the management of psoriasis. Their several benefits, *viz.* Enhanced skin penetration, flexibility, biocompatibility, and suitability for both hydrophilic and lipophilic drugs, make them well-suited for delivering therapeutic agents to the skin. Studies investigating the use of ethosome-based formulations for psoriasis treatment have demonstrated encouraging results. Ethosome-mediated delivery of anti-psoriatic drugs such as psoralen, acitretin, curcumin, glycyrrhetinic acid, mangiferin, diclofenac potassium, methotrexate, and many more has shown improved therapeutic efficacy, reduced side effects, and enhanced patient compliance compared to conventional formulations. Additionally, the ability of ethosomes to target the inflamed skin lesions characteristic of psoriasis while minimizing systemic exposure holds promise for achieving better treatment outcomes. Overall, ethosome-based pharmacotherapy represents a promising approach for addressing the challenges associated with psoriasis management, offering the potential for enhanced drug delivery, improved therapeutic outcomes, and better quality of life for patients with this chronic inflammatory skin condition. Through continued research and development, ethosomal formulations may offer a valuable addition to existing treatment options for psoriasis, ultimately benefiting both patients and healthcare providers.

REFERENCES

[1] Godin B, Touitou E. Ethosomes: new prospects in transdermal delivery. Crit Rev Ther Drug Carrier Syst 2003; 20(1): 63-102. [http://dx.doi.org/10.1615/CritRevTherDrugCarrierSyst.v20.i1.20] [PMID: 12911264]

[2] Touitou E, Godin B. Ethosomes for skin delivery. J Drug Deliv Sci Technol 2007; 17(5): 303-8. [http://dx.doi.org/10.1016/S1773-2247(07)50046-8]

[3] Nainwal N, Jawla S, Singh R, Saharan VA. Transdermal applications of ethosomes – a detailed review. J Liposome Res 2019; 29(2): 103-13. [http://dx.doi.org/10.1080/08982104.2018.1517160] [PMID: 30156120]

[4] Raszewska-Famielec M, Flieger J. Nanoparticles for topical application in the treatment of skin dysfunctions- An overview of dermo-cosmetic and dermatological products. Int J Mol Sci 2022; 23(24): 15980. [http://dx.doi.org/10.3390/ijms232415980] [PMID: 36555619]

[5] Ramadon D, McCrudden MTC, Courtenay AJ, Donnelly RF. Enhancement strategies for transdermal drug delivery systems: current trends and applications. Drug Deliv Transl Res 2022; 12(4): 758-91. [http://dx.doi.org/10.1007/s13346-021-00909-6] [PMID: 33474709]

[6] Akombaetwa N, Ilangala AB, Thom L, Memvanga PB, Witika BA, Buya AB. Current advances in lipid nanosystems intended for topical and transdermal drug delivery applications. Pharmaceutics 2023; 15(2): 656. [http://dx.doi.org/10.3390/pharmaceutics15020656] [PMID: 36839978]

[7] Emanet M, Ciofani G. Ethosomes as promising transdermal delivery systems of natural-derived active compounds. Adv NanoBiomed Res 2023; 3(10): 2300020. [http://dx.doi.org/10.1002/anbr.202300020]

[8] Kolay A, Parveen S, Dorai R, Hossain F, Chaudhuri P, Acharya M. Recent advancement in topical delivery methods for the treatment of psoriasis. J Pharm Negat Results 2022; 13(10): 2602-7. [http://dx.doi.org/10.47750/pnr.2022.13.S10.309]

[9] Jeong WY, Kwon M, Choi HE, Kim KS. Recent advances in transdermal drug delivery systems: a review. Biomater Res 2021; 25(1): 24. [http://dx.doi.org/10.1186/s40824-021-00226-6] [PMID: 34321111]

[10] Touitou E, Dayan N, Bergelson L, Godin B, Eliaz M. Ethosomes — novel vesicular carriers for enhanced delivery: characterization and skin penetration properties. J Control Release 2000; 65(3): 403-18. [http://dx.doi.org/10.1016/S0168-3659(99)00222-9] [PMID: 10699298]

[11] Ramakrishna GA, Shinkar DM, Saudagar RB. Ethosomes: Carrier for enhanced transdermal drug delivery system. J Adv Pharm Educ Res 2014; 4(4): 380-7. [http://dx.doi.org/10.51847/pd4yyUP]

[12] Chauhan N, Vasava P, Khan SL, *et al.* Ethosomes: A novel drug carrier. Ann Med Surg (Lond) 2022; 82: 104595. [http://dx.doi.org/10.1016/j.amsu.2022.104595] [PMID: 36124209]

[13] Kumar N, Dubey A, Mishra A, Tiwari P. Ethosomes: A novel approach in transdermal drug delivery system. Int J Pharm Life Sci 2020; 11(5): 6598-608.

[14] Shitole M, Nangare S, Patil U, Jadhav NR. Review on drug delivery applications of ethosomes: Current developments and prospects. Thaiphesatchasan 2022; 46(3): 251-65. Available from: https://digital.car.chula.ac.th/tjps/vol46/iss3/2
[http://dx.doi.org/10.56808/3027-7922.2568]

[15] Garg U, Jain K. Dermal and transdermal drug delivery through vesicles and particles: Preparation and applications. Adv Pharm Bull 2021; 12(1): 45-57.
[http://dx.doi.org/10.34172/apb.2022.006] [PMID: 35517881]

[16] Tamanna , Singh H. Nanotechnology: A novel approach for treatment of skin disorder. J Drug Deliv Ther 2021; 11(4-S): 271-7.
[http://dx.doi.org/10.22270/jddt.v11i4-S.4945]

[17] Verma NK, Singh AK, Mall PC, Yadav V, Jaiswal R. Ethosomal drug delivery system: A novel approach to transdermal drug delivery: A review. International Journal of Pharmaceutical Research and Development 2019; 1(2): 28-33.
[http://dx.doi.org/10.33545/26646862.2019.v1.i2a.12]

[18] Shelke S, Shahi S, Kale S, Patil V, Deshpande D. Ethosomes: A novel deformable carrier. World J Pharm Sci 2015; 3(9): 1830-9.

[19] Abu-Huwaij R, Zidan AN. Unlocking the potential of cosmetic dermal delivery with ethosomes: A comprehensive review. J Cosmet Dermatol 2024; 23(1): 17-26.
[http://dx.doi.org/10.1111/jocd.15895] [PMID: 37393573]

[20] Niu XQ, Zhang DP, Bian Q, *et al.* Mechanism investigation of ethosomes transdermal permeation. Int J Pharm X 2019; 1: 100027.
[http://dx.doi.org/10.1016/j.ijpx.2019.100027] [PMID: 31517292]

[21] Mohanty D, Mounika A, Bakshi V, Akiful Haque M, Keshari Sahoo C. Ethosomes: A novel approach for transdermal drug delivery. Int J Chemtech Res 2018; 11(8): 219-26.
[http://dx.doi.org/10.20902/IJCTR.2018.110826]

[22] Patrekar PV, Inamdar SJ, Mali SS, Mujib MT, Ahir AA, Hosmani AH. Ethosomes as novel drug delivery system: A review. Pharma Innovation J 2015; 4(9): 10-21.

[23] Celia C, Trapasso E, Cosco D, Paolino D, Fresta M. Turbiscan Lab® Expert analysis of the stability of ethosomes® and ultradeformable liposomes containing a bilayer fluidizing agent. Colloids Surf B Biointerfaces 2009; 72(1): 155-60.
[http://dx.doi.org/10.1016/j.colsurfb.2009.03.007] [PMID: 19376689]

[24] Pandey V, Golhani D, Shukla R. Ethosomes: versatile vesicular carriers for efficient transdermal delivery of therapeutic agents. Drug Deliv 2015; 22(8): 988-1002.
[http://dx.doi.org/10.3109/10717544.2014.889777] [PMID: 24580572]

[25] Thadanki ML, Thadanki M, Kishore BA. Review on Ethosomes: A novel approach of Liposomes. Int J Pharm Life Sci 2015; 6(1): 4171-6.

[26] Aggarwal D, Nautiyal U. Ethosomes: A review. Int J Pharm Med Res 2016; 4(4): 354-63.

[27] Pratima NA, Tiwari S. Ethosomes: A novel tool for transdermal drug delivery. IJRPS 2012; 2(1): 1-20.

[28] Fischer AH, Jacobson KA, Rose J, Zeller R. Hematoxylin and eosin staining of tissue and cell sections. CSH Protoc 2008: pdb.prot4986.
[http://dx.doi.org/10.1101/pdb.prot4986] [PMID: 21356829]

[29] Dwivedi D. Vesicular drug delivery system for the herbal treatment of skin disease. J Dev Drugs 2022; 11: 1-12.
[http://dx.doi.org/10.35248/2329-6631.22.11.177]

[30] Verma P, Pathak K. Therapeutic and cosmeceutical potential of ethosomes: An overview. J Adv Pharm Technol Res 2010; 1(3): 274-82.
[http://dx.doi.org/10.4103/0110-5558.72415] [PMID: 22247858]

[31] Ainbinder D, Paolino D, Fresta M, Touitou E. Drug delivery applications with ethosomes. J Biomed Nanotechnol 2010; 6(5): 558-68.
[http://dx.doi.org/10.1166/jbn.2010.1152] [PMID: 21329048]

[32] Ansari SA, Qadir A, Warsi MH, Mujeeb M, Aqil M, Mir SR *et al.* Ethosomes-based gel formulation of karanjin for treatment of acne vulgaris: *In vitro* investigations and preclinical assessment. 3 Biotech 2021; 11(11): 1-14.
[http://dx.doi.org/10.1007/s13205-021-02978-3]

[33] Petit RG, Cano A, Ortiz A, *et al.* Molecular sciences psoriasis: From pathogenesis to pharmacological and nano-technological-based therapeutics. Int J Mol Sci 2021; 22(9): 4983.
[http://dx.doi.org/10.3390/ijms22094983]

[34] Rahman M, Akhter S, Ahmad J, Ahmad MZ, Beg S, Ahmad FJ. Nanomedicine-based drug targeting for psoriasis: potentials and emerging trends in nanoscale pharmacotherapy. Expert Opin Drug Deliv 2015; 12(4): 635-52.
[http://dx.doi.org/10.1517/17425247.2015.982088] [PMID: 25439967]

[35] Xie J, Huang S, Huang H, *et al.* Advances in the application of natural products and the novel drug delivery systems for psoriasis. Front Pharmacol 2021; 12: 644952.
[http://dx.doi.org/10.3389/fphar.2021.644952] [PMID: 33967781]

[36] Saleem S, Iqubal MK, Garg S, Ali J, Baboota S. Trends in nanotechnology-based delivery systems for dermal targeting of drugs: an enticing approach to offset psoriasis. Expert Opin Drug Deliv 2020; 17(6): 817-38.
[http://dx.doi.org/10.1080/17425247.2020.1758665] [PMID: 32315216]

[37] Herman A, Herman A. Topically used herbal products for the treatment of psoriasis - Mechanism of action, drug delivery, clinical studies. Planta Med 2016; 82(17): 1447-55.
[http://dx.doi.org/10.1055/s-0042-115177] [PMID: 27574899]

[38] Huang TH, Lin CF, Alalaiwe A, Yang SC, Fang JY. Apoptotic or antiproliferative activity of natural products against keratinocytes for the treatment of psoriasis. Int J Mol Sci 2019; 20(10): 2558.
[http://dx.doi.org/10.3390/ijms20102558] [PMID: 31137673]

[39] Fattori V, Hohmann M, Rossaneis A, Pinho-Ribeiro F, Verri W. Capsaicin: Current understanding of its mechanisms and therapy of pain and other pre-clinical and clinical uses. Molecules 2016; 21(7): 844.
[http://dx.doi.org/10.3390/molecules21070844] [PMID: 27367653]

[40] Elkhawaga OY, Ellety MM, Mofty SO, Ghanem MS, Mohamed AO. Review of natural compounds for potential psoriasis treatment. Inflammopharmacology 2023; 31(3): 1183-98.
[http://dx.doi.org/10.1007/s10787-023-01178-0] [PMID: 36995575]

[41] Kasprzak-Drozd K, Niziński P, Hawrył A, *et al.* Potential of curcumin in the management of skin diseases. Int J Mol Sci 2024; 25(7): 3617.
[http://dx.doi.org/10.3390/ijms25073617] [PMID: 38612433]

[42] Palaniswamy D, Nithyanantham M, Raghu PS, Dwarampudi LP. Antipsoriatic activity and cytotoxicity of ethanolic extract of *Nigella sativa* seeds. Pharmacogn Mag 2012; 8(32): 268-72.
[http://dx.doi.org/10.4103/0973-1296.103650] [PMID: 24082629]

[43] Ahmed JH, Ibraheem AY, Al-Hamdi KI. Evaluation of efficacy, safety and antioxidant effect of *Nigella sativa* in patients with psoriasis: A randomized clinical trial. Journal of Clinical and Experimental Investigations 2014; 5(2): 186-93.
[http://dx.doi.org/10.5799/ahinjs.01.2014.02.0387]

[44] Jacob J, R G, P L, *et al.* Evaluation of antipsoriatic potential of the fruit rind of *Punica granatum L.*

Pharmacogn J 2019; 11(3): 466-8.
[http://dx.doi.org/10.5530/pj.2019.11.73]

[45] Sundarrajan S, Lulu S, Arumugam M. Deciphering the mechanism of action of *Wrightia tinctoria* for psoriasis based on systems pharmacology approach. J Altern Complement Med 2017; 23(11): 866-78. [http://dx.doi.org/10.1089/acm.2016.0248] [PMID: 28604055]

[46] Wang X, Yao Y, Li Y, Guo S, Li Y, Zhang G. Experimental study on the effect of luteolin on the proliferation, apoptosis and expression of inflammation-related mediators in lipopolysaccharide-induced keratinocytes. Int J Immunopathol Pharmacol 2023; 37: 03946320231169175. [http://dx.doi.org/10.1177/03946320231169175] [PMID: 37024790]

[47] Hung CH, Wang CN, Cheng HH, *et al.* Baicalin ameliorates imiquimod-induced psoriasis-like inflammation in mice. Planta Med 2018; 84(15): 1110-7. [http://dx.doi.org/10.1055/a-0622-8242] [PMID: 29763944]

[48] Wang A, Wei J, Lu C, *et al.* Genistein suppresses psoriasis-related inflammation through a STAT3–NF-κB-dependent mechanism in keratinocytes. Int Immunopharmacol 2019; 69: 270-8. [http://dx.doi.org/10.1016/j.intimp.2019.01.054] [PMID: 30743203]

[49] Mohd Nordin UU, Ahmad N, Salim N, Mohd Yusof NS. Lipid-based nanoparticles for psoriasis treatment: a review on conventional treatments, recent works, and future prospects. RSC Advances 2021; 11(46): 29080-101. [http://dx.doi.org/10.1039/D1RA06087B] [PMID: 35478537]

[50] Katare O, Raza K, Singh B, Dogra S. Novel drug delivery systems in topical treatment of psoriasis: Rigors and vigors. Indian J Dermatol Venereol Leprol 2010; 76(6): 612-21. [http://dx.doi.org/10.4103/0378-6323.72451] [PMID: 21079304]

[51] Witika BA, Mweetwa LL, Tshiamo KO, *et al.* Vesicular drug delivery for the treatment of topical disorders: current and future perspectives. J Pharm Pharmacol 2021; 73(11): 1427-41. [http://dx.doi.org/10.1093/jpp/rgab082] [PMID: 34132342]

[52] Tambe VS, Nautiyal A, Wairkar S. Topical lipid nanocarriers for management of psoriasis-an overview. J Drug Deliv Sci Technol 2021; 64: 102671. [http://dx.doi.org/10.1016/j.jddst.2021.102671]

[53] Cather JC, Crowley JJ. Use of biologic agents in combination with other therapies for the treatment of psoriasis. Am J Clin Dermatol 2014; 15(6): 467-78. [http://dx.doi.org/10.1007/s40257-014-0097-1] [PMID: 25373522]

[54] Bodade SS, Shaikh KS, Kamble MS, Chaudhari PD. A study on ethosomes as mode for transdermal delivery of an antidiabetic drug. Drug Deliv 2013; 20(1): 40-6. [http://dx.doi.org/10.3109/10717544.2012.752420] [PMID: 23311652]

[55] Zhu B, Jing M, Yu Q, Ge X, Yuan F, Shi L. Treatments in psoriasis: from standard pharmacotherapy to nanotechnology therapy. Postepy Dermatol Alergol 2022; 39(3): 460-71. [http://dx.doi.org/10.5114/ada.2021.108445] [PMID: 35950130]

[56] Singh S, Sharma N, Behl T, *et al.* Promising strategies of colloidal drug delivery-based approaches in psoriasis management. Pharmaceutics 2021; 13(11): 1978. [http://dx.doi.org/10.3390/pharmaceutics13111978] [PMID: 34834393]

[57] Raina N, Rani R, Thakur VK, Gupta M. New insights in topical drug delivery for skin disorders: From a nanotechnological perspective. ACS Omega 2023; 8(22): 19145–19167. [http://dx.doi.org/10.1021/acsomega.2c08016]

[58] Elmowafy M, Al-Sanea MM. Nanostructured lipid carriers (NLCs) as drug delivery platform: Advances in formulation and delivery strategies. Saudi Pharm J 2021; 29(9): 999-1012. [http://dx.doi.org/10.1016/j.jsps.2021.07.015] [PMID: 34588846]

[59] Zhao Z, Liu T, Zhu S, Pi J, Guo P, Qi D, *et al.* Natural medicine combined with nanobased topical delivery systems: a new strategy to treat psoriasis. Drug Deliv Transl Res 2022; 12(6): 1326–1338).

[http://dx.doi.org/10.1007/s13346-021-01031-3]

[60] Wollina U, Tirant M, Vojvodic A, Lotti T. Treatment of psoriasis: Novel approaches to topical delivery. Open Access Maced J Med Sci 2019; 7(18): 3018-25. [http://dx.doi.org/10.3889/oamjms.2019.414] [PMID: 31850114]

[61] Khan A, Qadir A, Ali F, Aqil M. Phytoconstituents based nanomedicines for the management of psoriasis. J Drug Deliv Sci Technol 2021; 64: 102663. [http://dx.doi.org/10.1016/j.jddst.2021.102663]

[62] Pradhan M, Alexander A, Singh MR, *et al.* Understanding the prospective of nano-formulations towards the treatment of psoriasis. Biomed Pharmacother 2018; 107: 447-63. [http://dx.doi.org/10.1016/j.biopha.2018.07.156] [PMID: 30103117]

[63] Garg T, Rath G, Goyal AK. Nanotechnological approaches for the effective management of psoriasis. Artif Cells Nanomed Biotechnol 2016; 44(6): 1374-82. [http://dx.doi.org/10.3109/21691401.2015.1037885] [PMID: 25919064]

[64] Zhang M, Hong S, Sun X, *et al.* Exploration of and insights into advanced topical nanocarrier systems for the treatment of psoriasis. Front Med (Lausanne) 2022; 9: 1017126. [http://dx.doi.org/10.3389/fmed.2022.1017126] [PMID: 36590975]

[65] Ahmad MZ, Mohammed AA, Algahtani MS, Mishra A, Ahmad J. Nanoscale topical pharmacotherapy in management of psoriasis: Contemporary research and scope. J Funct Biomater 2022; 14(1): 19. [http://dx.doi.org/10.3390/jfb14010019] [PMID: 36662067]

[66] Han R, Ho LWC, Bai Q, *et al.* Alkyl-terminated gold nanoparticles as a self-therapeutic treatment for psoriasis. Nano Lett 2021; 21(20): 8723-33. [http://dx.doi.org/10.1021/acs.nanolett.1c02899] [PMID: 34618470]

[67] Zhang YT, Feng N-P, Shen L-N, Zhao J-H. Evaluation of psoralen ethosomes for topical delivery in rats by using *in vivo* microdialysis. Int J Nanomedicine 2014; 9(1): 669-78. [http://dx.doi.org/10.2147/IJN.S57314] [PMID: 24489470]

[68] Petit RG, Cano A, Ortiz A, *et al.* Psoriasis: From pathogenesis to pharmacological and nano-technological-based therapeutics. Int J Mol Sci 2021; 22(9): 4983. [http://dx.doi.org/10.3390/ijms22094983] [PMID: 34067151]

[69] Kaur N, Kaur M, Mahajan M, Jain SK. Development, characterization and evaluation of nanocarrier based formulations of antipsoriatic drug "acitretin" for skin targeting. J Drug Deliv Sci Technol 2020; 60: 102010. [http://dx.doi.org/10.1016/j.jddst.2020.102010]

[70] Sahu R, Sharma NK. Formulation development and characterization of *Nigella sativa linn* loaded ethosomes and transethosomes gel for the treatment of psoriasis: A comparative assessment. Eur Chem Bull 2023; 12(5): 1113-25. [http://dx.doi.org/10.31838/ecb/2023.12.si5.0134]

[71] Guo T, Lu J, Fan Y, *et al.* TPGS assists the percutaneous administration of curcumin and glycyrrhetinic acid coloaded functionalized ethosomes for the synergistic treatment of psoriasis. Int J Pharm 2021; 604: 120762. [http://dx.doi.org/10.1016/j.ijpharm.2021.120762] [PMID: 34082000]

[72] Pleguezuelos-Villa M, Diez-Sales O, Manca ML, *et al.* Mangiferin glycethosomes as a new potential adjuvant for the treatment of psoriasis. Int J Pharm 2020; 573: 118844. [http://dx.doi.org/10.1016/j.ijpharm.2019.118844] [PMID: 31751638]

[73] Vijayakumar MR, Sathali AH, Arun K. Formulation and evaluation of diclofanac potassium ethosomes. Int J Pharm Pharm Sci 2010; 2(4): 82-6.

[74] Zhang Y, Xia Q, Li Y, *et al.* CD44 assists the topical anti-psoriatic efficacy of curcumin-loaded hyaluronan-modified ethosomes: A new strategy for clustering drug in inflammatory skin. Theranostics 2019; 9(1): 48-64.

[http://dx.doi.org/10.7150/thno.29715] [PMID: 30662553]

[75] Chandra A, Aggarwal G, Manchanda S, Narula A. Development of topical gel of methotrexate incorporated ethosomes and salicylic acid for the treatment of psoriasis. Pharm Nanotechnol 2019; 7(5): 362-74.
[http://dx.doi.org/10.2174/2211738507666190906123643] [PMID: 31490769]

[76] Negi P, Sharma I, Hemrajani C, *et al.* Thymoquinone-loaded lipid vesicles: a promising nanomedicine for psoriasis. BMC Complement Altern Med 2019; 19(1): 334.
[http://dx.doi.org/10.1186/s12906-019-2675-5] [PMID: 31771651]

[77] Fathalla D, Youssef EMK, Soliman GM. Liposomal and ethosomal gels for the topical delivery of anthralin: Preparation, comparative evaluation and clinical assessment in psoriatic patients. Pharmaceutics 2020; 12(5): 446.
[http://dx.doi.org/10.3390/pharmaceutics12050446] [PMID: 32403379]

[78] Korade S, Deshmukh MT, Shete RV. Formulation and evaluation of ethosomal gel containing clobetasol. EJPMR 2016; 3(9): 664-72.

[79] Li G, Fan C, Li X, *et al.* Preparation and *in vitro* evaluation of tacrolimus-loaded ethosomes. ScientificWorldJournal 2012; 2012: 1-6.
[http://dx.doi.org/10.1100/2012/874053] [PMID: 22629219]

[80] Arora D, Nanda S. Quality by design driven development of resveratrol loaded ethosomal hydrogel for improved dermatological benefits *via* enhanced skin permeation and retention. Int J Pharm 2019; 567: 118448.
[http://dx.doi.org/10.1016/j.ijpharm.2019.118448] [PMID: 31226472]

[81] Razavi H, Janfaza S. Ethosome: A nanocarrier for transdermal drug delivery. Arch Adv Biosci 2015; 6(2): 38-43.
[http://dx.doi.org/10.22037/jps.v6i2.8856]

CHAPTER 14

Transferosomes as a Drug Carrier for the Management of Psoriasis

Garima[1], **Pankaj Popli**[1], **Kashish Wilson**[2], **Deepak Sharma**[3] and **Meenakshi Dhanawat**[4,*]

[1] *Department of Pharmaceutics, Chitkara College of Pharmacy, Chitkara University, Rajpura, Punjab, India*

[2] *Department of Pharmaceutics, M. M. College of Pharmacy, Maharishi Markandeshwar (Deemed to be University), Ambala, Haryana, India*

[3] *Institute of Pharmacy, Assam Don Bosco University, Tapesi 782402, Assam, India*

[4] *Amity Institute of Pharmacy, Amity University Haryana, Amity Education Valley, Panchgaon, Manesar, Gurugram 122413, Haryana, India*

Abstract: The autoimmune condition psoriasis is typified by hyperproliferation of keratinocytes, lesions, and silver-white scales inside the epidermis. Environmental and genetic factors both contribute to its cause. For psoriasis, several medication targets and focused treatments have been discovered. To lessen the symptoms of this illness, numerous target-specific medicines have also been created. Psoriasis is being treated using a variety of techniques, such as herbal remedies, nano-carrier therapy, and conventional therapy. In this regard, delivery through the transdermal route is an intriguing choice because it is safe and convenient. Since transferosomes have a bilayered structure that makes it easier to encapsulate lipophilic, hydrophilic, and amphiphilic drugs with higher penetration efficiencies than regular liposomes, they are a popular option for transdermal medication delivery for psoriasis. Because of their flexibility, they can flex and sneak through small pores that are significantly smaller than their actual dimensions, while remaining intact as a whole vesicle. This chapter aims to explain the concept of transferosomes, their mode of action, various methods of preparation, and their current applications in psoriasis therapy.

Keywords: Autoimmune disease, Drug delivery, Psoriasis, Transferosomes, Transdermal.

INTRODUCTION

Psoriasis is an autoimmune skin disorder condition caused by environmental along with hereditary factors [1]. The skin ailment known as psoriasis is dry,

* **Corresponding author Meenakshi Dhanawat:** Amity Institute of Pharmacy, Amity University Haryana, Amity Education Valley, Panchgaon, Manesar, Gurugram 122413, Haryana, India; E-mail: meenakshi.itbhu@gmail.com

Anjali Sharma, Prerna Sharma, Roy Rillera Marzo & Ahmed A. Al Karmalawy (Eds.)

inflammatory, persistent, and incurable. T cells and enhanced cytokine secretion— such as IFN-γ, IL-20, IL-23, IL-17, IL-22, and others—which promote keratinocyte proliferation—are the conditions' mediators [2]. It might have an impact on the entire body. Thickened crimson plaques with silver-white scales on top are visible on the skin. It is distinguished by a recurrent episode of inflammation and hyperkeratosis [3]. This illness is accompanied by severe medical conditions like psoriatic arthritis, seronegative arthritis form, and cardiovascular disease [4]. The area's most frequently impacted by psoriasis are the scalp, fingertips, foot, elbows, knees, buttocks, beneath the breasts, gluteus, umbilicus, and hands [5]. Males and females can both have psoriasis. It can happen at any age, although it usually occurs in the second and fourth decades of life, from 20 to 40 years old [6]. The frequency is higher in females in comparison to males. Rarely, kids are also impacted. The global incidence of psoriasis is approximately 2% in underdeveloped countries, with an average prevalence rate of 4.6%. Psoriasis affects approximately 1.02% of the population, with incidence rates ranging from 0.44% to 2.2%. Phototherapy is a treatment option for psoriasis that involves using ultraviolet [UV] light, and medications can be administered through several ways, including topical and systemic routes [7]. The body reacts to UV radiation by going into an autoimmune state. The treatment is limited by the negative effects of phototherapy, which include the need for frequent visits to specialty medical centers, sunburn risk, increased costs, and skin cancer risks in the long run for PUVA [Psoralen Ultraviolet-B] [8]. In the 1990s, Cevc *et al.* presented transferosomes, a novel kind of carrier system. They are composed of phospholipids and the membrane-softening agent edge activator [EA] that helps the transferosomes' ultra-deformable characteristic [For example, sodium cholate, Span 80, and Tween 80] [9]. When they get to the skin pores, they can spontaneously pass through them by altering the flexibility of their membrane [10]. These highly deformable, self-optimizing lipid aggregates were effectively applied for the transdermal delivery of proteins and peptides, as well as sustained release of targeted medicinal agents, in a variety of phase I and phase II clinical trials and comprehensive preclinical testing [10]. Thus far, transferosomes have emerged as the most remarkable and inventive transdermal drug delivery system. The researcher's term, the underlying concept, the techniques for preparation and characterization, and the elements influencing the entry into or conduct of a study on transdermal medication delivery using elastic vesicles will all benefit from an understanding of the particular characteristics of the initial generation of elastic vesicles, or transferosomes [11]. We provide an outline of mechanisms of action, several preparations, and engaging in or carrying out studies on the existing features of the initial generation of elastic vesicles [transferosomes], which might be beneficial for the researcher's review of elastic vesicle-based transdermal delivery of medications. We provide a summary of the mechanisms of action, various preparations and characterization, with an emphasis on the most recent applications in the transdermal delivery of medications using current characterization techniques—elements influencing transferosome characteristics, along with a review including techniques and a focus on their latest uses in transdermal medication delivery.

MECHANISM OF ACTION OF TRANSFEROSOMES

Colloidal particles, or vesicles, are composed of amphiphilic molecules and consist of an aqueous compartment enclosed by a double layer that is concentric [12]. They are extremely valuable as vesicular drug delivery systems because of their capacity to transport hydrophilic medications, which are housed within the inner aqueous compartment, and hydrophobic medications, which are bound within the lipid bilayer [13]. Transferosomes are innovative drug carrier vesicles that are self-optimizing and entirely deformable [ultra-flexible]. Their ability to retain the integrity of the vesicle and their membrane flexibility are what primarily allows them to pass through the skin [14]. According to Cevc and Blume's research, transferosomes penetrate through the epidermis through a technique called hydrotaxis [xenophobia]. This is further clarified by the fact that, under a nonocclusive environment, moisture loss from the transferosomal formulation occurs after it is applied to the skin, explaining the moisture-seeking inclination in the direction of the deeper layers of the skin rather than a dry exterior landscape. Due to these channels, transferosomes that are ultra-deformable and slimy can cross the skin's moisture gradient [15]. Furthermore, the gradient evaporation leads to the development of the osmotic gradient. Furthermore, the body's heat-induced evaporation of skin surface water is what leads to the osmotic gradient to occur. This mechanism acts as a catalyst to enable the receptive transportation of medicinal substances across the skin from the application site toward the target region for local or systemic treatments at minimally harmful systemic concentrations (Fig. **1**) [16].

Transferosomes, then, are supramolecular structures made up of at least one kind of amphipathic agent and one type of bilayer-softening agent [edge activator], which significantly increases the flexibility and permeability of the lipid bilayer [17]. Some transferosomes contain small amounts of alcohol [propylene glycol or ethanol] in their formulations, which are utilized as cosolvents with strong solvating ability and to improve penetration. It has been suggested that ethanol can alter the polar head region of the lipid bilayer. Ethanol enhances the fluidity of the intercellular lipid matrix after penetration, which subsequently causes a decrease in the density of the lipid lamellae [18]. Transferosomes can penetrate the stratum corneum and get to their intended targets, which include blood circulation and the dermis. The vesicles' composition causes the transferosomal membrane to become deformable, which impacts its capacity to penetrate [19]. To find the most appropriate carriers that have optimum stability, deformability, and drug-carrying abilities, the ideal compositions of vesicles for each therapeutic agent must be determined through the use of specially designed experimental procedures.

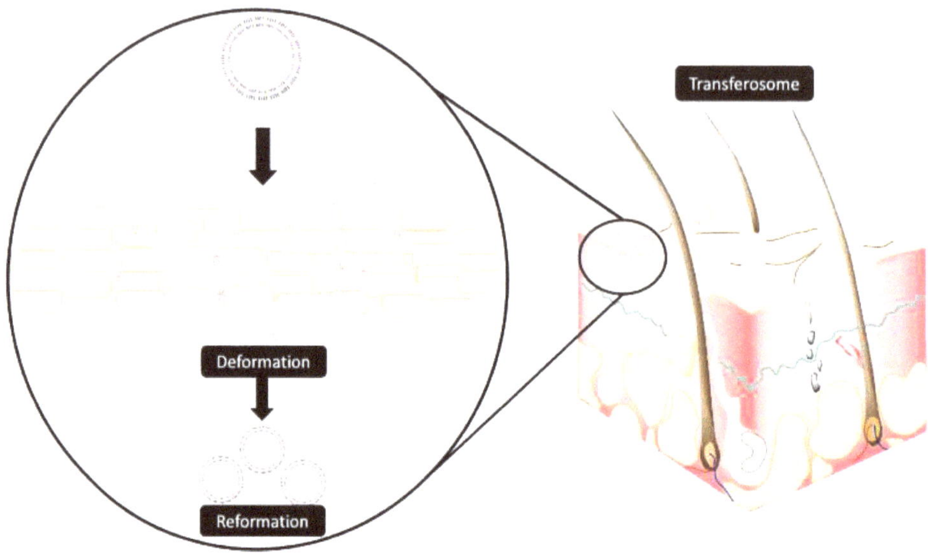

Fig. (1). Mechanism of permeation of transferosomes.

MATERIALS FOR TRANSFEROSOMES

Phospholipids, such as phosphatidylcholine, make up the majority of the mixed lipid aggregate that is self-adaptable and optimized, known as transferosomes. For an aqueous medium, these phospholipids assemble themselves in a lipid bilayer to create a vesicle structure [20]. The incorporation of an edge activator, a bilayer softening component, improves the lipid bilayer's flexibility and penetration. A single-chain surfactant is typically used as an edge activator which increases fluidity and flexibility of lipid bilayer by destabilizing it [21]. More recent elastic vesicles, first presented in 1998 by Van den Berg, use non-ionic surfactants as edge activators. It is possible to modify the membrane's elasticity of transferosomes by mixing adequate surface-active ingredients in defined ratios [22]. Transferosomes' superior flexibility and permeability enable them to adjust their form in response to external stressors, controlling the local concentrations of every component within the bilayer. This flexibility decreases the risk of vesicle rupture within the skin by enabling transferosomes to adhere to the inherent water gradient along the epidermis, especially when applied in non-occlusive settings [23].

Usually, phospholipids make up the majority of the component, with 10–25% surfactant added for flexibility. The hydrating medium is composed of a 6.5-7 pH saline phosphate buffer. For confocal scanning laser microscopy, dyes are frequently utilized (Table **1**) [24].

Table 1. Materials utilized in the formation of Transferosomes [25].

Materials Used	Materials	Properties
Phospholipid	Phosphorylcholine from soy, Phosphorylcholine from eggs, and Disteryl phosphatidylcholine	Formed vesicles
Surfactant	Tween 80, Span 80, sodium deoxycholate, and sodium chloride	Provide Flexibility
Alcohol	Methanol and Ethanol	Solvent
Buffering agent	Phosphate Buffer	Hydrating medium
Dye	Nil red, Rhodamine-123, Rhodamine-DHPE,	For research using Confocal Scanning Laser Microscopy

METHODS OF PREPARATION OF TRANSFEROSOMES

Numerous proprietary transferosome production procedures exist, but there is no established formula or standard methodology for its preparation [26]. For every therapeutic agent, specific studies must be conducted to determine, design, and optimize the ideal vesicle compositions and preparation conditions to produce the ideal carriers with the highest deformability, drug-carrying ability, and stable nature [27]. The conventional method of producing transferosomes is the thin film hydration strategy, also known as the rotary evaporation-sonication method. Additional modified methods for preparation include ethanol injection, centrifugation, suspension homogenization, reverse-phase evaporated water, vortexing-sonication, and the modified handshaking protocol [28]. Each method is generally described as follows:

Thin Film Hydration Technique/Rotary Evaporation-Sonication Method

A combination of volatile organic solvents, like methanol and chloroform, in a suitable [v/v] ratio, is used for dissolving the phospholipids and edge activator (the substances that form vesicles) in a round-bottom flask. This phase could involve the placement of lipophilic drugs. To create a thin layer, the organic solvent is evaporated over the lipid transition temperature while the air pressure is reduced utilizing a rotating vacuum evaporator. Once a thin film forms, hydration is carried out by spinning it in a buffer solution of an appropriate pH (*e.g.*, pH 7.4) over the required duration at the appropriate temperature. The hydrophilic drug inclusion undergoes completion at this movement. To create tiny vesicles, the resultant vesicles were sonicated in a probe sonicator after swelling at ambient temperature. The sonicated vesicles are homogenized by extrusion over a sandwich of 200 nm to 100 nm polycarbonate membrane [29].

Modified Handshaking Process

The underlying concept behind the modified handshaking method and the rotating evaporation-sonication method is identical. In the modified handshaking protocol, phospholipids, an edge activator, an organic solvent, and a lipophilic medicament are introduced into a round-bottom flask. Every excipient must be completely dissolved by the solvent to produce a clear, transparent solution. The organic solvent is subsequently eliminated *via* evaporation while shaking hands, in contrast to utilizing a spinning vacuum evaporator. At the same time, a water bath maintained at an elevated temperature [40–60 ◦C, for instance] partly submerges the round-bottom flask. A thin lipid layer then develops inside the flask's wall. Overnight, the solvent in the flask is allowed to evaporate entirely. Afterward, the resulting film is hydrated at a temperature above its phase transition temperature and gently shaken in the required buffering solution. The inclusion of a hydrophilic drug can be completed at this point [30].

Vortexing-Sonication Method

The drug, edge activator and phospholipids are incorporated and mixed in a phosphate buffer. After that, the above mixture is vortexed to generate a transferosomal suspension that is milky. Extrusion is performed *via* polycarbonate membranes that have been sonicated in a bath sonicator for a prescribed period at room temperature [22].

Reverse-Phase Evaporation Method

The phospholipids and edge activator are mixed in a combination of organic solvents [such as diethyl ether and chloroform] and then dispersed in a round-bottom flask. This phase involves the placement of the lipophilic drug. After the solvent evaporates, the lipid films are produced using a rotary evaporator. The lipid films are reconstituted in the organic phase, which is mostly made up of isopropyl ether and diethyl ether. After that, the aqueous and organic phases combine to form a two-phase system. Currently, the inclusion of hydrophilic drugs is underway. Following that, a bath sonicator is used to sonicate this system until a consistent w/o (water-in-oil) emulsion formation takes place. The organic solvent is continuously evaporated using a rotary evaporator, resulting in the formation of a thick gel which later develops into a vesicular suspension [31].

Ethanol Injection Method

The organic phase is produced when the phospholipid, edge activator, and lipophilic medicine are submerged in ethanol under magnetic stirring for the required length of time to generate a clear solution. The aqueous phase is created by dissolving the water-soluble components in the buffer consisting of phosphate. The hydrophilic drug insertion can be finished at this stage. Both solutions are between 45 and 50°C in temperature. The ethanolic phospholipid solution is subsequently added gradually while the aqueous solution is constantly agitated for a predetermined duration of time. The resultant dispersion is placed into a vacuum evaporator and sonicated to decrease the size of the particles to remove the ethanol [32].

CHARACTERIZATION OF TRANSFEROSOMES

Vesicle Size Distribution, Zeta Potential, Morphology, Surface Charge, and its Density

The size of vesicles and their distribution can be detected through a dynamic light scattering system, such as Malvern Zetasizer. Similarly, a Zetasizer is deployed to evaluate surface charge along with density [33]. However, the particle diameter of vesicles is assessed through the utilization of photon electron spectroscopy or Dynamic light scattering after samples preparation in distilled water, followed by filtration *via* 0.2 mm membrane. Moreover, these can be visualized using techniques such as phase contrast and transmission electron microscopy. Furthermore, the vesicle's stability was evaluated through differences in sizes and their structure over time, with dynamic light scattering measuring mean size and Transmission electron microscopy detecting structural alterations [34].

Entrapment efficiency

This represents the percentage of drugs trapped and detected through the initial separation of untrapped drugs using mini-column centrifugation. Subsequently, the vesicles were then broken up with either 0.1% Triton X-100 or 50% n-propanol. This could be calculated as the ratio of the amount of drug entrapped to the total amount added, multiplied by 100 [35].

$$EE = \frac{Amount\ of\ drug\ entrapped}{Total\ amount\ of\ drug\ added} \times 100$$

Drug Content

It can be assessed using an instrumental analytical technique, such as the modified HPLC method equipped with a column oven and a UV detector, autosampler, pump, and computerized analysis software tailored for specific requirements in the pharmacopeial drug analysis method [36].

Turbidity, Permeability Measurement, and Penetration Capacity

A nephelometer is utilized to assess the turbidity of the drug. However, the permeability study holds significance as a unique parameter for characterization [37]. For this deformability analysis, pure water is used as the standard. Transferosome formulation is run over several microporous filters with predetermined pore diameters. Using dynamic light scattering, the particle sizes and size distributions are measured following each filtering stage. Furthermore, fluorescence microscopy may be employed to assess transferosomes' capacity to penetrate [38].

Sealing Effect

The sealing of the skin is beneficial for drug permeation in traditional topical formulations, but it poses challenges for elastic vesicles. In the case of vesicles, the movement of water, known as hydrotaxis plays a significant role in driving permeation *via* the epidermis, traveling through the relatively dry top to regions that are deeper and more water-rich. Sealing prevents moisture from evaporating from the skin, which affects hydration levels [39].

In-vitro Skin Permeation Studies

A modified Franz diffusion cell having an effective diffusion area of 2.50 cm2 and a receiving compartment volume of 50 ml was employed for this research. Goat skin submerged in a phosphate buffer solution [pH 7.4] was used in *In-vitro* drug penetration investigations. A fresh goat's abdomen was obtained and then hydrated in a saline solution. After carefully wiping away the layer of adipose tissue with a cotton swab, the skin was cleaned with an isopropyl alcohol solution and maintained at a temperature between 0 °C and 40 °C. The experiment was then initiated by placing the tissue inside the Franz diffusion cell, applying a formulation equivalent to 10 mg of the drug to the skin, and covering the top of the diffusion cell [40].

Stability of Formulation

The formulations were then preserved in sealed glassware ampoules once the first proportion of the medication encapsulated in the formulation was determined. For several months, these ampoules were maintained at 4±2 degrees Celsius. To identify medication leakage, samples were extracted from each ampoule after thirty days and examined. Having the initial drug entrapment set at 100%, the percentage of drug loss was calculated. This evaluation pertains to the physical stability of the formulation [41].

APPLICATION OF TRANSFEROSOMES IN PSORIASIS

Transferosomes demonstrated the significant potential for the prolonged release and amelioration of the site-specific action of the administered drug. For example, Jain *et al.* formulated the transferosome and compared it with liposomes and ointments, concluding that the transferosome enhanced transdermal flux, extended-release duration, and improved the targeted delivery of bioactive molecules [42]. Similarly, it helps increase the solubility of medicines with low solubility. For instance, Gupta *et al.* utilized the transferosome to enhance the solubility of tacrolimus thus, results of kinetics and dynamics studies revealed that the utilization of transferosome demonstrated the promising permeation across the rat skin [43]. Moreover, transfersomes also ameliorated skin permeation. Alam *et al.* utilized a transferosome of betamethasone valerate; thus, the formulation revealed a significant result in diffusion through rat skin at a sustained rate for 10 hours. Furthermore, transfersomes are Biodegradable and biocompatible. Vohra *et al.* utilized the transferosome to deliver *Aloe vera* and vitamin E to treat psoriasis, thus, results demonstrated the skin compatibility and delivery of active constituents in a biodegradable and biocompatible manner [44]. Moreover, the transfersomes also demonstrated their application in the co-delivery of drugs for psoriasis therapy. Todke *et al.* utilized a transferosome for the concurrent administration of cyclosporine and Clobetasol propionate to treat the dermis and epidermis layers. The *ex vivo* results demonstrated the promising effects of the drugs, with clobetasol propionate delivered in the dermis and cyclosporine in the epidermis layer [45].

Transfersomes also takes part in delivering large molecules to treat psoriasis such as Motwani *et al.* utilized the transferosome to deliver vitamin E and *Aloe vera*, thus, its formulation delivered the drug and demonstrated the prolonged release of the drug of 12h, and also showed promising results in a reduction of the itchiness score in mice's skin lesions caused by oxazolone [46].

CONCLUSION

Compared to traditional vesicular systems, transferosomes are highly deformable carriers that enable the transport of a broad variety of medicinal substances across the barrier of skin with increased efficacy. The primary mechanism propelling transferosomes into the deeper skin layers is the osmotic gradient. When applied over the skin's surface, it is believed that elastic and ultra-deformable vesicles are more permeable and penetrate the stratum corneum at a greater rate than liposomes and niosomes. It is distinct and adaptable due to the inclusion of EA in its composition. Compared to conventional gels, there are extremely limited transferosomal formulations in the marketplace due to production costs, even though transferosomes' permeability is reported to be more effective in drug delivery. To boost medication delivery *via* the skin, more research is necessary to create protocols that integrate this technology with other permeation augmentation methods.

REFERENCES

[1] Zeng J, Luo S, Huang Y, Lu Q. Critical role of environmental factors in the pathogenesis of psoriasis. J Dermatol 2017; 44(8): 863-72. Available from: https://pubmed.ncbi.nlm.nih.gov/28349593/ [http://dx.doi.org/10.1111/1346-8138.13806] [PMID: 28349593]

[2] Nayak N, Somanna P, Patil AB, Radhakrishnan A. Progress in novel ultradeformable vesicular drug carrier in the topical and transdermal treatment of psoriasis. Ther Deliv 2020; 11(12): 807-19. Available from: https://pubmed.ncbi.nlm.nih.gov/33267650/ [http://dx.doi.org/10.4155/tde-2020-0081] [PMID: 33267650]

[3] Caro-Chang LA, Fung MA. The role of eosinophils in the differential diagnosis of inflammatory skin diseases. Hum Pathol 2023; 140: 101-28. Available from: https://pubmed.ncbi.nlm.nih.gov/37003367/ [http://dx.doi.org/10.1016/j.humpath.2023.03.017] [PMID: 37003367]

[4] Dogra S, Mahajan R. Psoriasis: Epidemiology, clinical features, co-morbidities, and clinical scoring. Indian Dermatol Online J 2016; 7(6): 471-80. Available from: https://pubmed.ncbi.nlm.nih.gov/27990381/ [http://dx.doi.org/10.4103/2229-5178.193906] [PMID: 27990381]

[5] Armstrong AW, Jayade S, Rege S, *et al.* Evaluating treatment choice in patients with moderate to severe psoriasis in the united states: Results from a US patient survey. Dermatol Ther (Heidelb) 2024; 14(2): 421-39. Available from: https://link.springer.com/article/10.1007/s13555-023-01089-6 [http://dx.doi.org/10.1007/s13555-023-01089-6] [PMID: 38252376]

[6] Swanbeck G, Inerot A, Martinsson T, Wahlström J. A population genetic study of psoriasis. Br J Dermatol 1994; 131(1): 32-9. Available from: https://pubmed.ncbi.nlm.nih.gov/8043420/ [http://dx.doi.org/10.1111/j.1365-2133.1994.tb08454.x] [PMID: 8043420]

[7] Zhang P, Wu MX. A clinical review of phototherapy for psoriasis. Lasers Med Sci 2018; 33(1): 173-80. Available from: https://pubmed.ncbi.nlm.nih.gov/29067616/ [http://dx.doi.org/10.1007/s10103-017-2360-1] [PMID: 29067616]

[8] Finlay AY, Ortonne JP. Patient satisfaction with psoriasis therapies: an update and introduction to biologic therapy. J Cutan Med Surg 2004; 8(5): 310-20. Available from: https://pubmed.ncbi.nlm.nih.gov/15868312/ [http://dx.doi.org/10.1177/120347540400800502] [PMID: 15868312]

[9] Albalawi W, Alharbi S, Alanazi F, *et al.* Elegant, flexible vesicular nanocarriers for the efficient skin delivery of topically applied drugs. Curr Nanosci 2023; 19(4): 493-508. [http://dx.doi.org/10.2174/1573413718666211230111538]

[10] Opatha SAT, Titapiwatanakun V, Chutoprapat R. Transfersomes: A promising nanoencapsulation technique for transdermal drug delivery. Pharmaceutics [Internet]. 2020 Sep 1 [cited 2024 Apr 8];12(9):1–23. Available from: /pmc/articles/PMC7559928/ [http://dx.doi.org/10.3390/pharmaceutics12090855]

[11] Benson HAE. Transfersomes for transdermal drug delivery. Expert Opin Drug Deliv 2006; 3(6): 727-37. Available from: https://pubmed.ncbi.nlm.nih.gov/17076595/ [http://dx.doi.org/10.1517/17425247.3.6.727] [PMID: 17076595]

[12] Verma S. Singh; S K, Syan N, Mathur P, Valecha V. Nanoparticle vesicular systems: A versatile tool

for drug delivery. J Chem Pharm Res 2010; 2(2): 496-509.

[13] Supraja B, Mulangi S. An updated review on pharmacosomes, a vesicular drug delivery system. J Drug Deliv Ther 2019; 9(1-s): 393-402. [http://dx.doi.org/10.22270/jddt.v9i1-s.2234]

[14] Chaurasiya P, Ganju E, Upmanyu N, Ray SK, Jain P, Kiran H. Transfersomes: A novel technique for transdermal drug delivery. J Drug Deliv Ther 2019; 9(1): 279-85. [http://dx.doi.org/10.22270/jddt.v9i1.2198]

[15] Oyarzún P, Gallardo-Toledo E, Morales J, Arriagada F. Transfersomes as alternative topical nanodosage forms for the treatment of skin disorders. Nanomedicine (Lond) 2021; 16(27): 2465-89. Available from: https://pubmed.ncbi.nlm.nih.gov/34706575/ [http://dx.doi.org/10.2217/nnm-2021-0335] [PMID: 34706575]

[16] Björklund S, Engblom J, Thuresson K, Sparr E. A water gradient can be used to regulate drug transport across skin. J Control Release 2010; 143(2): 191-200. Available from: https://pubmed.ncbi.nlm.nih.gov/20074596/ [http://dx.doi.org/10.1016/j.jconrel.2010.01.005] [PMID: 20074596]

[17] Rajan R, Jose S, Mukund VPB, Vasudevan DT. Transferosomes - A vesicular transdermal delivery system for enhanced drug permeation. J Adv Pharm Technol Res [Internet]. 2011 [cited 2024 Apr 8];2(3):138. Available from: /pmc/articles/PMC3217704/

[18] Benson HAE, Grice JE, Mohammed Y, Namjoshi S, Roberts MS. Topical and transdermal drug delivery: from simple potions to smart technologies. Curr Drug Deliv [Internet]. 2019 Feb 4 [cited 2024 Apr 8];16(5):444. Available from: /pmc/articles/PMC6637104/

[19] Sapkota R, Dash AK. Liposomes and transferosomes: A breakthrough in topical and transdermal delivery. https://doi.org/104155/tde-2020-0122 [Internet]. 2021 Feb 15 [cited 2024 Apr 8]; 12(2):145–58. Available from: https://www.future-science.com/doi/10.4155/tde-2020-0122 [http://dx.doi.org/10.4155/tde-2020-0122]

[20] Transferosome: latest updates | international journal of pharmaceutical sciences and research [Internet]. [cited 2024 Apr 8]. Available from: https://ijpsr.com/bft-article/transferosome-latest-updates/

[21] (1) (PDF) Transfersomes: a promising approach for transdermal drug delivery system [internet]. [cited 2024 Apr 8]. Available from: Available from: https://www.researchgate.net/publication/286451763_TRANSFERSOMES_A_PROMISING_APPROACH_FOR_TRANSDERMAL_DRUG_DELIVERY_SYSTEM

[22] Naik US. The synthesis and characterisation of novel ultra-flexible lipidic vesicles using propanol. 2013 [cited 2024 Apr 8]; Available from: https://www.uclan.ac.uk/research/index.php

[23] Fernández-García R, Lalatsa A, Statts L, Bolás-Fernández F, Ballesteros MP, Serrano DR. Transferosomes as nanocarriers for drugs across the skin: Quality by design from lab to industrial scale. Int J Pharm 2020; 573: 118817. Available from: https://pubmed.ncbi.nlm.nih.gov/31678520/ [http://dx.doi.org/10.1016/j.ijpharm.2019.118817] [PMID: 31678520]

[24] Rajkumar J, Sree Lakshmi RK, Vineesha S, Rajkumar J. A new approach to transdermal drug delivery using transfersomes-based nanoencapsulation: a research update. Asian J Pharm Res Dev [Internet]. 2022 Feb 15 [cited 2024 Apr 8];10(1):64–70. Available from: https://ajprd.com/index.php/journal/article/view/1082 [http://dx.doi.org/10.22270/ajprd.v10i1.1082]

[25] (1) (PDF) "Transferosomes-a review" [Internet]. [cited 2024 Apr 8]. Available from: https://www.researchgate.net/publication/337077339_TRANSFEROSOMES-A_REVIEW [http://dx.doi.org/10.20959/wjpps201610-7845]

[26] Rizwan M, Aqil M, Talegaonkar S, Azeem A, Sultana Y, Ali A. Enhanced transdermal drug delivery techniques: an extensive review of patents. Recent Pat Drug Deliv Formul 2009; 3(2): 105-24.

Available from: https://pubmed.ncbi.nlm.nih.gov/19519571/
[http://dx.doi.org/10.2174/187221109788452285] [PMID: 19519571]

[27] Witwer KW, Buzás EI, Bemis LT, Bora A, Lässer C, Lötvall J, *et al.* Standardization of sample collection, isolation and analysis methods in extracellular vesicle research. J Extracell Vesicles [Internet]. 2013 [cited 2024 Apr 8];2(1). Available from: /pmc/articles/PMC3760646/

[28] Chaurasiya P, Ganju E, Upmanyu N, Ray SK, Jain P. Transfersomes: a novel technique for transdermal drug delivery. J Drug Deliv Ther 2019; 9(1): 279-85. Available from: https://jddtonline.info/index.php/jddt/article/view/2198
[http://dx.doi.org/10.22270/jddt.v9i1.2198]

[29] Jeevajothi M, Sinha P, Rathnam G, Ubaidulla U, Nagar J, Gandhi Salai R. Review on background of future prospects of transfersome in drug delivery system. Int J Pharm Res Appl [Internet]. [cited 2024 Apr 8];6:277. Available from: www.ijprajournal.com

[30] Kodi SR, Reddy MS, Shruti K. Transferosomes: A novel topical approach. J Drug Deliv Ther 2023; 13(2): 126-31. Available from: https://jddtonline.info/index.php/jddt/article/view/5952/5247
[http://dx.doi.org/10.22270/jddt.v13i2.5952]

[31] Shukla T, Upmanyu N, Prakash Pandey S, Gosh D. Lipid nanocarriers. Lipid Nanocarriers Drug Target. 2018 Jan 1; 1–47.
[http://dx.doi.org/10.1016/B978-0-12-813687-4.00001-3]

[32] Pathan RA, Bhandari U. Preparation & characterization of embelin–phospholipid complex as effective drug delivery tool. J Incl Phenom Macrocycl Chem 2011; 69(1-2): 139-47. Available from: https://link.springer.com/article/10.1007/s10847-010-9824-2
[http://dx.doi.org/10.1007/s10847-010-9824-2]

[33] (1) (PDF) particle size distribution and zeta potential based on dynamic light scattering: techniques to characterise stability and surface distribution of charged colloids [Internet]. [cited 2024 Apr 8]. Available from: https://www.researchgate.net/publication/328577330_Particle_Size_Distribution_and_Zeta_Potential_Based_on_Dynamic_Light_Scattering_Techniques_to_Characterise_Stability_and_Surface_distribution_of_Charged_Colloids

[34] Ottaviani MF, Matteini P, Brustolon M, Turro NJ, Jockusch S, Tomalia DA. Characterization of starburst dendrimers and vesicle solutions and their interactions by CW- and Pulsed-EPR, TEM, and dynamic light scattering. J Phys Chem B 1998; 102(31): 6029-39. Available from: https://pubs.acs.org/doi/abs/10.1021/jp980715c
[http://dx.doi.org/10.1021/jp980715c]

[35] Singh B, Mehta G, Kumar R, Bhatia A, Ahuja N, Katare O. Design, development and optimization of nimesulide-loaded liposomal systems for topical application. Curr Drug Deliv 2005; 2(2): 143-53. Available from: https://pubmed.ncbi.nlm.nih.gov/16305415/
[http://dx.doi.org/10.2174/1567201053585985] [PMID: 16305415]

[36] Siddiqui MR, AlOthman ZA, Rahman N. Analytical techniques in pharmaceutical analysis: A review. Arab J Chem 2017; 10: S1409-21.
[http://dx.doi.org/10.1016/j.arabjc.2013.04.016]

[37] Lipinski CA, Lombardo F, Dominy BW, Feeney PJ. Experimental and computational approaches to estimate solubility and permeability in drug discovery and development settings 1PII of original article: S0169-409X(96)00423-1. The article was originally published in Advanced Drug Delivery Reviews 23 (1997) 3–25. 1. Adv Drug Deliv Rev 2001; 46(1-3): 3-26. Available from: https://pubmed.ncbi.nlm.nih.gov/11259830/
[http://dx.doi.org/10.1016/S0169-409X(00)00129-0] [PMID: 11259830]

[38] Pawar AY, Jadhav KR, Chaudhari LH. Transfersome: A novel technique which improves transdermal permeability. Asian J Pharm 2016; 10(04): 425. Available from: https://www.asiapharmaceutics.info/index.php/ajp/article/view/875

[39] Sharma G, Goyal H, Thakur K, Raza K, Katare OP. Novel Elastic Membrane Vesicles (EMVs) and

ethosomes-mediated effective topical delivery of aceclofenac: a new therapeutic approach for pain and inflammation. Drug Deliv 2016; 23(8): 3135-45. Available from: https://pubmed.ncbi.nlm.nih.gov/26960815/
[http://dx.doi.org/10.3109/10717544.2016.1155244] [PMID: 26960815]

[40] Rapalli VK, Sharma S, Roy A, Singhvi G. Design and dermatokinetic evaluation of Apremilast loaded nanostructured lipid carriers embedded gel for topical delivery: A potential approach for improved permeation and prolong skin deposition. Colloids Surf B Biointerfaces 2021; 206: 111945. Available from: https://pubmed.ncbi.nlm.nih.gov/34216849/
[http://dx.doi.org/10.1016/j.colsurfb.2021.111945] [PMID: 34216849]

[41] (1) Drug carrier transfersomes: a novel tool for transdermal drug delivery system | Request PDF [Internet]. [cited 2024 Apr 8]. Available from: https://www.researchgate.net/publication/305387042_Drug_carrier_transfersomes_a_novel_tool_for_transdermal_drug_delivery_system

[42] Gupta A, Aggarwal G, Singla S, Arora R. Transfersomes: A novel vesicular carrier for enhanced transdermal delivery of sertraline: development, characterization, and performance evaluation. Sci Pharm [Internet]. 2012 [cited 2024 Apr 8];80(4):1061. Available from: /pmc/articles/PMC3528046/

[43] Parkash V, Maan S, Chaudhary V, Jogpal V, Mittal G, Jain V. Implementation of design of experiments in development and optimization of transfersomal carrier system of tacrolimus for the dermal management of psoriasis in albino wistar rat. J Bioequivalence Bioavailab 2018; 10(5)
[http://dx.doi.org/10.4172/0975-0851.1000385]

[44] (1) (PDF) Nano-transferosomes of *Aloe-vera* and vitamin-E for management of psoriasis: an archetype in herbal drug technology final year b pharmacy student at HKCP final year b pharmacy student at VIVA institute of Pharmacy Associate professor at VIVA Institute of Pharmacy [Internet]. [cited 2024 Apr 8]. Available from: https://www.researchgate.net/publication/370897078_Nano-Transferosomes_of_Aloe-Vera_and_Vitami-
-
E_for_Management_of_Psoriasis_An_Archetype_in_Herbal_Drug_Technology_Final_year_B_Pharmacy_Student_at_HKCP_Final_year_B_Pharmacy_Student_at_VIVA_institute_

[45] Todke P, Polaka S, Raval N, *et al.* 'Transfersome-embedded-gel' for dual-mechanistic delivery of anti-psoriatic drugs to dermal lymphocytes. J Microencapsul 2022; 39(6): 495-511. Available from: https://pubmed.ncbi.nlm.nih.gov/35993180/
[http://dx.doi.org/10.1080/02652048.2022.2116119] [PMID: 35993180]

[46] (1) (PDF) Nano-transfersomes of vitamin-E and *Aloe-vera* for the management of psoriasis [Internet]. [cited 2024 Apr 8]. Available from: Available from: https://www.researchgate.net/publication/362229728_Nano-Transfersomes_of_Vitamin-E_and_Al-
e-Vera_for_the_Management_of_Psoriasis

CHAPTER 15

Emulsomes-Based Pharmacotherapy for the Management of Psoriasis

Vishnu Mittal[1], **Devkant Sharma**[2,*] and **Anjali Sharma**[3]

[1] *Adesh Institute of Pharmacy and Biomedical Sciences, Adesh University, Bathinda 151101, Punjab, India*

[2] *Department of Pharmaceutics, Ch. DeviLal College of Pharmacy, Jagadhai 135003, Haryana, India*

[3] *Department of Pharmaceutics, Guru Gobind Singh College of Pharmacy Yamunanagar 135001, Haryana, India*

Abstract:

Background: Psoriasis is an inflammatory, autoimmune skin condition that is driven by T cells & is characterized by abnormal keratinization, hyperkeratosis, angiogenesis, and inflammation of the skin's surface. There are now many different pharmacotherapies for it; nevertheless, standard formulation-based pharmacotherapy can only partially improve treatment outcomes. Recent developments in nanomedicine based on nanotechnology may make pharmacotherapeutic drugs for psoriasis more safe and effective.

Objective: The objective is to offer a comprehensive overview of the development & utilization of emulsomes for targeted delivery of anti-psoriatic agents. This addresses the various drugs, the pathophysiology of psoriasis in short, and the therapeutic issues that come with it. Below, we have discussed the collective reports of several medications operating on distinct psoriasis molecular targets as well as the function of nanomedicine in their efficient targeting.

Methods: The formulation techniques involved in preparing emulsomes loaded with anti-psoriatic drugs highlight the key parameters considered for their optimization. Various methods for characterizing emulsomes, such as particle size analysis, encapsulation efficiency determination, & surface morphology examination, are elaborated. The *in vitro* & *in vivo* experimental methods employed to assess drug release, skin permeation, and therapeutic efficacy are also detailed.

Results: Emulsomes-based formulations demonstrated superior encapsulation efficiency, sustained drug release, and enhanced skin penetration, leading to improved therapeutic outcomes in psoriasis management. Experimental findings and comparative analyses reveal the advantages of emulsomes over conventional drug delivery systems.

* **Corresponding author Devkant Sharma:** Department of Pharmaceutics, Ch. DeviLal College of Pharmacy, Jagadhai 135003, Haryana, India; E-mail: devkant2088@gmail.com

Anjali Sharma, Prerna Sharma, Roy Rillera Marzo & Ahmed A. Al Karmalawy (Eds.)

Conclusion: Emulsomes-based pharmacotherapy presents a promising approach for targeted and efficient management of psoriasis. The chapter focuses on emphasizing emulsomes' potential to revolutionize psoriasis treatment paradigms and highlighting future research directions in this field.

Keywords: Drug delivery, Emulsomes, Lipid-based nanocarriers, Psoriasis, Targeted therapy.

INTRODUCTION

Psoriasis typically manifests as scaly and irritated patches on areas such as the knees, elbows, or scalp, although it can appear on other parts of body as well. Psoriasis symptoms may sometimes cycle, peaking for a few weeks or months and then fading or going into remission for extended periods of time [1]. Psoriasis may be treated in a variety of methods, and the kind and severity of your condition will determine the course of your care. While moderate and severe psoriasis may need medication, injections, or light therapies, mild psoriasis is often effectively treated using creams or ointments [2]. Controlling frequent triggers, such as skin injuries and stress, may also aid in the management of symptoms [3].

Psoriasis patients are at risk for developing additional severe illnesses, such as:

- Psoriatic arthritis is a persistent kind of arthritis characterized by joint pain, swelling, and stiffness.
- Cardiovascular events, such as strokes and heart attacks.
- Psychological challenges like depression, anxiety, and low self-esteem.
- A person's risk of developing certain malignancies, such as obesity, osteoporosis, uveitis (an inflammatory condition of the middle part of the eye), liver disease, and kidney disease may also increase if they have psoriasis [4].

Types of Psoriasis

Psoriasis is classified into many categories, which include:

Plaque Psoriasis

The most prevalent type manifests as elevated, red skin patches coated in silvery-white scales. The patches often form on the head, torso, and limbs, particularly the knees and elbows, and they normally grow symmetrically throughout the body [5].

Pustular Psoriasis

This kind is characterized by pustules, which are pus-filled lumps encircled by red skin. Although the hands and feet are often affected, there is a variant that affects the whole of the body. Stress, certain substances, diseases, and drugs may all cause symptoms.

Inverse Psoriasis

This variety manifests as red, smooth patches in skin folds, such as those under breasts, in crotch, or under armpits. Sweating and rubbing may exacerbate it [6].

Guttate Psoriasis

This kind of condition resembles little red spots and commonly affects the chest or limbs. It usually manifests in youngsters or young adults. Upper respiratory tract infections, such as strep throat, can cause outbreaks.

Erythrodermic Psoriasis

With red, scaly skin covering the majority of the body, this uncommon but severe type of psoriasis is characterized. It may be brought on by taking certain drugs, including corticosteroids, or by getting a terrible sunburn. People with poorly treated psoriasis often develop erythrodermic psoriasis, which may be quite dangerous [7].

Symptoms of Psoriasis

While each individual experiences psoriasis differently, some typical symptoms include:

- Typically found on elbows, knees, scalp, torso, palms, & soles of feet, areas of thickened, reddened skin covered in silver-white scales that may itch or cause a burning sensation.
- Dry, cracked skin that may bleed.
- Thickened nails with small dents and grooves.
- Poor sleep quality [8].

Achilles heel discomfort, back or neck pain, and stiff, swollen, or painful joints are some of the symptoms of psoriatic arthritis, a similar disorder that affects certain people. See your doctor right away if you have psoriatic arthritis symptoms because if you don't get treatment, the condition may cause irreparable harm. Psoriasis symptoms might appear and go [9]. There can be periods when your symptoms worsen, known as flare-ups, and then periods when you feel better [10].

Causes of Psoriasis

Immune cells get activated and release chemicals when you have psoriasis, which triggers the skin's fast cell growth. This explains why the condition causes scaly, irritated skin in those who have it. Some external factors may increase the chances of developing psoriasis, including:

- Infections, particularly those caused by HIV and streptococci.
- Tobacco use.
- Being overweight [11].

CURRENT CHALLENGES IN PSORIASIS MANAGEMENT

Treatments for Mild Psoriasis

The boundaries between mild and moderate-to-severe psoriasis are not widely agreed upon. Generally speaking, less than 3% to 5% of body's surface is affected with mild psoriasis. For moderate psoriasis, calcineurin inhibitors, keratolytics, calcium analogs, topical corticosteroids, and targeted phototherapy are among the current treatment possibilities. The position and severity of the lesions [12]. These are the existence of comorbidities, and the preferences of the individual patient all play a role in the treatment plan selection. For individuals with mild or localized psoriasis, topical corticosteroids are often first line of treatment. By downregulating inflammatory pathways, they function by lowering inflammation, preventing cell division, and narrowing blood arteries [13]. To reduce side effects, the location of the lesions should be taken into consideration while choosing the strength and formulation of corticosteroids. Unless patient suffers from renal impairment, they may be used extensively. Irritation and a burning feeling are possible side effects, although they normally go away with time. Tacrolimus and pimecrolimus are examples of topical calcineurin inhibitors that are mostly used to treat psoriatic lesions in the face and intertrigonous regions [14]. The chance of these adverse effects may be decreased by first administering topical corticosteroids, since they can be more noticeable in places with significant inflammation. After about two months of therapy, it may result in a considerable improvement with a low chance for carcinogenicity. Blisters and a burning feeling are examples of adverse effects that may be avoided with the right treatment plan [15].

Treatments for Moderate-to-Severe

When psoriasis affects 3% to 5% to 10% of the body's surface area, it is normally classified as moderate, while severe psoriasis usually affects 10% or more of the body's surface area. The mainstay of therapy for moderate-to-severe psoriasis is the use of systemic drugs; topical therapies may not be adequate in some cases, or the illness may be localized [16]. For these individuals, a combination of oral medicines, phototherapy, and biologics is advised by both American and European standards. When it comes to effectiveness, biologics have outperformed oral drugs or phototherapy. Topical treatments are not usually utilized as stand-alone treatments, however they may be used as supplementary therapy for moderate-to-severe psoriasis [17].

Phototherapy

For treating moderate-to-severe psoriasis, phototherapy methods including narrowband and broadband UV-B, as well as PUVA, have been employed. Narrowband UV-B therapy is preferred due to its superior safety profile and greater efficacy compared to broadband UV-B. Narrowband UV-B, being more effective with longer remission periods and lower risk of skin cancer, is often preferred over broadband UV-B [18]. Combining systemic retinoids with narrowband UV-B may further reduce the risk of skin cancer while enhancing effectiveness. In PUVA therapy, UV-A radiation is administered following the use of psoralens like methoxalen to suppress DNA synthesis. Gastrointestinal distress, burning, itching, hypertrichosis, and photoaging are possible side effects [19]. For palmoplantar psoriasis, topical PUVA therapy which involves immersing hands and feet in psoralen-infused water and then exposure to UV-A radiation is often used. The primary obstacle associated with phototherapy is that patients have to travel for in-office treatments. Although it's a practical choice, space and insurance restrictions may apply to home phototherapy [20].

Oral Systemic Treatments

Oral medications were often utilized to treat moderate-to-severe plaque psoriasis prior to development of biologics. Methotrexate, apremilast, acitretin, and cyclosporine are the oral therapy choices for plaque psoriasis. With the exception of cyclosporine, oral therapies often have lower efficacies than biologics [21]. For individuals who choose non-injectable therapy or have restricted access to biologics, oral medicines may still be taken into consideration. The adverse effect profiles of the oral alternatives vary greatly, and since each oral medication has a different set of warnings and contraindications, choosing one requires considerable thought [22].

Challenges in the Current Treatment of Psoriasis

Reduced effectiveness in a patient who reacted well to a therapy at first is known as secondary failure. The emergence of neutralizing antibodies in patients is one potential explanation for the decline in efficacy. It has been shown that combining biologic medicines with methotrexate extends the duration of biologic therapeutic response in various immune-mediated disorders. Numerous research on biologic change in the therapy of psoriasis have been reported to far. Ineffectiveness was the most common cause of first therapy discontinuation. Patients who changed biologic agents showed gains in PASI scores that were similar to those of patients who were not exposed to biologics [23]. In one research, psoriasis patients receiving biologic drug treatments in the US were asked to share their real-world switching behaviors. After 12 months, they discovered that the total switching rates were 14.4%, and after 24 months, they were 26.0%. Although the half-life of biologic medicines may be used as a guide, tailored strategies are often needed depending on the severity of the patient's illness, how they responded to previous treatments, and the advice of experts [24].

The high cost of biologic medicines is a key problem as well. Patients and healthcare systems are burdened financially by these drugs, which are often costly. Most psoriasis sufferers who responded to a study said they need a more affordable course of therapy. However, the creation of biosimilars presents the possibility of lower medication prices since the patents for several biologic drugs are about to expire. Their accessibility, affordability, and capacity to offer patients more treatment alternatives may all be improved by their availability. The effects of TNF-α inhibitor biosimilars were comparable to those of the original product [25].

Pathophysiology of Psoriasis

Psoriasis is a complex pathophysiology that includes inflammation and immunologic changes in the skin, aberrant differentiation of epidermal keratinocytes, and hyperproliferation of epidermal cells. T lymphocytes, on the other hand, are primarily composed of lymphocyte infiltration and exhibit specific vascular changes in endothelial cells within the dermal microvasculature. These changes include limited neoangiogenesis, dilation of capillaries, and high l venule formation in endothelia, all of which contribute to the visible redness of psoriatic skin [26]. Through the interaction of LFA-1 and ICAM-1, an activated T cell expands, enters the bloodstream, and expels itself *via* diapedesis in the endothelium at the site of skin inflammation. The reactions of one cytokine are downregulated by the other. The ultimate consequence of this is the development of psoriatic plaque due to keratinocyte proliferation, which also causes an increase in other inflammatory cells' migration and activity as well as vascular abnormalities [27].

Epidemiology

The prevalence of psoriasis varies greatly across people worldwide. About 2% of people in the United States are affected by this. There have been reports of a high prevalence of psoriasis in the Faroe Islands, where 2.8% of the population has the condition. Nearly both genders are equally affected by psoriasis. According to a monozygotic twin survey, if one of the index twins has psoriasis, the other twin has a 70% risk of getting the condition as well [28]. After examining a group of 2147 individuals, Henseler and Christophers concluded that there are two forms of psoriasis: type I and type II. Type II induces beyond the age of forty years, but type I induces at or before that age. Type I induction occurs in almost 75% of instances. Compared to Type II, Type I is more caustic. When comparing patients with early onset to those with later onset, there is a high correlation between psoriatic illness and the human leukocyte antigen, or Cw6 [29].

Use of Nanomedicines in Psoriasis Medication Treatment

Nanomedicines, which are also known as nanotherapeutics, have special properties that allow them to interact with skin and change its barrier, especially in cases of psoriasis. This makes them a flexible carrier. Lipid-based and polymeric nanocarriers are two general categories for the variety of nanocolloidal drug carriers that make up these nanotherapeutics. Depending on their structure, vesicles may range in size from nanometers to several hundred micrometers, from unilamellar to multilamellar [30]. Liposomes have the ability to encapsulate pharmaceuticals that are hydrophilic or lipophilic in aqueous cores or bilayers, respectively. These possess several admirable qualities, including as improved biocompatibility, controlled-release medication delivery rate, and greater encapsulation efficiency [31]. Numerous liposomal characteristics, such as their smaller size, flexibility, and malleability, have been linked to increased efficacy in the administration of antipsoriatic drugs. The soft vesicular nanocarriers known as ethosomes are mostly made up of stabilizers, phospholipids, and ethanol. The vesicles' high ethanol content contributes to their easy penetration into stratum corneum [32].

These are suitable for administering medications to treat various skin conditions, such as dermatitis & psoriasis. The nanoparticulate carriers known as aquasomes are made of self-assembling, three-layered structures. Aquasomes have been shown to be a more effective carrier than simple nanoparticles because to their physiological chemical characteristics, which also improve protection of labile biological molecules. Microemulsions, which consist of lipids, surfactants, and cosurfactants, are isotropic dispersions that have a greater medication penetration rate because of their surface area and ability to partition across skin layers. These are being used more often to provide medications topically to treat psoriasis. One kind of polymeric carrier that ranges in size from 1 to 1000 μm is the microsphere [33]. These provide longer-lasting medication administration and decrease the frequency of doses while increasing patient compliance. Additionally, it has the capacity to improve the specificity of medication targeting. Topical formulations based on microspheres have shown to offer regulated medication distribution and long-lasting therapeutic efficacy [34]. These have been effectively used as a topical psoriasis therapy. Due to their resistance to oxidation, they are more stable than liposomes and ethosomes. With fewer side effects and improved patient compliance, niosomes have been utilized extensively in the treatment of psoriasis. The elastic vesicles known as transfersomes facilitate easy penetration through the skin's stratum corneum. Studies in the literature have shown how effective nanomedicines may be in treating a variety of skin conditions [35].

EMULSOMES: CONCEPT AND CHARACTERISTICS

Emulsomes

A distinct kind of lipoid vesicle system known as emulsomes has an outer phospholipid bilayer and an inside solid fat core. Compared to liposomes, which are more unstable, emulsomes are more stable. Emulsomes may help you avoid the issues with oxidation, hydrolysis sensitivity, and aggregation that might arise with other vesicular delivery methods like liposomes. Emulsions and liposomes combine to form emulsomes. This method is being studied as a carrier for drugs that are hard to disintegrate. The active ingredient is contained within a vesicular structure by emulsomes [36].

Emulsomes is a novel lipid based vesicular system comprising of lipid core composed of solid fat, which is surrounded by phospholipid bilayer. The solid core lipid is made up of material which remains in solid state at room temperature and core is stabilized by phospholipid bilayer and cholesterol. Vesicular drug delivery system has proven advantages in drug delivery on prolonged existence of drug in systemic circulation without causing any toxic effect with increased therapeutic efficacy and controlled drug release, which conventional drug delivery systems fails to meet [37]. Unlike emulsion, emulsomes does not have fluid core, instead possess solid fatty core which can prolonged the release of drug incorporated. Phospholipid bilayer can be tailored/modified with certain ligands which are specific for certain types of receptors and can therefore use for tissue targeting [38]. Emulsomes possess various advantages over other types of vesicular/lipid based drug delivery systems and are as follows:

- High drug loading of lipophilic drugs.
- Improved stability in the gastrointestinal tract after oral administration.
- Prolonged/sustained release of drug encapsulated.
- Possibility of surface modification for use in targeting.
- Improved drug absorption and drug bioavailability.
- Reduced toxic effect of drug with improved pharmacological activity
- Relative benefit compared to other lipid drug delivery methods [39].

Emulsomes enhance solubility & bioavailability of hydrophobic drugs exhibit poor water solubility. Triglycerides form the core of these emulsomes. Given their distinctive properties, phospholipids are particularly well-suited as excipients for drugs with limited water solubility. Technology based on emulsomes showed exceptional targeting capability. The drug's complimentary localization in target cells may induce toxicity, but the formulations might significantly lessen it by prolonging the duration of its effectiveness at comparatively modest dosages [40]. Emulsomes offer a controlled and sustained drug release profile. In contrast to liposomes, emulsomes exhibit an extended drug release duration of up to 24 hours, whereas liposomes typically release the drug over a period of only 6 hours. Additionally, emulsomes are nano-sized vesicles, distinguishing them from other vesicular delivery systems such as Niosomes, pharmacosomes, & ethosomes. Furthermore, pre-clinical research often shows that excipients used in emulsome production alter animal model epithelial permeability. In comparison to other conventional lipid formulations, emulsomes are more affordable [41]. The internal lipid core of emulsomes differentiates them from liposomes, while the liposome's inner core is composed of an aqueous compartment. Compared to other vesicular drug delivery techniques, they also have a high drug loading capacity. Specific lipid combinations may be used to create stable lipid particles for the emulsomes interior core using specific emulsification and manufacturing techniques. A diameter of between 50 and 250 nm has been reached [42]. The difference between emulsomes and liposomes are show in Table **1**.

Table 1. Difference between emulsomes and liposomes [43, 44].

Emulsomes	Liposomes
They contain solid core consisting of triglycerides	They are composed of aqueous core
High drug loading as compared to other vesicular drug delivery systems	Relatively low drug loading as compared to emulsomes
Prolonged release of drug can be achieved upto 24 hours	Prolonged release of drug can be upto 6 hours
More stable in GIT due to presence of triglycerides, which is susceptible to hydrolysis by gastric pH & enzymes	Less stable in GIT

Structure of Emulsomes

Emulsomes are vesicular drugs delivery system. Structurally emulsomes resembles with liposomes as both are composed of outer covering of phospholipid bilayer but differs in composition of core material. Liposomes are composed of aqueous core whereas emulsomes are made up of solid lipid core [45].

Phospholipids

Phospholipids form one or more layer over the core material (triglycerides) to stabilize the emulsion (O/W). This layer on contact with aqueous environment tries to align itself to mask hydrophobic portion from aqueous bulk and attain minimum surface area. By this phenomena hydrophilic head groups are exposed towards aqueous bulk while shielding solid lipid by forming layer over solid lipids and encapsulate as core of vesicle. The number of bilayers envelop is variable and depends upon properties of phospholipid used. Along with above mentioned naturally occurring phospholipids, synthetic phospholipids are also used. All these phospholipids have different gel to fluid phase transition temperature [46].

Cholesterol

As discussed above, the phospholipid bilayer has to be rigid enough so that it can stay in circulatory system for long time. Cholesterol privides rigidity to the bilayer and are usually used in concentration of 50% of that total phospholipid used. Cholesterol molecules incorporate into phospholipid bilayer and act as part of envelop rather than core.

Solid Lipids

Emulsomes are unique drug delivery systems because of their solid lipid core, which is a necessary component. Lipids with a solid phase at room temperature (25 °C) make up the core. These lipids are nearly entirely made of nonpolar moieties and may be either single compounds or mixtures. The most prevalent kind of fatty acid esters used as the foundational substance for emulsome production are triglycerides. Fats extracted from natural sources are often only accessible as a triglyceride combination, and around 25 °C, they display a solid or liquid crystal phase after melting [47]. Other solid triglycerides that form core material at 25 °C include hydrogenated vegetable oils, polyunsaturated fatty acids, and esters of monounsaturated fatty acids. Triglycerides may also be combined with other triglycerides to create mixes. Another need for core material is that it must melt at a temperature between 25 and 37 degrees Celsius in order to transition from the solid to the fluid phase when delivered and to release the medicine that has been trapped when it comes into contact with physiological temperature of 37 degrees Celsius [48].

Charge Inducers

These are employed to give vesicles a surface charge. They are added to the phospholipid bilayer to raise the vesicles' zeta potential and stabilize them. Moreover, adding these charge particles to emulsomes causes phospholipid bilayers to develop that have opposing charges, which increases the quantity of hydrophilic medicines in the space created between the phospholipid bilayer and the core. Greater aqueous space forms between bilayers as a consequence of this action. Reducing particle aggregation, which is hindered by repulsive interactions between the vesicles, is another benefit of generating charge [39].

Methods of Preparation of Emulsomes

Some commonly used methods of preparation of emulsomes are shown in Figure **1** & discussed below:

Lipid Film Formation (Hand Shaking Method)

By using this technique, an aqueous solution hydrates inner wall of a Round Bottom Flask (RBF), forming a dry film of lipids, drug, and other materials. An organic solvent is used in RBF to dissolve the prescribed quantity of lipids, cholesterol, and medication. The necessary mechanical energy for the operation is applied by shaking the film by hand or by subjecting it to a steam of nitrogen that is saturated with water for a certain amount of time, after which it swells in the aqueous medium without shaking.

Reserve Phase Evaporation

In this method, two steps are involved: the first is the preparation of an oil-in-water emulsion, and the second is the addition of buffers in the excess organic phase. The lipid and aqueous phases are combined through mechanical agitation or sonication. This technique is applicable for encapsulating both small and large molecules, with an achievable encapsulation efficiency typically ranging between 60% and 65% [40].

High-Pressure Extrusion Technique

This method is basically used to formulate unilamellar vesicles by forcefully passing through a small orifice. Filter membrane is used in this method and is generally made up of polycarbonate having pore size of 0.8 to 1.0 pm. Multilamellar vesicles are passed through filter membrane under high pressure after 5-10 passes through membrane unilamellar vesicles of size range 60-180 nm are obtained. Some researchers had also used micro fluidizer to obtain nanosized vesicles. By doing this multilayers of phospholipid bilayer are removed to obtain nanosized unilamellar vesicles.

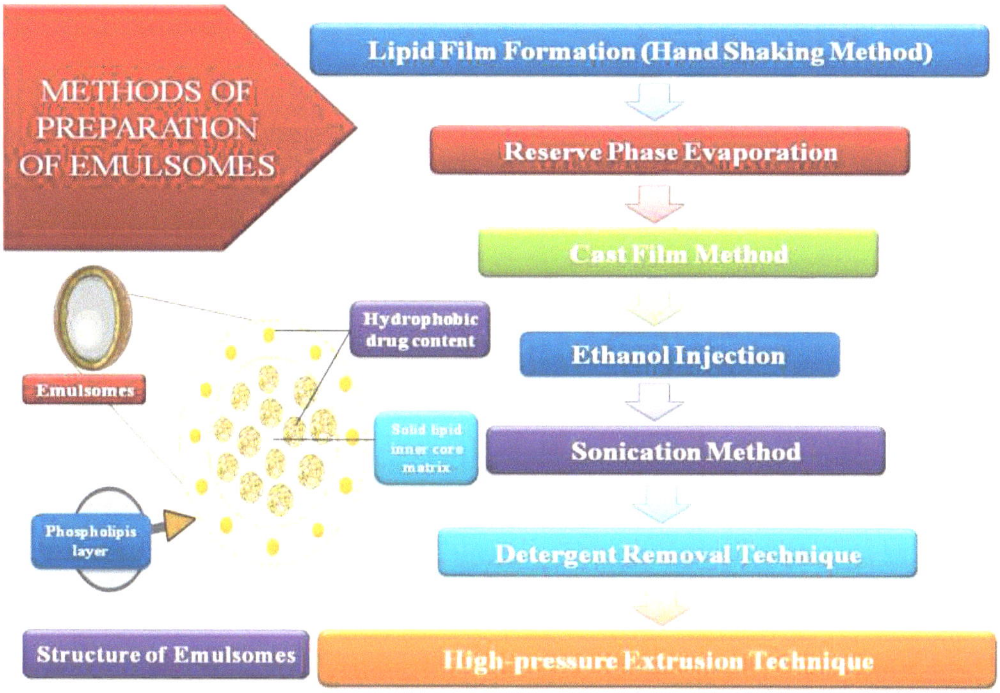

Fig. (1). Emulsomes and their methods of preparation.

Sonication Method

With a few little changes, this approach is quite similar to the lipid film hydration method. A dry film is produced along the inner wall of a round-bottom flask after phospholipids, cholesterol, and solid lipids are first dissolved in chloroform and the solvent is then evaporated. After that, phosphate-buffered saline with a pH of 7.4 is used to hydrate the dry film causing the phospholipid to swell and form a milky emulsion containing large multilamellar vesicles. Subsequently, this emulsion undergoes sonication using a sonicator (either probe or bath type) for a specific duration to achieve uniformly dispersed nanosized emulsome vesicles [41].

Cast Film Method

Using this technique, solid lipids like triglycerides are blended with phospholipids to create emulsomes. After that, the combination is suspended in an aqueous solution at a temperature below the solid-to-liquid transition point. The end product is an emulsion made up of liquid particles with diameters between 10 and 250 nm. Ideally, weight % is used to establish the size range instead of particle count. Using a stream of inert gases or a rotating evaporator, the solvent is removed at low pressure. The resultant dry film is then agitated with an aqueous solution to hydrate it. The medicine to be encapsulated may be added to the organic solution or the aqueous solution, depending on the drug's characteristics [42].

Ethanol Injection

Ethanol evaporates to form vesicles. By this method continuous vesicles of uniform size can be obtained. Phospholipids, solid lipid and cholesterol was dissolved in ethanol and filled in syringe, through this syringe solution is injected in aqueous solution with pressure at constant rate. Narrow distributed vesicles of nanosized range are obtained without extrusion or sonication.

Detergent Removal Technique

In this method lipids are mixed in detergent to obtain a micelle mixture, then detergent is removed from the mixture by various methods resulting in micelle formation which attract phospholipid molecules from bulk and further lipid molecules come together to form layer. Detergent can be removed by dialysis, column chromatography or adsorption [43].

Applications of Emulsomes in Various Medical Fields

The phospholipid multilayer around the solid lipid core of emulsomes allows for the encapsulation of lipophilic medications, whose medicinal applications may be limited because of their insoluble nature.

Drug Targeting

One of most useful features of emulsomes is alteration/tailoring of phospholipid bilayer which makes them suitable candidate for surface coating with specific ligand. These ligands have some free ending that specifically binds to surface over expressed receptors. So, by coating emulsomes with specific ligands like O-Palmitoyl Amylopectin, O-Palmitoyl Mannan can be used for tissue targeting. After administration in body emulsomes get coated with certain serum factor known as opsonin, which is recognized by reticulo-endothelial system and are taken up. This process of clearing particles coated with opsonin is called as opsonisation. Due to this feature emulsomes can be used to treat tumors and other infections of liver and spleen [44].

Anti-Fungal Therapy

Amphotericin B is drug of choice for diagnosis of fungal infection and leishmaniasis. Amphotericin B is a problematic drug having serious lethal effect of hepatotoxicity due to which its use is limited. But emulsomes as a carrier have certain advantages which reduce its hepatotoxic effect and prove to be efficient carrier of Amphotericin B for effective diagnosis. When it comes to kidney damage, lipid-based AmB formulations outperform traditional AmB formulations.

Anti-Inflammatory Action

A novel NSAID for pain relief is lornoxicam. It belongs to family of oxicams. Its half-life in plasma is about three hours [45]. Lornoxicam is an emulsomal nanoparticle-based musculoskeletal and joint pain treatment applied topically *via* soy lecithin. It is used to treat ankylosing spondylitis, osteoarthritis, and rheumatoid arthritis.

Anti-Neoplastic Therapy

Anti-neoplastic treatment may have significant adverse effects. Emulomes may change how a drug is metabolized, extending its half-life and circulation while reducing adverse effects. Methotrexate (MTX) and curcumin are the two medications most often utilized to create emulsomes. MTX is an anti-folate medication used to treat human osteosarcoma, lymphoma, choriocarcinoma, and leukemia [46].

Anti-viral Therapy

The emulsomes had a net negative charge from DMPG, whereas they had a neutral surface charge from DPPC. Zidovudine ester prodrug zidovudine palmitate (AZT-P) may be produced and added to emulsomes. The amphiphilic compound AZT-P integrates more readily into nano formulation. DMPG and other negatively charged PL bilayers boost the assimilation of AZT-P in comparison to neutrally charged emulsomes. Trilaurin and tristearin-based positively charged emulsomes should shield body from lysosomal breakdown & guarantee medication is absorbed as intended [47]. It is possible for cationic emulsomes to keep drug concentrations in the liver up for a minimum of six hours. Eliminate lamivudine with more bioavailability in the lymphatic system by using an emulsome or other lipid-based carrier technology. Anti-HIV medications might be administered more effectively using an emulsome filled with lamivudine. It could be a more effective therapeutic technique for HIV treatment than the current method of delivering medications [48].

Autoimmunity

The inclusion of a vaccine within an immune-enhancing membrane carrier like emulsomes helps maintain the antigenic integrity of the vaccine while also boosting its immunogenicity. Additionally, the surface modification of emulsomes' phospholipid bilayer with a bioadhesive polymer led to increased mucoadhesion of the emulsomes. Emulsomes might be added to mucosal vaccinations as adjuvants. Oral and nasal anti-CD3 treatment increases the Th2 response, which in turn activates regulatory T cells that bind to latency-associated peptides (LAP+) and suppresses arthritis. This kind of non-invasive and mucosal treatment for rheumatoid arthritis has been shown to be beneficial and safe [49].

Biotechnology

Emulsomes may be used to study immune response because of their low toxicity, enhanced stability, and immunological selectivity. They might be utilized to find out more about the immunological responses that antigens trigger.

Dermal Therapy

Dithranol has been used for treatment of psoriasis (an autoimmune skin disorder) but drug is having side effects. However, dithranol incorporation in emulsomes results in reduced side effect with enhanced skin permeation. Psoriasis patients have been treated with dithranol, often referred to as anthralin. On the other hand, encapsulating dithranol in lipid core of emulsomes greatly improves drug retention in skin tissues by increasing permeability across the skin. A range of compritol-based emulsomes may be produced *via* the formulation by design (FbD) method. Because more PLs provide more multilamellar barriers, the amount of PLs in the skin decreased the rate of penetration. Emulsomes demonstrated superior pharmacodynamics compared to commercial treatments in a mousetail model antipsoriatic research [50 - 55].

MECHANISMS OF ACTION OF EMULSOMES IN PSORIASIS MANAGEMENT

Emulsomes have enormous potential for achieving high skin permeability flux and drug retention, as well as possibly improved antipsoriatic action and almost no skin irritation. The medicine was made accessible in the skin portal with little latency time thanks to the emulsomes that were produced, which also increased the pharmacodynamics activity. Therefore, the carrier system has a great deal of potential to enhance both length & start of the drug's activity. There isn't a perfect medication available right now to completely treat psoriasis. Presently, the primary approach to treatment primarily aims at alleviating symptoms, halting disease progression, and improving the patient's overall well-being. Various therapeutic options are available for psoriasis [56, 57]. Pharmacological interventions for psoriasis encompass topical, systemic, and phototherapy modalities. Because of the skin's barrier function, traditional topical therapies including ointments, lotions, and gels minimal absorption and poor penetration. When drug-loaded nanocarriers were administered locally, there were less systemic adverse effects and greater permeability and effectiveness at lower dosages [58, 59]. The contact with skin improves as the particle size decreases. Smaller particles (less than 20 nm) may pass through undamaged skin, while bigger particles can pass through sick or defective skin because of a weakened barrier. There are still particles on the stratum corneum layer that range in size from 50 to 100 nm [60, 61].

These days, these nanocarriers finding more and more application as anti-psoriasis drug delivery systems due to their high biocompatibility, natural decay, non-toxicity, and biodegradability; they also quickly exit the body without causing any negative inflammatory reactions [62]. The nanocarriers exhibit consistent performance, suitable porosity, an optimal pore size distribution, interconnectivity, ease of processing, malleability into desirable shapes, and other attributes. each enhances their standing [63, 64].

EXPERT OPINION

Innovative nanomedicines, liposomes and polymeric nanoparticles, have shown the capacity to enhance the therapeutic advantages of anti-psoriatic medications by augmenting their effectiveness while minimizing their toxicities [65]. Even while the findings on animal models utilizing drugs based on nanomedicine to target psoriasis *via* alternative routes are promising, a limitation is the absence of adequate data in a clinical scenario, necessitating more clinical trials on the effectiveness & security of nanomedicines in the treatment of psoriasis [66, 67].

FUTURE PERSPECTIVES AND CHALLENGES

When it comes to the formulation of medication substances with variable oral bioavailability and low water solubility, emulsomes provide a viable solution [68]. The majority of emulsome development is still empirical, and there aren't many *in vitro* models that can be used to predict an increase in oral bioavailability [69, 70]. Since skin acts as an impermeable barrier to exogenous molecules and is in constant contact with the outside world, evidence suggests that using nanotechnology in subcutaneous systems could be a viable strategy in the future due to its higher potency, increased absorption of active ingredients to the site of action, & minimal toxicity. This calls for the development of novel therapeutics that can effectively and non-toxically penetrate the skin's natural barrier to deliver drugs to the surface. Additionally, determining the prevalence of PSO is important since it informs and conveys the epidemiologic burden of the disease to medical professionals, patients, researchers, legislators, and other stakeholders in an effort to improve the lives of those who suffer from this illness. The increased prevalence seen in other countries may be, at least in part, explained by increased knowledge about PSO or longer lifespans [71, 72]. The psoriatic burden may rise further because of factors including aging populations and the fact that PSO mostly affects adults. PSO is a difficult condition for which novel medications have been developed recently. These reasons include cost, dose regimens, and side effect characteristics. A growing body of evidence indicates that HaCaT functions. This understanding and recognition of HaCaT's importance in PSO led to the development of numerous useful drugs for PSO treatment. This review also looks at the mechanisms that lead to the development of the condition and the new therapeutic approaches that have been developed as a result of the analysis of inflammatory psoriatic pathways. The continued development of NPs and their medical applications portend bright possibilities for the delivery of healthcare to the public [73, 74].

CONCLUSION

Skin conditions like psoriasis are caused by a range of autoimmune biological mechanisms, such as those involving keratinocytes, dendritic cells, T cells, *etc.* Psoriasis may be treated in a number of ways, but none of them is entirely safe, highly successful, or highly complied with by patients. Drugs like methotrexate and cyclosporine that are now on the market suppress the disease and lessen its symptoms, but do not totally cure psoriasis. Hence, the administration of antipsoriatic drugs has shifted to a more modern technique, particularly the use of nanocarriers. Treatments using nanotechnology have increased patient compliance and effectiveness without causing unfavourable side effects. They have potential use in the treatment of neurological disorders, cancer, and respiratory ailments. A patient's acuity for their condition, the severity of the disease, and how it affects their life all influence the treatment that is best for managing their psoriasis. Unfortunately, it has been discovered that none of the treatment approaches now in use has the potential to be safe, successful, or a full cure for psoriasis. Antipsoriatic medications given in clinical settings nowadays are only useful in stopping the disease's development. The lack of safer and possibly successful psoriasis treatments has highlighted the necessity to create and improve nanomedicine-based treatments in order to increase the treatment's clinical acceptability and promise. Drug delivery systems mediated by nanotechnology (NDDS) are essential for the accurate administration of several treatments, including anti-psoriatic medications. Despite being a relatively young field under nano biotechnology, nanomedicine seems to have many applications for NDDS in pharmacotherapy. By using drug carriers to facilitate the administration of loaded treatments, such as anti-psoriatic medications, it has increased the benefit/risk ratio and/or decreased drug toxicity, hence improving the therapeutic potential of pharmaceuticals. Compared to traditional drug delivery systems, these intelligent delivery methods enable the administration of lower dosages and fewer dose intervals for the same therapies.

REFERENCES

[1] Mahil SK, Capon F, Barker JN. Update on psoriasis immunopathogenesis and targeted immunotherapy. Semin Immunopathol 2016; 38(1): 11-27.
[http://dx.doi.org/10.1007/s00281-015-0539-8] [PMID: 26573299]

[2] World Health Organization. Global report on psoriasis. World Health Organization; 2016.

[3] Parisi R, Iskandar IYK, Kontopantelis E, Augustin M, Griffiths CEM, Ashcroft DM. National, regional, and worldwide epidemiology of psoriasis: systematic analysis and modelling study. BMJ 2020; 369: m1590.
[http://dx.doi.org/10.1136/bmj.m1590] [PMID: 32467098]

[4] Raharja A, Mahil SK, Barker JN. Psoriasis: a brief overview. Clin Med (Lond) 2021; 21(3): 170-3.
[http://dx.doi.org/10.7861/clinmed.2021-0257] [PMID: 34001566]

[5] Barker J. Psoriasis. In: Hoeger P, Kinsler V, Yan A, *et al.,* Eds., Harper's Textbook of Pediatric Dermatology. 2019.
[http://dx.doi.org/10.1002/9781119142812.ch28]

[6] Gold LS, Lebwohl MG, Sugarman JL, *et al.* Safety and efficacy of a fixed combination of halobetasol and tazarotene in the treatment of moderate-to-severe plaque psoriasis: Results of 2 phase 3 randomized controlled trials. J Am Acad Dermatol 2018; 79(2): 287-93.
[http://dx.doi.org/10.1016/j.jaad.2018.03.040] [PMID: 29614243]

[7] Soleymani T, Hung T, Soung J. The role of vitamin D in psoriasis: a review. Int J Dermatol 2015; 54(4): 383-92.
[http://dx.doi.org/10.1111/ijd.12790] [PMID: 25601579]

[8] Armstrong AW, Puig L, Joshi A, *et al.* Comparison of biologics and oral treatments for plaque psoriasis. JAMA Dermatol 2020; 156(3): 258-69.
[http://dx.doi.org/10.1001/jamadermatol.2019.4029] [PMID: 32022825]

[9] Lee HJ, Kim M. Challenges and future trends in the treatment of psoriasis. Int J Mol Sci 2023; 24(17): 13313.
[http://dx.doi.org/10.3390/ijms241713313] [PMID: 37686119]

[10] Puig L. Induction phase, primary endpoint, time to decide on primary failure, and therapeutic goals in biologic treatment of psoriasis. J Eur Acad Dermatol Venereol 2013; 27(2): e257-60.
[http://dx.doi.org/10.1111/j.1468-3083.2012.04585.x] [PMID: 22632099]

[11] Barker J. Psoriasis. In: Hoeger P, Kinsler V, Yan A, Eds. Harper's Textbook of Pediatric Dermatology. 2019.
[http://dx.doi.org/10.1002/9781119142812.ch28]

[12] Gold LS, Lebwohl MG, Sugarman JL, *et al.* Safety and efficacy of a fixed combination of halobetasol and tazarotene in the treatment of moderate-to-severe plaque psoriasis: Results of 2 phase 3 randomized controlled trials. J Am Acad Dermatol 2018; 79(2): 287-93.
[http://dx.doi.org/10.1016/j.jaad.2018.03.040] [PMID: 29614243]

[13] Soleymani T, Hung T, Soung J. The role of vitamin D in psoriasis: a review. Int J Dermatol 2015; 54(4): 383-92.
[http://dx.doi.org/10.1111/ijd.12790] [PMID: 25601579]

[14] Armstrong AW, Puig L, Joshi A, *et al.* Comparison of biologics and oral treatments for plaque psoriasis. JAMA Dermatol 2020; 156(3): 258-69.
[http://dx.doi.org/10.1001/jamadermatol.2019.4029] [PMID: 32022825]

[15] Lee HJ, Kim M. Challenges and future trends in the treatment of psoriasis. Int J Mol Sci 2023; 24(17): 13313.
[http://dx.doi.org/10.3390/ijms241713313] [PMID: 37686119]

[16] Puig L. Induction phase, primary endpoint, time to decide on primary failure, and therapeutic goals in biologic treatment of psoriasis. J Eur Acad Dermatol Venereol 2013; 27(2): e257-60.
[http://dx.doi.org/10.1111/j.1468-3083.2012.04585.x] [PMID: 22632099]

[17] Porter C, Woods A, Mendelow M, Purvis C, Feldman S. Unmet needs in psoriasis patients. J Drugs Dermatol 2022; 21(8): 839-44.
[http://dx.doi.org/10.36849/JDD.6589] [PMID: 35946978]

[18] Kocsis D, Horváth S, Kemény Á, *et al.* Drug delivery through the psoriatic epidermal barrier—A "Skin-On-A-Chip" permeability study and *ex vivo* optical imaging. Int J Mol Sci 2022; 23(8): 4237.
[http://dx.doi.org/10.3390/ijms23084237] [PMID: 35457056]

[19] Eita AS, M A Makky A, Anter A, Khalil IA. Repurposing of atorvastatin emulsomes as a topical antifungal agent. Drug Deliv 2022; 29(1): 3414-31.
[http://dx.doi.org/10.1080/10717544.2022.2149898] [PMID: 36428290]

[20] Islek Z, Ucisik MH, Keskin E, *et al.* Antileishmanial activity of BNIPdaoct-and BNIPdanon-loaded emulsomes on leishmania infantum parasites. Frontiers in Nanotechnology 2022; 3(101): 773741.
[http://dx.doi.org/10.3389/fnano.2021.773741]

[21] Jacquin-Porretaz C, Cordonnier M, Nardin C, *et al.* Increased levels of interleukin-17A exosomes in psoriasis. Acta Derm Venereol 2019; 99(12): 0.
[http://dx.doi.org/10.2340/00015555-3300] [PMID: 31449317]

[22] Amselem AS, Yogev A, Zawoznik E, Friedman D. International symposium on the control and release of bioactive materials 1994; 1369.

[23] Amselem AS, Zawoznik E, Yogev A, Friedman D. Emulsomes, a new type of lipid assembly Handbook of Nonmedical Applications of Liposomes. In: Barenholz Y, Lasic DD, Eds. III. Florida: CRC Press 1996; pp. 209-23.

[24] Vyas SP, Subhedar R, Jain S. Development and characterization of emulsomes for sustained and targeted delivery of an antiviral agent to liver. J Pharm Pharmacol 2006; 58(3): 321-6.
[http://dx.doi.org/10.1211/jpp.58.3.0005] [PMID: 16536898]

[25] Kumar R, Seth N, Hari kumar SL. Emulsomes: an emerging vesicular drug delivery system. J Drug Deliv Ther 2013; 3(6): 133-42.
[http://dx.doi.org/10.22270/jddt.v3i6.665]

[26] Jain S, Jain V, Mahajan SC. Lipid based vesicular drug delivery systems. Adv Pharm.
[http://dx.doi.org/10.1155/2014/574673]

[27] Patel M, Jain S. AN INCLUSIVE review on novel drug delivery strategies for an effectual delivery of bio-active drug molecules in the treatment of acne. Journal of Advanced Scientific Research. 2020;11(04 Suppl 9):01-15.

[28] Aldawsari H, Ahmed O, Alhakamy N, Neamatallah T, Fahmy U, Badr-Eldin S. Lipidic nano-sized emulsomes potentiates the cytotoxic and apoptotic effects of raloxifene hydrochloride in MCF-7 human breast cancer cells: factorial analysis and *in vitro* anti-tumor activity assessment. Pharmaceutics 2021; 13(6): 783.
[http://dx.doi.org/10.3390/pharmaceutics13060783] [PMID: 34073780]

[29] Pandey K, Nimisha . An overview on promising nanotechnological approaches for the treatment of psoriasis. Recent Pat Nanotechnol 2020; 14(2): 102-18.

[http://dx.doi.org/10.2174/1872210514666200204124130] [PMID: 32013854]

[30] Amalnath S, Ganesh NS, Chandy V. A well explained review on: emulsomes as vesicular drug delivery system. World J Pharm Pharm Sci.

[31] Banerjee G, Nandi G, Mahato SB, Pakrashi A, Basu MK. Drug delivery system: targeting of pentamidines to specific sites using sugar grafted liposomes. J Antimicrob Chemother 1996; 38(1): 145-50.
[http://dx.doi.org/10.1093/jac/38.1.145] [PMID: 8858467]

[32] Moghbel A, Zand Moghaddam A, Rezaee S, *et al.* High performance liquid chromatography determination of methotrexate in plasma. Iran J Pharm Res 2003; 2: 149-52.

[33] Yu YQ, Yang X, Wu XF, Fan YB. Enhancing permeation of drug molecules across the skin *via* delivery in nanocarriers: novel strategies for effective transdermal applications. Front Bioeng Biotechnol 2021; 9: 646554.
[http://dx.doi.org/10.3389/fbioe.2021.646554] [PMID: 33855015]

[34] Torchilin VP. Multifunctional nanocarriers. Adv Drug Deliv Rev 2011; 63(4-5): 302-15.
[PMID: 17092599]

[35] Motta S, Monti M, Sesana S, *et al. In vitro* and *in vivo* evaluation of a corticosteroid-loaded emulsomes-based hydrogel for skin application. Int J Pharm 2016; 505(1-2): 83-90.

[36] Kaur R, Thakur K, Choudhary A, *et al.* Nanocarrier-based strategies for the treatment and management of psoriasis: A review of recent advances and future prospects. Int J Pharm 2019; 572: 118802.

[37] Jain A, Jain SK, Ganesh N, *et al.* Emulsomes: a promising drug delivery system for poorly soluble drugs. Int J Pharm Investig 2013; 3(3): 150-6.

[38] Lee WJ, Park YM, Lee MH. Advances in topical delivery of nanocarriers for the treatment of psoriasis. Int J Nanomedicine 2020; 15: 1839-57.

[39] Pandita D, Ahuja A, Lather V. Transdermal delivery of anti-psoriatic agent *via* ethanolic liposomes. Drug Deliv 2016; 23(7): 2507-17.

[40] Hauss DJ. Oral lipid-based formulations. Adv Drug Deliv Rev 2007; 59(7): 667-76.
[http://dx.doi.org/10.1016/j.addr.2007.05.006] [PMID: 17618704]

[41] Zhao X, Ma X, Dupius JH, *et al.* Negatively charged phospholipids accelerate the membrane fusion activity of the plant-specific insert domain of an aspartic protease. J Biol Chem 2022; 298(1): 101430.
[http://dx.doi.org/10.1016/j.jbc.2021.101430] [PMID: 34801553]

[42] Kumar , *et al.* Preparation and characterization techniques in niosomal vesicular systems- a review. J Pharm Biomed Sci 2011; 5: 1-8.

[43] Sudhamani T, Priyadarisini N. Radhakrishna. Proniosomes-A promising drug carriers. Int J Pharm Tech Res 2010; 2: 1446-54.

[44] Ruwizhi N, Aderibigbe BA. The efficacy of cholesterol-based carriers in drug delivery. Molecules 2020; 25(18): 4330.
[http://dx.doi.org/10.3390/molecules25184330] [PMID: 32971733]

[45] Veldurthi R, Abbaraju K, Sailaja. Formulation and evaluation of etoricoxib niosomes by thin film hydration technique and ether injection method. Nano Biomedicine and Engineering.
[http://dx.doi.org/10.5101/nbe.v9i3.p242-248]

[46] Lombardo D, Kiselev MA. Methods of liposomes preparation: formation and control factors of versatile nanocarriers for biomedical and nanomedicine application. Pharmaceutics 2022; 14(3): 543.
[http://dx.doi.org/10.3390/pharmaceutics14030543] [PMID: 35335920]

[47] Ameta RK, Soni K, Bhattarai A. Recent advances in improving the bioavailability of hydrophobic/lipophilic drugs and their delivery *via* self-emulsifying formulations. Colloids and

Interfaces 2023; 7(1): 16.
[http://dx.doi.org/10.3390/colloids7010016]

[48] Vedanshu, Malviya. Preparation and evaluation of emulsomes as a drug delivery system for bifonazole. Indian Journal of Pharmaceutical Education and Research.
[http://dx.doi.org/10.5530/ijper.55.1.12]

[49] Singh B, Kumar R, Ahuja N. Optimizing drug delivery systems using systematic "design of experiments." Part I: fundamental aspects. Crit Rev Ther Drug Carrier Syst 2005; 22(1): 27-105. b
[http://dx.doi.org/10.1615/CritRevTherDrugCarrierSyst.v22.i1.20] [PMID: 15715503]

[50] Bakhaidar RB, Naveen NR, Basim P, *et al.* Response Surface Methodology (RSM) powered formulation development, optimization and evaluation of thiolated based mucoadhesive nanocrystals for local delivery of simvastatin. Polymers (Basel) 2022; 14(23): 5184.
[http://dx.doi.org/10.3390/polym14235184] [PMID: 36501579]

[51] Dubey S, Vyas PS. Emulsomes for lipophilic anticancer drug delivery: development, optimization and *in vitro* drug release kinetic study. International Journal of Applied Pharmaceutics.
[http://dx.doi.org/10.22159/ijap.2021v13i2.40339]

[52] Moghassemi S, Hadjizadeh A. Nano-niosomes as nanoscale drug delivery systems: An illustrated review. J Control Release 2014; 185: 22-36.
[http://dx.doi.org/10.1016/j.jconrel.2014.04.015] [PMID: 24747765]

[53] Ghasemiyeh P, Mohammadi-Samani S. Potential of nanoparticles as permeation enhancers and targeted delivery options for skin: advantages and disadvantages. Drug Des Devel Ther 2020; 14: 3271-89.
[http://dx.doi.org/10.2147/DDDT.S264648] [PMID: 32848366]

[54] Hu G, Guo M, Xu J, *et al.* Nanoparticles targeting macrophages as potential clinical therapeutic agents against cancer and inflammation. Front Immunol 2019; 10: 1998.
[http://dx.doi.org/10.3389/fimmu.2019.01998] [PMID: 31497026]

[55] Zhou X, Chen Z. Preparation and performance evaluation of emulsomes as a drug delivery system for silybin. Arch Pharm Res 2015; 38(12): 2193-200.
[http://dx.doi.org/10.1007/s12272-015-0630-7] [PMID: 26152876]

[56] Dubey S, Vyas SP. Emulsomes for lipophilic anticancer drug delivery: development, optimization and *in vitro* drug release kinetic study. International Journal of Applied Pharmaceutics 2021; 13(2): 114-21.
[http://dx.doi.org/10.22159/ijap.2021v13i2.40339]

[57] Gupta S, Vyas SP. Development and characterization of amphotericin B bearing emulsomes for passive and active macrophage targeting. J Drug Target 2007; 15(3): 206-17.
[http://dx.doi.org/10.1080/10611860701195395] [PMID: 17454358]

[58] Gupta S, Dube A, Vyas SP. Antileishmanial efficacy of amphotericin B bearing emulsomes against experimental visceral leishmaniasis. J Drug Target 2007; 15(6): 437-44.
[http://dx.doi.org/10.1080/10611860701453836] [PMID: 17613662]

[59] Paliwal R, Paliwal SR, Mishra N, Mehta A, Vyas SP. Engineered chylomicron mimicking carrier emulsome for lymph targeted oral delivery of methotrexate. Int J Pharm 2009; 380(1-2): 181-8.
[http://dx.doi.org/10.1016/j.ijpharm.2009.06.026] [PMID: 19576973]

[60] Redondo-Morata L, Giannotti MI, Sanz F. Influence of cholesterol on the phase transition of lipid bilayers: a temperature-controlled force spectroscopy study. Langmuir 2012; 28(35): 12851-60.
[http://dx.doi.org/10.1021/la302620t] [PMID: 22873775]

[61] Jain R, Naik S, Paliwal R, *et al.* Optimization and characterization of amphotericin-B-loaded emulsomes for parenteral delivery. Pharm Dev Technol 2020; 25(5): 609-16.

[62] Shiv B, Sharma M. Liposome based drug delivery for the management of psoriasis - A comprehensive review. Current Pharmaceutical Biotechnology.

[http://dx.doi.org/10.2174/1389201024666221213144228] [PMID: 36518042]

[63] Latif MS, Nawaz A, Asmari M, Uddin J, Ullah H, Ahmad S. Formulation development and *in vitro/in vivo* characterization of methotrexate-loaded nanoemulsion gel formulations for enhanced topical delivery. Gels 2022; 9(1): 3.
[http://dx.doi.org/10.3390/gels9010003] [PMID: 36661771]

[64] Ucisik MH, Küpcü S, Schuster B, Sleytr UB. Characterization of CurcuEmulsomes: nanoformulation for enhanced solubility and delivery of curcumin. J Nanobiotechnology 2013; 11(1): 37.
[http://dx.doi.org/10.1186/1477-3155-11-37] [PMID: 24314310]

[65] Neslihan Gursoy R, Benita S. Self-Emulsifying Drug Delivery Systems (SEDDS) for improved oral delivery of lipophilic drugs. Biomed Pharmacother 2004; 58(3): 173-82.
[http://dx.doi.org/10.1016/j.biopha.2004.02.001] [PMID: 15082340]

[66] Gupta R, Gupta M, Mangal S, Agrawal U, Vyas SP. Capsaicin-loaded vesicular systems designed for enhancing localized delivery for psoriasis therapy. Artif Cells Nanomed Biotechnol 2016; 44(3): 825-34.
[PMID: 25465045]

[67] Foulkes AC, Warren RB. Brodalumab in psoriasis: evidence to date and clinical potential. Drugs Context 2019; 8: 1-11.
[http://dx.doi.org/10.7573/dic.212570] [PMID: 31024633]

[68] Reich, K.; Leonardi, C.; Langley, R.G.; *et al.* Inflammatory bowel disease among patients with psoriasis treated with ixekizumab: A presentation of adjudicated data from an integrated database of 7 randomized controlled and uncontrolled trials. J. Am. Acad. Dermatol. 2017, 76, 441–448.E2.
[http://dx.doi.org/10.1016/j.jaad.2016.10.027] [PMID: 28027825]

[69] Dávila-Seijo P, Dauden E, Descalzo MA, *et al.* Infections in moderate to severe psoriasis patients treated with biological drugs compared to classic systemic drugs: findings from the biobadaderm registry. J Invest Dermatol 2017; 137(2): 313-21.
[http://dx.doi.org/10.1016/j.jid.2016.08.034] [PMID: 27677836]

[70] Beck KM, Koo J. Brodalumab for the treatment of plaque psoriasis: up-to-date. Expert Opin Biol Ther 2019; 19(4): 287-92.
[http://dx.doi.org/10.1080/14712598.2019.1579794] [PMID: 30831036]

[71] Hazlewood GS, Barnabe C, Tomlinson G, Marshall D, Devoe DJA, Bombardier C. Methotrexate monotherapy and methotrexate combination therapy with traditional and biologic disease modifying anti-rheumatic drugs for rheumatoid arthritis: A network meta-analysis. Cochrane Libr 2016; 2016(8): CD010227.
[http://dx.doi.org/10.1002/14651858.CD010227.pub2] [PMID: 27571502]

[72] Cather JC, Crowley JJ. Use of biologic agents in combination with other therapies for the treatment of psoriasis. Am J Clin Dermatol 2014; 15(6): 467-78.
[http://dx.doi.org/10.1007/s40257-014-0097-1] [PMID: 25373522]

[73] Ormerod AD. Switching biologics for psoriasis. Br J Dermatol 2010; 163(4): 667-9.
[http://dx.doi.org/10.1111/j.1365-2133.2010.09999.x] [PMID: 20854399]

[74] Özkur E, Kıvanç Altunay İ, Oğuz Topal İ, *et al.* Switching biologics in the treatment of psoriasis: a multicenter experience. Dermatology 2021; 237(1): 22-30.
[http://dx.doi.org/10.1159/000504839] [PMID: 31865339]

CHAPTER 16

Nanoemulsions-Based System for the Management of Psoriasis

Minky Mukhija[1,*], Sonia Kamboj[1], Monga Jyoti[2], Prabhjot Singh Bajwa[3] and Bhuwan Chandra Joshi[4]

[1] *Department of Pharmacognosy, Ch. Devi Lal College of Pharmacy, Jagadhri, Haryana, India*

[2] *Department of Pharmaceutical Chemistry, Ch. Devi Lal College of Pharmacy, Jagadhri, Haryana, India*

[3] *Department of Pharmaceutics, Ch. Devi Lal College of Pharmacy, Jagadhri, Haryana, India*

[4] *Faculty of Pharmacy Maharaja Agrasen Himalayan Garhwal University Pauri Garhwal, Uttarakhand 246169, India*

Abstract: The word "psoriasis" comes from the Ancient Greek word "*psora*," which means "itch." Severe itching is a common symptom of psoriasis, a chronic, non-contagious, inherited skin condition. It is an immune-mediated condition characterised by both hyperproliferation and inadequate keratinocyte differentiation in the epidermis of the skin. Although only affecting 2-3% of the population, this immune-mediated skin condition has a major harmful effect on the patient's quality of life. Although they have demonstrated poor efficacy and lack aesthetic value, topical psoriatic therapies such as emollients, coal tar, and dithranol are safer. Many strategies have been investigated by modern medicine to treat this condition (such as injectables, oral medication, and steroid-based lotions). However, none of these approaches have proven successful, as they lack an ideal and safe carrier that can deliver the anti-psoriatic medication to the patient safely and effectively, thereby achieving the greatest possible therapeutic impact. Researchers are working with nanotechnology to overcome the shortcomings of traditional treatments, aiming to improve the effectiveness of anti-psoriatic drug delivery and reduce its unfavourable side effects.

Utilising a colloidal model, nanoemulsion is a technique that applies high surface area active substances in the form of nanosized droplets to the skin's afflicted area. A number of advantages over traditional delivery methods are provided by nanoemulsions, which include decreased drug degradation and loss, avoided hazardous side effects, and higher drug bioavailability. Compared to coarse emulsions, nanoemulsions exhibit greater kinetic stability, prevent cream separation, significantly influence topical systems, and have a higher solubilization capacity.

* **Corresponding author Minky Mukhija:** Department of Pharmacognosy, Ch. Devi Lal College of Pharmacy, Jagadhri, Haryana, India; E-mail: minkymukhija@gmail.com

Anjali Sharma, Prerna Sharma, Roy Rillera Marzo & Ahmed A. Al Karmalawy (Eds.)

Significant research on nanoemulsion-loaded antipsoriatic medicines has previously been done. Many antipsoriatic drugs, including Capsaicin, Aceclofenac, Turmeric oil, Calcipotriol, Betamethasone Dipropionate, salicylic acid, Clobetasol propionate and others have been loaded into nanoemulsion using various preparation methods.

Keywords: Antipsoriatic medicine, Nanoemulsions, Psoriasis, Skin disease.

INTRODUCTION

Psoriasis is a skin condition characterized by relapsing and remitting. Although temporary remission is possible with treatment, there is no known cure for the condition. The illness is currently understood to be an inflammatory systemic immune-mediated condition that has multiple comorbidities. Heart disease, depression, and psoriatic arthritis are a few of them [1, 2]. The development of psoriasis is linked to the interleukin (IL)23/IL17 axis, which plays a significant role. The condition has three main histologic features: epidermal hyperplasia, dilated and prominent blood vessels in the dermis, and an inflammatory infiltrate of leucocytes, mainly into the dermis [3]. Biological therapies (tumour necrosis factor (TNF), IL-17, and IL-23 inhibitors), phototherapy (narrowband ultraviolet B radiation (NB-UVB) and psoralen and ultraviolet A radiation (PUVA)), standard systemic therapies (methotrexate, ciclosporin, and acitretin), and topical agents (vitamin D analogues and corticosteroids) are some of the options available for treating psoriasis [2, 3].

According to estimates from the Global Burden of Disease Study, 5.6 million Disability-Adjusted Life Years (DALYs) across all age groups were caused by psoriasis in 2016 [4]. Compared to inflammatory bowel disease, this is at least three times more. Additionally, metabolic syndrome, non-alcoholic fatty liver, cardiovascular disease, respiratory conditions, autoimmune diseases like Hashimoto's thyroiditis and autoimmune hepatitis, multiple sclerosis, and psychiatric disorders are all more common in people with psoriasis [5]. Compared to people without psoriasis, those with severe psoriasis had an increased overall mortality rate and a reduced life expectancy of 3.5 and 4.4 years, respectively, for men and women [5, 6].

Pathogenesis of Psoriasis

Psoriasis is a skin condition that results from various factors, including genetics. Studies have shown that genetics plays a significant role in individuals with early-onset plaque psoriasis, especially those under 40 years old. Heritability is estimated at 60-90%, and over 60 susceptibility loci have been identified through genome-wide association studies [4].

Psoriatic skin lesions overexpress antimicrobial peptides, such as LL-37, which activate dendritic cells, leading to inflammation. While it was initially thought that T-helper (Th)1 overactivation caused psoriasis, it has been discovered that Th17 cells play a more crucial role in the development of the condition. IL-23, mainly produced by dendritic cells, maintains their development [4, 7]. Th17 cells produce cytokines such as IL-17A, IL-17F, and IL-22, which lead to keratinocyte proliferation, TNF-α, chemokine (C-X-C motif) ligand (CXCL)1, and CXCL8 production. Psoriatic lesions are characterized by an increased number of dendritic cells and T cells [8].

Cytokines produced by the psoriasis condition create systemic inflammation, which can result in comorbidities such as metabolic syndrome, obesity, diabetes, and cardiovascular disease. Psoriasis is caused by a combination of abnormal antimicrobial activity, altered Toll-like receptor expression, and defective extracellular matrix deposition. Adipokines, proteins released by adipocytes, including leptin, adiponectin, and resistin, are vital components in regulating both innate and adaptive immunity, promoting healthy physiological function [9]. The pathogenesis of psoriasis is illustrated in Fig. (**1**).

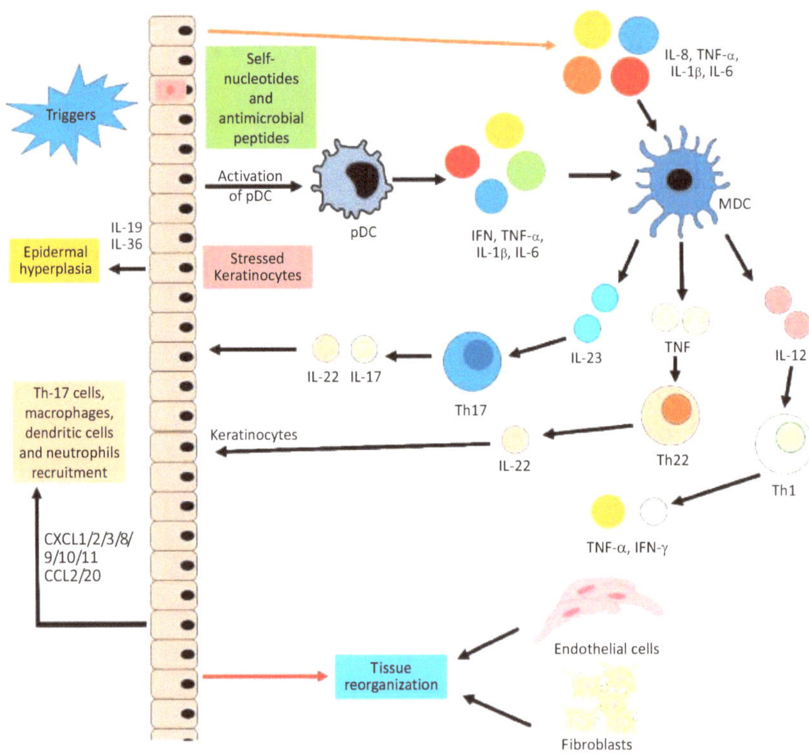

Fig. (1). Pathogenesis of psoriasis.

During the development of psoriasis, keratinocytes, T cells, and dendritic cells (DCs) establish a close relationship [10]. Keratinocytes release cytokines in response to environmental stimuli, bacteria, or some drugs, while simultaneously releasing antimicrobial peptides (AMPs) such as LL37, which binds to nucleic acid DNA or RNA to form a complex. Another important autoantigen in psoriasis is ADAMTS-like protein 5 (ADAMTSL5), which stimulates CD8+ cells and is selectively expressed by melanocytes in the epidermis [11, 12].

TREATMENT STRATEGIES FOR PSORIASIS

Modern System of Medicine (Allopathy)

Psoriasis is a complex medical condition. The primary drawback of this treatment strategy is patient noncompliance, which can be attributed to medication side effects or a low rate of remission. Both reasons highlight the flaw in the therapeutic strategy. The development of the drug delivery system with the aid of contemporary technologies can improve this. The severity of the condition serves as a baseline for choosing the best course of treatment. Topical therapy is recommended for mild to moderate symptoms, and oral or biologics are recommended for moderate to severe conditions [13].

Topical therapy: Such as creams, gels, and ointments, is preferred for treating skin problems. Intimate touch with the diseased area can be achieved in this way, ensuring greater effectiveness and avoiding systemic negative effects. Some medications used to treat psoriasis are Coal Tar, which is frequently combined with UV-B therapy as a dressing regimen [14, 15]. Anthralin (Dithranol), works well for scalp and localized plaque psoriasis. However, due to its staining ability and tendency to cause skin irritation at high doses, its use is dwindling [16]. Salicylic acid, which has keratolytic and anti-inflammatory properties, is most commonly utilized in this category [17].

Radiation: A common treatment for stable psoriatic lesions is phototherapy. While many light and laser sources are used for treatment, UV radiation is the most commonly utilized.

The UV radiation-assisted phototherapies vary depending on the UV radiation wavelength that is used. Two forms of UV light are used: UV-A, which has a wavelength of 320–400 nm (long-wave); UV-B, which has a wavelength of 290–320 nm (short-wave or broadband); and UV-B, which has a wavelength of 311 nm (narrowband). The first-line treatment for stable plaque psoriasis, which affects more than 10% of the body surface, is currently UV-B narrow band. The most common form of treatment, called PUVA therapy, combines UV-A with a photosensitizing medication (psoralen). PUVA can be administered systemically (oral/injectables) or topically (bath/cream) [18]. In this case, ultraviolet light activates the psoralen, which then binds to DNA to limit DNA synthesis. The primary hazards associated with these treatments are erythema, skin cancer, and early skin aging [19].

A recent advancement in this category is the use of high-intensity excimer lasers (308 nm), in addition to UV radiation therapy. Compared to standard UV radiation therapy, this laser enables the treatment of damaged keratinocytes, allowing for higher doses to be administered during the treatment session. Erythema, blistering, and hyperpigmentation in the treated areas are reported as side effects [20].

Oral Therapy: By preventing the formation of deoxyribonucleic acid in the proliferating epidermal cells, the folic acid antagonist methotrexate (MTX) inhibits both immunosuppressive and antiproliferative effects [21]. It is applied topically, orally, and parenterally (intramuscularly, dermally, and subcutaneously). It is currently regarded as "the gold standard" for the treatment of psoriasis. Because it is more likely to cause nephrotoxicity and hepatotoxicity in patients receiving systemic treatment, frequent monitoring of its pharmacokinetic profile is crucial [22]. Acitretin, which is a retinoid of the second generation, is used to treat severe psoriasis. It attaches itself to RAR-α, β and γ to suppress the release of cytokines and restore normal keratinocyte differentiation and proliferation [23]. To increase effectiveness, it can be used either alone or in conjunction with ultraviolet-B (UV-B) or Psoralen ultraviolet A (PUVA) phototherapy. It frequently causes alopecia, cheilitis, mucous membrane dryness, and elevated cholesterol levels among other side effects. Because it can cause teratogenicity in women, it should not be used [24]. One of the most widely used antipsoriatic medications in Europe is FAE. It is primarily used in conjunction with monomethyl and dimethyl fumarate. It increases apoptosis, suppresses the generation of cytokines, and downregulates NF-κ B's transcriptional activity. Patients with moderate to severe psoriasis are advised to use it. Headache, eosinophilia, severe diarrhea, and a decrease in lymphocytes are a few of the side effects that cause treatment to be stopped [25, 26].

Biologics: The medications that are presently available lack specificity, have observable adverse effects, and are unable to produce remission. Consequently, novel approaches, such as the development of safe and efficient biologics that provide immunosuppressive therapy through the use of specific antibodies, are made possible by recombinant DNA technology. The therapeutic protein and peptide group II, which includes these antibodies, has specific targeting activity [27].

Alefacept, a dimeric protein, was the first biologic to be approved by the FDA to treat psoriasis. The medication was taken off the market in 2011 because it was not expected to produce long-term remission and because it was too expensive [28, 29]. A human IgG1 monoclonal antibody called utekinumab (Stelara) has been licensed by the US to treat moderate-to-severe psoriasis. By sharing the p40 subunit of the IL-12 and IL-23 subunits in the Th1 and Th17 signaling pathways, it demonstrates its function [30]. The medication proved to be safe in the short term and effective. It was also easy to use. Headache and respiratory infection are the side effects that have been documented [31].

Human recombinant TNF protein etanercept (Enbrel), chimeric IgG1 monoclonal antibody infliximab (Remicade), and human monoclonal antibody of the IgG1 isotype adalimumab (Humira) are other examples of this treatment strategy.

Alternative Systems of Medicine (ASM)

The traditional therapy used in alternative medical systems takes a holistic approach to the patient's well-being. Ayurveda, Yoga, Naturopathy, Unani, Siddha, and Homeopathy make up the majority of it. All of these medical systems treat patients with herbal remedies and inorganic salts, emphasizing a restricted diet to minimize negative effects.

Ayurvedic system: Ayurvedic treatment offers several external and internal medications, or Panchakarma processes. For some patients, leech therapy is also recommended [32]. Here are a few of the Ayurvedic products that are offered by the top Ayurvedic outsourcing companies, primarily Kottakkal Arya Vaidhya Sala, Oushadhi, and Himalaya. The *Ayyappala* coconut skin oil is one of Kottakkal Arya Vaidya Sala's primary products. The main components of the composition are *Wrightia tinctoria*, *Azadirachta indica*, and coconut oil (*Cocos nucifera*). These same ingredients are also used to create the gel, which is sold under the name Kottakal Psorakot gel. Manjishthadi kwatham is the product that can be taken orally [33]. Talekt, which is a syrup or pill form, is the Himalaya product that is sold. The two main components of the mixture are neem and turmeric. The dried stem of *Rubia cordifolia* is used in the formulation of Manjishtha capsules. In inflammatory, skin, and blood disorders, it is recommended for use.

Yoga and Naturopathy: Yoga primarily focuses on deep breathing techniques that support immunity, stress relief, and body purification. This is based on the fundamental idea that eliminating toxins improves the oxygen supply to all of the organs [34]. When metabolic problems are linked to psoriasis, naturopathy may be appropriate. The condition is treated with freshly extracted carrot, cucumber, and grape juice for one week [35], with a primary focus on food.

Unani System: The goal of Unani, a Greek medical system, is to restore the body's humors, or blood, lymph, and hormones. By enhancing immunity and cytokine modulation, the treatment aims to purify the blood and restore normal function to skin cells. A paste made of sulfur, borax, camphor, and sesame oil is administered topically to the lesion for treatment. The herbal ingredients in the oral formulation (tablets/syrup) are very diverse. *Vetivera zizanoides*, *Rosa damascene*, *Santalum album*, *Zizyphus jujuba*, *Pterocarpus santalinus*, *Acacia arabica*, *Coriandrum sativum*, *Cinnamomum glabra*, *Lactuca sativa*, and so on are a few of them [36].

Siddha System: One of the earliest traditional medical systems, siddha, has its roots in Tamil Nadu, South India. The five fundamental qualities of this therapeutic approach are suvai, gunam, veeryam, pirivu, and mahimai [37]. The National Institute of Siddha, Chennai, approved the use of a herbo mineral formulation called "Gandhaga Mezhugu" as a treatment for psoriasis (Kalajagapadai). Sulfur is a prominent element in this waxy internal composition, which also includes ginger and white onion [38].

Homeopathy System: The natural method of therapy known as homeopathy uses a highly diluted form of the natural ingredient. A person's mind, body, spirit, and emotions are taken into account while choosing the right medication for illness management and prevention. Medication regimens are recommended based on the patient's psychological state and type of psoriasis. A moisturizing cream and Lycopodium C200 (diluted to 200 times potency) can be used to treat scalp psoriasis. Sulfur-containing cream and oral sulphur at M concentration (1000 dilution) are used to treat generalized psoriasis. *Arsenicum album* at M potency, combined with 10% urea cream or Lycopodium at M potency, is used to treat nail psoriasis. There are many more therapy choices available, and each patient's choice of treatment is unique [39].

Traditional Chinese System of Medicine (TCM): The "blood aspect" is connected to TCM treatment. According to TCM, the buildup of a poisonous material in the body and the intense heat involved cause impure blood to form. Psoriasis is caused by this blood warming. As a result, TCM treatment encourages blood flow, cleansing, and feeding, which causes the body to feel cold [40]. Topical (cream, oil, lotion, ointment) and oral (powder, tablet, and decoction) formulations are available for the therapy. The two topical formulations for psoriasis that are most frequently used are *Indigo naturalis* composite ointment and *Yinxieling ointment* [41]. In cases of plaque psoriasis, oral remedies such as Herose capsules and decoction *HuoXueSanYu* [42] are recommended. The two injectables used to treat psoriasis are *Fructus psoraleae* (Buguzhi) and *Radix sophorae* (Kushen). The most popular TCM is Huangquin, or *Scutellaria* *baicalensis*.

Despite the fact that every therapeutic agent now in use has been shown to be effective in treating psoriasis pharmacologically, treatment strategies are hindered by the absence of suitable drug delivery mechanisms. The primary drawback of the traditional dose form can be solved by developing a formulation that makes use of innovative methods. Additionally, the therapeutic alternatives that are currently accessible are linked to both unsuitable visual appearance and associated toxicities, which might result in low patient compliance with prolonged use. Numerous negative consequences, including hepatotoxicity, renal toxicity, hypertension, hyperlipidemia, and skin cancer, are associated with phototherapy and systemic drugs. Furthermore, the conventionally formulated psoriasis medications currently on the market are linked to issues including higher dosage frequency, more adverse effects, and a lower long-term safety profile.

The development of the delivery system in an appropriate polymer and solvent to avoid the pitfalls of the traditional dosage form is one of the innovative drug delivery approaches.

PSORIASIS TREATMENT WITH NANOEMULSIONS: A NEW COLLOIDAL DRUG DELIVERY METHOD

Oil, water, and surfactant combine to form a nanoemulsion, a type of colloidal carrier system. These nanoemulsions' excellent kinetic stability, low viscosity, and optical clarity make them suitable for a range of dermatological uses [43]. One may refer to droplets as nanoemulsions if they are as small as 500 nm [44, 45]. Nanoemulsions are made up of incredibly tiny and uniform-sized droplets. Nanoemulsions can be used to create a variety of dosage forms, including liquids, creams, sprays, gels, foams, and aerosols. Additionally, a variety of delivery methods, such as oral, intravenous, topical, intranasal, ophthalmic, and pulmonary, can be used to provide them. Compared to coarse emulsions, nanoemulsions have a higher solubilization capacity, are more kinetically stable, prevent cream separation, and have a substantial effect on topical systems [46, 47]. Compared to other conventional formulations, nanoemulsions offer several advantages such as higher drug bioavailability, decreased drug loss and degradation, avoided toxic side effects, increased drug accumulation in the target region, enhanced patient compliance, adaptability, and flexibility in drug handling. Because of its small droplet size, which inhibits common destabilising processes including creaming, sedimentation, and coalescence, nanoemulsions have long-term physical stability. Nanoemulsions are a good option as a carrier for anti-psoriatic medications since macroemulsions typically exhibit inherent creaming, flocculation, sedimentation, and coalescence.

METHODS OF PREPARATION OF NANOEMULSION

Essentially, there are two ways to prepare a nanoemulsion. High-energy emulsification techniques provide extremely disruptive pressures that cause the water and oil phases to separate and intermix, forming droplets the size of nanometers. In contrast, low-energy emulsification techniques such as phase inversion, heat, and stirring [48].

High Pressure Homogenization

This is an extremely effective technique for creating nanoemulsions, involving the forceful entrance of water and oil, as well as the high-pressure passage of cosurfactants and surfactants through a tiny aperture. An emulsion may be diluted when it initially forms with a large volume fraction of dispersed phase. Surfactants are applied in excess to prevent coalescence [49, 50].

Microfluidisation

By using a pressure pump to introduce water and oil through a small hole into a mixing area, they can mix with other materials that have high shear and become minute droplets, which can then be utilised to make a nanoemulsion [51].

Sonication

This popular technique uses a probe sonicator submerged in a mixture of water and surfactants, along with cosurfactants, to provide mechanical force that causes the dispersion to condense into tiny droplets [52].

Phase Inversion Temperature Technique

This method involves mixing water, oil, and surfactants at room temperature. Then, the temperature is raised, and the surfactant is incorporated into the oily phase. Phase inversion results in stable nanoemulsions by preventing coalescence caused by temperature changes [53].

Solvent Displacement Method

By mixing an organic phase containing oil that has been dissolved in a solvent with an aqueous phase that contains surfactants at room temperature, one can create nanoemulsions using this approach. By allowing an organic solvent to diffuse and then evaporate under vacuum, a nanoemulsion is prepared. By using the proper solvent-to-oil ratio, small droplets of nanoemulsion can be created [49].

Spontaneous Emulsification

To create o/w nanoemulsions, water is added to the oil and surfactant solution at a steady temperature and gently stirred. Surfactant structure, concentration, bulk and interfacial viscosity, and phase transition region all affect how a nanoemulsion is prepared [48, 54, 55].

COMPONENTS IN THE TOPICAL NANOEMULSION FORMULATIONS FOR ANTIPSORIATIC DRUGS

Oil Phase

Examples of oil phases that can be chosen are castor oil, coconut oil, corn oil, cottonseed oil, evening primrose oil, fish oil, jojoba oil, lard oil, linseed oil, mineral oil, olive oil, peanut oil, PEG-vegetable oil, perflurochemicals, pine nut oil, safflower oil, sesame oil, soybean oil, squalene, sunflower oil and wheatgerm oil. This oil phase aids in the drug's permeation. Antipsoriatic medications are often lipophilic and have a log P value of 3, which qualifies them for emulsion encapsulation. Antipsoriatic medications are occasionally encapsulated in a blend of oils [49].

Surfactant

The choice of surfactant is utilised to reduce interfacial tension and create stable emulsions with the necessary particle size while also guaranteeing the least amount of skin irritation. Surfactants can be classified into four categories: anionic, cationic, zwitterionic, and nonionic. Tween, Cremophor, Transcutol P, Plurol Oleique, Plurol Isostearique, Labrasol, Lecithin, and Organogels are examples of surfactants that are often employed [55].

Co-surfactant

Cosurfactants are typically employed to reduce interfacial tension by altering the interfacial film's curvature and fluidity. Cosurfactants, such as ethanol, isopropanol, isopropyl myristate, and propylene glycol (PG), are short- and medium-chain alcohols and derivatives of polyglyceryl [49].

Other Excipients

Antioxidants (ascorbic acid, α-tocopherol), tonicity modifiers (xylitol, sorbitol, glycerol), pH-adjusting agents (NaOH, HCl), preservatives, penetration enhancers, aqueous-phase ingredients (sodium chloride, buffer salts), and viscosity-enhancing substances (such as gelatin, Aerosil®, and Carbopol®) are incorporated into the formulation to reduce fluidity and achieve the desired final consistency [56].

CHARACTERIZATION OF NANOEMULSION

Drug-excipients compatibility studies: Fourier Transform Infrared Spectroscopy (FTIR) is utilised to determine the excipients, and UV Spectrophotometry investigations can be performed to establish the drug-excipient physicochemical compatibility and interactions. Drug-excipient interactions suggest that a 1:1 ratio between the drug and the excipient maximises the likelihood of an interaction and facilitates the identification of incompatibilities more easily [52].

Globule size distribution & polydispersity index: With the aid of a Zeta sizer and photon correlation spectroscopy (PCS), the mean globule size of the nanoemulsion can be ascertained. The mean diameter of the particle at 25 °C and a 90° angle (n=10) is revealed by this analytical result. The PCS analysis produces two key results: the polydispersity index, which measures the width of a globule size distribution, and the mean diameter (z-average), which is a light intensity-weighed size of the bulk population [57].

Zeta potential: A Laser Doppler Anemometer that is attached to the Zeta Sizer apparatus can be used to determine the electrophoretic mobility. An appropriate quantity of sample (50-100μL) should be diluted with 5mL of water (0.45μm) and then injected into the instrument's electrophoretic cell, which has a potential set at ±150mV. The instrument software can utilise the Smoluchosky equation to compute the values of zeta potential [52].

Morphology by transmission electron microscope (TEM): The intrinsic matrix and form of each globule can be seen with the aid of TEM. A copper grid coated with holes in carbon was given a drop of the appropriately diluted sample, which was then left for ten minutes. After that, keep the grid inverted and apply a drop of phosphotungstic acid (PTA) to the grid for 10 seconds. After removing extra PTA by absorbing it on filter paper, examine the grid under a specific magnification [58].

pH: A pH metre can be used to determine the formulation's pH [59].

Viscosity: Using a spindle that rotates at a maximum of 100 rotations per minute for 10 minutes, a Brookfield viscometer can be used to measure the viscosity of the nanoemulgel [60].

Drug content: To ascertain the drug content of the nanoemulgel, sonicate 5g of the material to dissolve it in 25ml of phosphate buffer solution at pH 7.4.

Following sonication, filter the mixture, dilute the filtrate appropriately, and then use a UV-visible spectrophotometer to measure absorbance at 273 nm to determine the percentage of drug concentration [61].

Spreadability: By measuring the spreading diameter of the nanoemulgel between two glass slides, one can conduct a spreadability test. Weigh approximately 0.5g of the sample and place it in the centre of the glass plate (in a circle). Place another glass plate on top of the first one, push between the two slides, and after five minutes, measure the gel's spreadability in centimetres [57].

***In-Vitro* Release:** The dialysis membrane bag method can be used for *in-vitro* release experiments. For eight hours, the dialysis membrane is immersed in phosphate buffer at pH 7.4. Take a 3 mL drug-loaded nanoemulgel and submerge it in 200 mL of phosphate buffer solution (pH 7.4) using a dialysis membrane. To keep a sink condition, remove a 5 mL sample from the dissolution setup every 8 hours and replace it with an equivalent volume of phosphate buffer (pH 7.4). Utilising a UV spectrophotometer set to 290 nm, analyse the samples, determine the amount of medicine released, and compare the results to the commercially available standard dose form [62, 63].

EXAMPLES OF ANTIPSORIATIC DRUGS LOADED INTO NANOEMULSION

Numerous nanoemulsion formulations have been innovatively developed to address the challenges associated with psoriasis treatment. Notably, researchers have harnessed the potential of diverse natural oils, including kalonji oil, turmeric oil, fish oil, olive oil, and babchi oil, as functional ingredients within these formulations. The research community has diligently conducted comprehensive *ex vivo* and *in vivo* studies to assess the efficacy and performance of these prepared formulations thoroughly. A compilation of these studies is presented to provide an overview of the advancements in nanoemulsion-based approaches for psoriasis management.

Md. Sajid Ali and colleagues developed and assessed a nanoemulsion containing 15% turmeric oil, 42% Smix (at a 1:1 ratio), and 43% distilled water. The formulation process utilized the titration method. The resulting formulation underwent evaluations for physical stability, irritation potential, and *in vivo* inflammatory activity. It was determined to be practically non-irritating in the organotypic HET-CAM model. Furthermore, the optimized nanoemulsion exhibited a 70.35% inhibition of carrageenan-induced paw edema in terms of its anti-inflammatory activity [64].

For the purpose of treating psoriasis, Md. Sarfaraz Alam and associates created and evaluated a nanoemulsion containing Clobetasol Propionate (CP). Eucalyptus oil, Tween 20, ethanol, and distilled water were used as the oil phase, surfactant, co-surfactant, and aqueous phase, respectively, in the aqueous phase titration procedure used to create the nanoemulsions. Investigating if adding CP to nanoemulsions could improve CP delivery and, in turn, antipsoriatic activity was the main goal of this work. The outcomes showed that the activity of NTPDase (Nucleoside triphosphate diphosphohydrolases) in lymphocytes was considerably enhanced by the CP-loaded nanoemulsion. This membrane protein is in charge of breaking down extracellular ATP (adenosine triphosphate), which is involved in inflammation, cell division, and proliferation. Importantly, *in vivo* irritation studies revealed no irritation despite the high amount of surfactant used in the formulation [65].

Rajitha P and colleagues formulated a nanoemulsion loaded with methotrexate using the low-energy self-emulsification method. The oil phase was Chaulmoogra oil, while the surfactant and co-surfactant were Tween 80 and ethanol, respectively. The resultant nanoemulsion had a pH that was suitable for skin, a negative surface charge, and an average particle size of 34 nm. Methotrexate's release mechanism was shown by *in vitro* release tests to have a non-Fickian diffusion mechanism and zero-order kinetics. In comparison to a control drug solution, *ex vivo* skin permeation investigations utilising pig skin in a Franz diffusion cell device showed better skin penetration and retention of the drug in deep skin layers. Superior anti-psoriatic efficacy was found in *in vivo* anti-psoriatic tests conducted on an imiquimod psoriatic model. Comparing the nanoemulsion to oral methotrexate tablets, the latter demonstrated less serum and tissue accumulation and better skin retention [66].

Mittal S. and colleagues used high-pressure homogenization in conjunction with the spontaneous emulsification method to create and evaluate a nanoemulsion. In the oil phase, two distinct oils—fish oil and linseed oil—were used, together with Tween 80 as the surfactant and transcutol-P as the co-surfactant. By adding 1% Carbopol 934, the optimised nanoemulsion was further processed into a nanoemulsion gel. When mice treated with nanoemulsion gels were compared to a commercially available ointment in an *in vivo* investigation employing an Imiquimod-induced psoriasis-like inflammatory model, the results showed much greater anti-psoriatic effectiveness [67].

Mohammed S. Algahtani and collaborators formulated and assessed a nanoemulsion formulation of curcumin with the objective of enhancing its solubility and skin penetrability upon topical application. The curcumin nanoemulsion was optimized through a low-energy emulsification method and subsequently transformed into a nano-emulgel using crosslinked polyacrylic acid (carbopol 934) as a gelling agent. For achieving high loading, transcutol-HP (105.40±3.84 mg/g) and acconon-MC8-2 (104.73±2.85 mg/g) were investigated as potential solubilizers for curcumin. The nano-emulgel formulation demonstrated faster and earlier healing in psoriatic mice compared to both curcumin and betamethasone-17-valerate gel, indicating its potential in providing effective treatment for psoriasis [68].

Kaur A and her team developed and optimized a nanoemulsion-based gel loaded with Clobetasol Propionate (CP) and Calcipotriol (CT) for the topical treatment of psoriasis. The chosen ingredients, Capmul MCM C8 EP, Cremophor RH 40, and Labrafil 1944 CS, were used as the oil, surfactant, and co-surfactant, respectively, in a weight ratio of 5:3:2. The spontaneous emulsification technique was used to create the nanoemulsion. When compared to free drugs, both from the nanoemulsion and the gel, the nanoemulsion showed higher drug absorption in HaCaT cell lines, which was correlated with an enhancement in the penetration of both medications in the stratum corneum (SC) and viable layer. As compared to free medications and a commercial formulation, the nanoemulsion gel exhibited noticeably greater anti-psoriatic effectiveness in psoriatic BALB/c mice that were induced with imiquimod. Crucially, despite the formulation's greater penetration into the skin, it caused very little skin irritation [69].

Rashid SA and colleagues formulated a methotrexate-olive oil-loaded nanoemulsion with the primary goal of this project being to develop an effective delivery system. The formulation process involved the use of high shear homogenization. Olive oil served as the oil phase, while Tween 80 and PEG 400 were utilized as the surfactant and co-surfactant, respectively. The formulated nanoemulsion underwent assessment for various parameters, including thermodynamic stability, physicochemical characterization, drug release kinetics, entrapment efficiency, and *in vitro*/*in vivo* skin permeation analysis. *In vivo* studies conducted on rabbit skin revealed that the enhanced skin permeation of the methotrexate-loaded nanoemulsion was not attributable to structural changes in the intercellular lipid layers of the stratum corneum [70].

Fulvic acid (FA) and thymoquinone (TQ) were combined in a nanoemulsion formulation which Khan R and his colleagues developed and evaluated. Using kalonji oil as the oil phase and Tween 80 and Transcutol-P as the co-surfactant and surfactant, respectively, the nanoemulsion was prepared by aqueous titration. Next, utilising Carbopol 971, the nanoemulsion formulation was formed into a gel. After undergoing *in vitro* testing, the optimised nanoemulsion gel (NEG) showed improved TQ skin penetration and dissolution rate. The development of a dual-targeted synergistic nanoemulsion gel for the treatment of psoriasis is aided by this research in the pharmaceutical industry. Using BALB/c mice as an animal model, *in vivo* experiments demonstrated TQ's potent anti-psoriatic properties. These findings were validated by molecular docking studies, which showed a strong binding affinity for both targets, TNF-α and IL-6 [71].

Along with her team, Khatoon K. developed a unique nanoemulsion gel that combined three different natural bioactives: resveratrol, thymoquinone, and curcumin. The oil phase of the nanoemulsion system was oleic acid, the surfactant was Tween 20, and the co-surfactant was PEG 200. The formulation that was optimised demonstrated a droplet size of 76.20 ± 1.67 nm, a viscosity of 137.9 ± 4.07 mp, a PDI of 0.12 ± 0.05, and a RI of 1.403 ± 0.007. The nanoemulsion gel was prepared using carbopol 940 (0.5% w/v) as the gelling agent, and it showed a good textural profile. In the HET-CAM test, the optimised formulation showed a substantial anti-angiogenic effect and a higher percentage of growth inhibition on A-431 cells. Research carried out *in vivo* using a model of Balb/c mice demonstrated enhanced anti-psoriatic conditions, suggesting that the triple natural bio-actives combination in the nanoemulgel formulation is beneficial in managing psoriasis [72].

Algahtani MS and collaborators formulated and evaluated an imiquimod and curcumin nanoemulgel. Initially, a nanoemulsion was developed using oleic acid as the oil phase, Tween 20 as the surfactant, and Trascutol HP as the cosurfactant. For nano-encapsulation, low-energy emulsification was used. To produce a nanoemulgel delivery system, the optimised imiquimod-loaded nanoemulsion was then uniformly disseminated in carbopol 934 hydrogel. After topical administration, the imiquimod nanoemulgel showed a significant improvement ($p < 0.05$) in skin permeability and deposition profile. The *in vivo* efficacy of imiquimod and curcumin nanoemulgel was evaluated by topically applying different formulations of imiquimod gel and imiquimod nanoemulgel to BALB/c mice for 10 days. In contrast to the imiquimod nanoemulgel and imiquimod gel formulations, the results demonstrated that the combination of curcumin and imiquimod in the nanoemulgel system prevented the emergence of psoriasis-like symptoms [73].

An active natural oil-based nanoemulsion containing tacrolimus for the treatment of psoriasis was developed and evaluated by Sahu S and colleagues. After the preparation and characterization of the nanoemulsion, 1.5% w/v Carbopol 980 was used as a gelling agent to incorporate the nanoemulsion into a gel system. Using polyethylene glycol 400 as the cosurfactant, Kalonji oil as the oil phase, and Cremophor RH 40 as the surfactant, the nanoemulsion was created by the spontaneous emulsification method. The proposed formulation was tested in a BALB/c mouse psoriasis model for efficacy, skin penetration, release profile, and cell line analysis. Higher suppression of A-431 cell lines by the nanoemulsion and better skin layer penetration by the nanoemulsion gel were found in *in vitro* effectiveness testing. The anti-inflammatory effect of Kalonji oil also contributed to the suppression of various pro-inflammatory cytokines, indicating its potential role in treating psoriasis [74].

Ramanunny AK and colleagues formulated and evaluated a non-aqueous nanoemulsion of Alpinia galanga extract. The formulation utilized Palmester 3595 as the oil phase, Cremophor RH 40 as surfactant and Transcutol P® as the co-surfactant, and glycerin as the non-aqueous polar continuous phase. The composition was optimized using a three-level, four-factor Box-Behnken design (BBD), leading to a 10-fold increase in the flux. Mice treated with both low and high doses of the nanoemulsion showed significant ($p < 0.05$) amelioration of psoriasis, indicating the potential therapeutic efficacy of the formulated non-aqueous nanoemulsion containing Alpinia galanga extract [75].

Alam MS and collaborators formulated and tested a nanoemulsion topical gel containing betamethasone dipropionate. Eucalyptus oil and babchi oil were employed for the preparation of the nanoemulsion, which was created using the aqueous phase-titration method. Tween 20 was used as surfactant and ethanol was used as co-surfactant. To transform the nanoemulsion into a gel, a nanoemulsion gel was formulated using 3% carbopol 934 and acetate buffer solution to mimic the pH of the skin. The *in vitro* skin permeation of betamethasone dipropionate through rat abdominal skin was assessed using the Franz diffusion cell [76].

Sharma M and team manufactured and tested a nanoemulsion formulation of Retinol utilizing the probe sonication method. Soybean oil was employed as the oil phase, and a surfactant combination of SPAN 20 and SPAN 80 in an 8:2 ratio served as the surfactant. The formulation underwent evaluation for various parameters, including pH, viscosity, conductivity, particle size analysis, % drug content, and % *in vitro* drug release at different time intervals, with experimental values recorded for each parameter [77].

Wang Y and colleagues formulated and assessed a nanoemulsion of Calcipotriol using exopolysaccharides produced by the marine bacterial strain FYS (*Bacillus halotolerans*) as an emulsifier. Soybean oil was chosen as the oil phase, and PEG 400 served as the co-surfactant. The nanoemulsion formulations were prepared using ultrasound and optimized through the response surface method. The study encompassed the examination of size distribution, microstructure, stability, and *in vitro* drug release of the nanoemulsion. The therapeutic effect of the nanoemulsion on psoriasis vulgaris was investigated through animal experiments and *in vivo* characterization of histomorphology [78].

Pund S and team formulated and evaluated a leflunomide nanoemulgel. Capryol 90, Cremophor EL, and Transcutol HP were selected as the oil, surfactant, and co-solvent, respectively. The formulated nanoemulsion was then incorporated into a gel using Pluronic F127 as a gelling agent. Comprehensive mechanical characterization was conducted using a Texture Analyzer, measuring parameters such as hardness, adhesiveness, and springiness index. The *in vitro* cytotoxicity of LFD nanoemulgel in human HaCaT, melanoma A375, and SK-MEL-2 cell lines showed a significantly enhanced therapeutic response [79].

Raza K and colleagues formulated and evaluated a nanoemulsion of dithranol (anthralin). Emulsomes were prepared using a thin film hydration technique and optimized for composition using Formulation by Design (FbD). Nanoemulsion formulations were then prepared using a similar thin film hydration technique. The drug, cholesterol, compitrol, and phospholipon 90H were dissolved in chloroform, which was evaporated to form a film. The film was hydrated using a buffer, and the resulting dispersion was achieved using an ultrasonicator. The optimized formulations significantly enhanced antipsoriatic activity in a mouse-tail model compared to a marketed product. Furthermore, the chosen formulation demonstrated significant skin retention and enhanced medication penetration. Compared to the commercial product, the formulation was discovered to be non-irritating, stable, and biocompatible [80].

A functional excipient-based fluticasone propionate nanoemulgel was developed and tested by Jain S and colleagues to treat psoriasis. Using Capmul® MCM EP (oil), Cremophor® RH 40 (surfactant), and Labrafil® 1944 CS (co-surfactant) as well as Babchi oil as a functional excipient, a nanoemulsion was first prepared. *Aloe vera* (1.5% w/v) was then added as a gelling agent to turn the final product into a gel. *Ex vivo* tests revealed enhanced skin penetration and around a 4-fold rise in the fluticasone propionate retention from the nanoemulgel in deeper skin layers when compared to the free drug in the gel. Additionally, *in vivo* investigations showed that the nanoemulgel had greater anti-psoriatic potential than the commercially available formulation (Flutivate®). The created nanoemulgel was shown to cause very little skin irritation, indicating that it is safe for use [81].

Pioglitazone was formulated as a nanoemulsion by Espinoza LC and coworkers. Castor oil served as the oil phase, labrasol® as the surfactant, and propylene glycol and transcutol® P as co-surfactants in the formulation. The formulations were evaluated for a number of characteristics, including zeta potential, mean droplet size, and pH. Diffusion membranes made of human skin from an abdominal lipectomy of a 38-year-old healthy woman were used in *ex vivo* skin permeation tests at the Hospital of Barcelona, SCIAS, Barcelona, Spain. An arachidonic acid (AA)-induced mouse ear inflammation model was used for *in vivo* investigations. In the *in vivo* investigations, the produced formulation showed good anti-inflammatory activity by reducing the expression of inflammatory cytokines, namely IL-6, IL-1β, and TNF-α [82].

Chitosan gels loaded with Apremilast Nanoemulsion were developed by Ahmed MM and colleagues. Eucalyptus oil (EO) was used as the oil phase in the formulation, and Tween-80 and Transcutol-HP (THP) were used as the co-surfactant and surfactant, respectively. After characterising the prepared formulation, it was optimised for even greater improvement. 2% w/v of the optimised formulation was added to the chitosan gel. Following development, the gel formulation was assessed for a number of characteristics, such as pH, spreadability, *in vitro* diffusion, and investigations on wound healing and anti-inflammatory properties. Studies conducted *in vivo* revealed enhanced anti-inflammatory and wound healing properties, as well as a reduction in the percentage of wound size as compared to the control group. This suggests the potential effectiveness of the Apremilast Nanoemulsion-Loaded Chitosan Gel for wound healing and anti-inflammatory applications [83]. Oil Phase, surfactant and co-surfactant used in the nanoemulsion-based antipsoriatic formulation are shown in Table **1**.

Table 1. Oil phase, surfactant and co-surfactant used in the nanoemulsion-based antipsoriatic formulation.

S. No.	Drug	Oil Phase	Surfactant Used	Co Surfactant
1	Turmeric oil	Turmeric oil	Tween 20, Tween 80, Lecithin and Labrasol	Isopropyl alcohol
2	clobetasol propionate	eucalyptus oil	Tween 20	ethanol
3	methotrexate	Chaulmoogra oil	Tween 80	Ethanol
4	tacrolimus	fish oil and linseed oil	tween 80	transcutol-P
5	curcumin	Labrafac PG (Propylene glycol dicaprylocaprate), in combination with Transcutol HP (Diethylene glycol monoethyl ether)	Tween 20 (Polyoxyethylene sorbitan monolaurate)	Solutol HS15 (Polyethylene glycol (15)-hydroxy stearate),
6	clobetasol propionate (CP) and calcipotriol	Capmul MCM C8 EP	Cremophor RH 40	Labrafil 1944 CS
7	Methotrexate	olive oil	Tween 80	PEG 400
8	Thymoquinone (TQ) and Fulvic acid (FA)	kalonji oil	Tween 80	Transcutol-P

(Table 1) cont.....

S. No.	Drug	Oil Phase	Surfactant Used	Co Surfactant
9	curcumin, thymoquinone, and resveratrol	oleic acid	Tween 20	PEG 200
10	Imiquimod and Curcumin	oleic acid	Tween 20	Transcutol HP
11	Tacrolimus and Kalonji oil (functional expectant)	Kalonji oil	Cremophor RH 40	polyethylene glycol 400
12	*Alpinia galanga* extract	Palmester 3595	Cremophor RH 40	Transcutol P
13	betamethasone dipropionate.	eucalyptus oil and babchi oil	Tween 20	Ethanol
14	Retinol	Soybean oil	8:2 ratio of SPAN 20 & 80	Propylene glycol
15	Calcipotriol	Soybean oil	Exopolysaccharides	PEG 400
16	leflunomide	Capryol 90	Cremophor EL	Transcutol HP
17	dithranol (anthralin),	Compitrol	-	-
18	fluticasone propionate	Capmul® MCM EP babchi oil (functional excipient)	S Cremophor® RH 40	Labrafil® 1944 CS
19	Pioglitazone	castor oil	labrasol®	transcutol® P and propylene glycol
20	apremilast	eucalyptus oil	Tween-80	transcutol-HP

CONCLUSION

Finding the best psoriasis treatment plan continues to be a difficult task, despite great advancements in our knowledge of the disease's mechanism of action and the development of efficacious therapies. There are numerous psoriasis treatments available, but there is no consistent method that works for moderate to severe cases of the disease. Because psoriasis is a chronic condition, people must take medication constantly. Therefore, expanding the prescription of medications and constantly attempting to enhance treatment research are imperative, regardless of the approaches, medications employed, or delivery therapy viewpoint. Since nanoemulsions are a novel carrier, they undoubtedly have the ability to address several problems related to antipsoriatic therapy. Better medication bioavailability, reduced drug loss and degradation, avoidance of harmful side effects, increased drug accumulation in the target area, enhanced patient compliance, adaptability, and flexibility in drug handling are all demonstrated by nanoemulsion formulations. Nanoemulsions have a larger solubilization capacity, are more kinetically stable, prevent cream separation, and have a substantial impact on topical systems when compared to coarse emulsions. Many medications are incorporated into nanoemulsion formulations, which are utilized to treat psoriasis and exhibit higher bioavailability.

Although a great deal of research has been conducted on preclinical and formulation development, relatively little clinical research has been conducted to determine the clinical safety of such innovative nanocarrier-based systems. However, assessing the benefit-to-risk ratio of the medications contained in nanocarriers needs to be the main goal of future studies.

REFERENCES

[1] Reid C, Griffiths C. Psoriasis and treatment: past, present and future aspects. Acta Derm Venereol 2020; 100(3): 70-80.
[http://dx.doi.org/10.2340/00015555-3386] [PMID: 31971601]

[2] Raho G, Koleva DM, Garattini L, Naldi L. The burden of moderate to severe psoriasis: an overview. PharmacoEconomics 2012; 30(11): 1005-13.
[http://dx.doi.org/10.2165/11591580-000000000-00000] [PMID: 22994598]

[3] Rahman M, Alam K, Ahmad MZ, *et al.* Classical to current approach for treatment of psoriasis: a review. Endocr Metab Immune Disord Drug Targets 2012; 12(3): 287-302.
[http://dx.doi.org/10.2174/187153012802002901] [PMID: 22463723]

[4] Raharja A, Mahil SK, Barker JN. Psoriasis: a brief overview. Clin Med (Lond) 2021; 21(3): 170-3.
[http://dx.doi.org/10.7861/clinmed.2021-0257] [PMID: 34001566]

[5] Kumar R, Priyadarshi RN, Anand U. Non-alcoholic fatty liver disease: growing burden, adverse outcomes and associations. J Clin Transl Hepatol 2020; 8(1): 76-86.
[http://dx.doi.org/10.14218/JCTH.2019.00049] [PMID: 32274348]

[6] Manolis AA, Manolis TA, Melita H, Manolis AS. Psoriasis and cardiovascular disease: the elusive link. Int Rev Immunol 2019; 38(1): 33-54.
[http://dx.doi.org/10.1080/08830185.2018.1539084] [PMID: 30457023]

[7] Takahashi T, Yamasaki K. Psoriasis and antimicrobial peptides. Int J Mol Sci 2020; 21(18): 6791.
[http://dx.doi.org/10.3390/ijms21186791] [PMID: 32947991]

[8] Ferrari SM, Ruffilli I, Colaci M, Antonelli A, Ferri C, Fallahi P. CXCL10 in psoriasis. Adv Med Sci 2015; 60(2): 349-54.
[http://dx.doi.org/10.1016/j.advms.2015.07.011] [PMID: 26318079]

[9] Ryan C, Kirby B. Psoriasis is a systemic disease with multiple cardiovascular and metabolic comorbidities. Dermatol Clin 2015; 33(1): 41-55.
[http://dx.doi.org/10.1016/j.det.2014.09.004] [PMID: 25412782]

[10] Lappas M, Permezel M, Rice GE. Leptin and adiponectin stimulate the release of proinflammatory cytokines and prostaglandins from human placenta and maternal adipose tissue *via* nuclear factor-kappaB, peroxisomal proliferator-activated receptor-γ and extracellularly regulated kinase 1/2. Endocrinology 2005; 146(8): 3334-42.
[http://dx.doi.org/10.1210/en.2005-0406] [PMID: 15905315]

[11] Albanesi C. Immunology of psoriasis. Clinical Immunology. Elsevier 2019; pp. 871-8.
[http://dx.doi.org/10.1016/B978-0-7020-6896-6.00064-8]

[12] Hawkes JE, Gonzalez JA, Krueger JG. Autoimmunity in psoriasis: evidence for specific autoantigens. Curr Dermatol Rep 2017; 6(2): 104-12.
[http://dx.doi.org/10.1007/s13671-017-0177-6]

[13] Ramanunny AK, Wadhwa S, Singh SK, Sharma DS, Khursheed R, Awasthi A. Treatment strategies against psoriasis: Principle, perspectives and practices. Curr Drug Deliv 2020; 17(1): 52-73. [http://dx.doi.org/10.2174/1567201816666191120120551] [PMID: 31752655]

[14] Slutsky JB, Clark RA, Remedios AA, Klein PA. An evidence-based review of the efficacy of coal tar preparations in the treatment of psoriasis and atopic dermatitis. J Drugs Dermatol 2010; 9(10): 1258-64. [PMID: 20941951]

[15] Schoket B, Horkay I, Kósa Á, *et al.* Formation of DNA adducts in the skin of psoriasis patients, in human skin in organ culture, and in mouse skin and lung following topical application of coal-tar and juniper tar. J Invest Dermatol 1990; 94(2): 241-6. [http://dx.doi.org/10.1111/1523-1747.ep12874576] [PMID: 2299199]

[16] Runne U, Kunze J. Short-duration ('minutes') therapy with dithranol for psoriasis: a new out-patient regimen. Br J Dermatol 1982; 106(2): 135-9. [http://dx.doi.org/10.1111/j.1365-2133.1982.tb00922.x] [PMID: 7059509]

[17] Fluhr JW, Cavallotti C, Berardesca E. Emollients, moisturizers, and keratolytic agents in psoriasis. Clin Dermatol 2008; 26(4): 380-6. [http://dx.doi.org/10.1016/j.clindermatol.2008.01.015] [PMID: 18691519]

[18] Zhang P, Wu MX. A clinical review of phototherapy for psoriasis. Lasers Med Sci 2018; 33(1): 173-80. [http://dx.doi.org/10.1007/s10103-017-2360-1] [PMID: 29067616]

[19] Lebwohl M, Feldman SR, Walther R, Shelk J, Morgan P, Gutkin SW. Clinical management of psoriasis: principles and practice. Cutis 2001; 67(1) (Suppl.): 1-15. [PMID: 11210296]

[20] Feldman SR, Duffin KC. Treatment of psoriasis in adults. [Internet]. 2017. Available from: https://www.uptodate.com/contents/treatment-of-psoriasis-in-adults

[21] Weinstein GD, Goldfaden G, Frost P. Methotrexate. Arch Dermatol 1971; 104(3): 236-43. [http://dx.doi.org/10.1001/archderm.1971.04000210010003] [PMID: 5096831]

[22] Warren RB, Griffiths CEM. Systemic therapies for psoriasis: methotrexate, retinoids, and cyclosporine. Clin Dermatol 2008; 26(5): 438-47. [http://dx.doi.org/10.1016/j.clindermatol.2007.11.006] [PMID: 18755362]

[23] Saurat J-H. Retinoids and psoriasis: Novel issues in retinoid pharmacology and implications for psoriasis treatment. J Am Acad Dermatol 1999; 41(3): S2-6. [http://dx.doi.org/10.1016/S0190-9622(99)70358-0] [PMID: 10459139]

[24] Sue Lee C, Koo J. A review of acitretin, a systemic retinoid for the treatment of psoriasis. Expert Opin Pharmacother 2005; 6(10): 1725-34. [http://dx.doi.org/10.1517/14656566.6.10.1725] [PMID: 16086658]

[25] García-Caballero M, Marí-Beffa M, Medina MÁ, Quesada AR. Dimethylfumarate inhibits angiogenesis *in vitro* and *in vivo*: a possible role for its antipsoriatic effect? J Invest Dermatol 2011; 131(6): 1347-55. [http://dx.doi.org/10.1038/jid.2010.416] [PMID: 21289642]

[26] Mrowietz U, Christophers E, Altmeyer P. Treatment of severe psoriasis with fumaric acid esters: scientific background and guidelines for therapeutic use. Br J Dermatol 1999; 141(3): 424-9. [http://dx.doi.org/10.1046/j.1365-2133.1999.03034.x] [PMID: 10584060]

[27] Usmani SS, Bedi G, Samuel JS, *et al.* THPdb: Database of FDA-approved peptide and protein therapeutics. PLoS One 2017; 12(7): e0181748. [http://dx.doi.org/10.1371/journal.pone.0181748] [PMID: 28759605]

[28] Jenneck C, Novak N. The safety and efficacy of alefacept in the treatment of chronic plaque psoriasis.

Ther Clin Risk Manag 2007; 3(3): 411-20.
[http://dx.doi.org/10.2147/tcrm.2007.3.3.411] [PMID: 18488075]

[29] Krueger GG, Papp KA, Stough DB, *et al.* A randomized, double-blind, placebo-controlled phase III study evaluating efficacy and tolerability of 2 courses of alefacept in patients with chronic plaque psoriasis. J Am Acad Dermatol 2002; 47(6): 821-33.
[http://dx.doi.org/10.1067/mjd.2002.127247] [PMID: 12451365]

[30] Zaghi D, Krueger GG, Callis Duffin K. Ustekinumab: a review in the treatment of plaque psoriasis and psoriatic arthritis. J Drugs Dermatol 2012; 11(2): 160-7.
[PMID: 22270196]

[31] Gniadecki R, Bang B, Bryld LE, Iversen L, Lasthein S, Skov L. Comparison of long-term drug survival and safety of biologic agents in patients with psoriasis vulgaris. Br J Dermatol 2015; 172(1): 244-52.
[http://dx.doi.org/10.1111/bjd.13343] [PMID: 25132294]

[32] Psoriasis. Central Council for Research in Ayurvedic Sciences. Available from: http://www.ccras.nic.in/sites/default/files/viewpdf/faq/PSORIASIS.%20pdf

[33] Ayyappala Coconut Skin Oil Highlight. Kottakkal Shop. Available from: https://www.kottakkal.shop/blogs/healing-with-kottakkalayurveda/ayyappala-coconut-skin-oil-highlight.

[34] Yoga for Psoriasis: Deep Breathing. Psoriasis Self-Management. Available from: http://www.psoriasisselfmanagement.com/detoxification-ideas/yoga-for-psoriasis-deep-breathing/

[35] Naturopathy Treatment for Psoriasis. Naturopathy Cure. Available from: http://www.naturopathycure.com/naturopathy-treatment-for-psoriasis.php

[36] Ahmad DZ. Role of Unani (Greek) therapy in the treatment of psoriasis -Case series. IOSR J Dent Med Sci 2016; 15(9): 24-7.
[http://dx.doi.org/10.9790/0853-1509122427]

[37] Saranya MS, Mustafa MM. Anti-bacterial activity of siddha polyherbomineral drug Gandhagarasayanam. Int J Curr Res Biol Med 2017; 2(10): 19-23.

[38] National Institute of Siddha. Available from: http://nischennai.org/siddha-success-stories- nis-psoriasis-kaalaanjagapadai.html

[39] Nwabudike LC. Psoriasis and homeopathy. 2011.

[40] Meng S, Lin Z, Wang Y, Wang Z, Li P, Zheng Y. Psoriasis therapy by Chinese medicine and modern agents. Chin Med 2018; 13(1): 16.
[http://dx.doi.org/10.1186/s13020-018-0174-0] [PMID: 29588654]

[41] Wang M, Sui S, Gong A, Guan Y, Kuang X. Efficacy of Yinxieling ointment on 675 cases. Zhongchengyao 1990; 12(11): 21.

[42] Shi Q, Shengshun T, Zhiping S, An ZJ, Yi YJ, Ping L. Clinical study on Huoxuesanyuxiaoyin decoction for treating psoriasis vulgaris with blood stasis syndrome. Zhong Yao Cai 2005; 5: 442-4.

[43] Puglia C, Rizza L, Drechsler M, Bonina F. Nanoemulsions as vehicles for topical administration of glycyrrhetic acid: Characterization and *in vitro* and *in vivo* evaluation. Drug Deliv 2010; 17(3): 123-9.
[http://dx.doi.org/10.3109/10717540903581679] [PMID: 20136625]

[44] Solans C, Izquierdo P, Nolla J, Azemar N, Garcia-Celma MJ. Nano-emulsions. Curr Opin Colloid Interface Sci 2005; 10(3-4): 102-10.
[http://dx.doi.org/10.1016/j.cocis.2005.06.004]

[45] Jafari SM, He Y, Bhandari B. Optimization of nano-emulsions production by microfluidization. Eur Food Res Technol 2007; 225(5-6): 733-41.
[http://dx.doi.org/10.1007/s00217-006-0476-9]

[46] Usón N, Garcia MJ, Solans C. Formation of water-in-oil (W/O) nano-emulsions in a water/mixed non-

ionic surfactant/oil systems prepared by a low-energy emulsification method. Colloids Surfaces A Physicochem Eng Asp. 2004;250(1-3 SPEC. ISS.): 415-421.

[47] Baboota S, Shakeel F, Ahuja A, Ali J, Shafiq S. Design, development and evaluation of novel nanoemulsion formulations for transdermal potential of celecoxib. Acta Pharm 2007; 57(3): 315-32. [http://dx.doi.org/10.2478/v10007-007-0025-5] [PMID: 17878111]

[48] Nastiti C, Ponto T, Abd E, Grice J, Benson H, Roberts M. Topical nano and microemulsions for skin delivery. Pharmaceutics 2017; 9(4): 37. [http://dx.doi.org/10.3390/pharmaceutics9040037] [PMID: 28934172]

[49] Somagoni J, Boakye CHA, Godugu C, *et al.* Nanomiemgel--a novel drug delivery system for topical application--*in vitro* and *in vivo* evaluation. PLoS One 2014; 9(12): e115952. [http://dx.doi.org/10.1371/journal.pone.0115952] [PMID: 25546392]

[50] Khurana B, Arora D, Narang RK. Topical delivery of nanoemulsion for antipsoriatic drugs. J Drug Deliv Ther 2018; 8(5-s): 1-11. [http://dx.doi.org/10.22270/jddt.v8i5-s.1914]

[51] Behera J, Keservani RK, Yadav A, Tripathi M, Chadoker A. Methoxsalen loaded chitosan-coated microemulsion for effective treatment of psoriasis. Int J Drug Deliv. 2010;2(2):159–67. [http://dx.doi.org/10.5138/ijdd.2010.0975.0215.02025]

[52] Vicentini FTMC, Depieri LV, Polizello ACM, *et al.* Liquid crystalline phase nanodispersions enable skin delivery of siRNA. Eur J Pharm Biopharm 2013; 83(1): 16-24. [http://dx.doi.org/10.1016/j.ejpb.2012.08.011] [PMID: 23010565]

[53] Shinde G, Rajesh KS, Prajapati N, Murthy RSR. Formulation, development and characterization of nanostructured lipid carrier (NLC) loaded gel for psoriasis. Pharm Lett 2013; 5: 13-25.

[54] Ali S, Alam S, Imam F, Siddiqui MR. Topical nanoemulsion of turmeric oil for psoriasis: characterization, *ex vivo* and *in vivo* assessment. Int J Drug Deliv 2012; 4: 184-97.

[55] Kaur A, Katiyar SS, Kushwah V, Jain S. Nanoemulsion loaded gel for topical co-delivery of clobitasol propionate and calcipotriol in psoriasis. Nanomedicine 2017; 13(4): 1473-82. [http://dx.doi.org/10.1016/j.nano.2017.02.009] [PMID: 28259803]

[56] Salim N, Ahmad N, Musa SH, Hashim R, Tadros TF, Basri M. Nanoemulsion as a topical delivery system of antipsoriatic drugs. RSC Advances 2016; 6(8): 6234-50. [http://dx.doi.org/10.1039/C5RA14946K]

[57] Wohlrab J, Goebel A, Scherer D, Bingham D, Reinhard HH. A topical tacrolimus, microemulsion for plaque-type psoriasis therapy. Drug Development & Delivery 2012; p. 12.

[58] Lei W, Yu C, Lin H, Zhou X. Development of tacrolimus-loaded transfersomes for deeper skin penetration enhancement and therapeutic effect improvement *in vivo.* Asian Journal of Pharmaceutical Sciences 2013; 8(6): 336-45. [http://dx.doi.org/10.1016/j.ajps.2013.09.005]

[59] Sah AK, Jain SK, Pandey RS. Microemulsion based hydrogel formulation of methoxsalen for the effective treatment of psoriasis. Asian J Pharm Clin Res 2011; 4: 140-5.

[60] Baroli B, López-Quintela MA, Delgado-Charro MB, Fadda AM, Blanco-Méndez J. Microemulsions for topical delivery of 8-methoxsalen. J Control Release 2000; 69(1): 209-18. [http://dx.doi.org/10.1016/S0168-3659(00)00309-6] [PMID: 11018558]

[61] Raza K, Negi P, Takyar S, Shukla A, Amarji B, Katare OP. Novel dithranol phospholipid microemulsion for topical application: development, characterization and percutaneous absorption studies. J Microencapsul 2011; 28(3): 190-9. [http://dx.doi.org/10.3109/02652048.2010.546435] [PMID: 21395406]

[62] Setya S, Talegaonkar S, Razdan BK. Nanoemulsions: formulation methods and stability aspects. World J Pharm Pharm Sci 2014; 3(2): 2214-28.

[63] Prabu SL, Sharvana SP, Aravindan S, Bhuvaneswari A, Manikandan V. Nanoemulgel for transdermal delivery of cyclobenzaprine hydrochloride: design, characterization and *in-vitro* studies. PLoS One 2017; 12(5): e0178286.
[PMID: 28542563]

[64] Imam FI, Alam MS, Siddiqui MR, Ali MS. Topical nanoemulsion of turmeric oil for psoriasis: characterization, *ex vivo* and *in vivo* assessment. Int J Drug Deliv. 2012;4(2):184–97.
[http://dx.doi.org/10.5138/ijdd.v4i2.575]

[65] Alam MS, Ali MS, Alam N, Siddiqui MR, Shamim M, Safhi MM. *In vivo* study of clobetasol propionate loaded nanoemulsion for topical application in psoriasis and atopic dermatitis. Drug invention today. 2013 Mar 1; 5(1): 8-12.
[http://dx.doi.org/10.1016/j.dit.2013.02.001]

[66] Rajitha P, Shammika P, Aiswarya S, Gopikrishnan A, Jayakumar R, Sabitha M. Chaulmoogra oil based methotrexate loaded topical nanoemulsion for the treatment of psoriasis. J Drug Deliv Sci Technol 2019; 49: 463-76.
[http://dx.doi.org/10.1016/j.jddst.2018.12.020]

[67] Mittal S, Ali J, Baboota S. Enhanced anti-psoriatic activity of tacrolimus loaded nanoemulsion gel *via* omega 3 - Fatty acid (EPA and DHA) rich oils-fish oil and linseed oil. J Drug Deliv Sci Technol 2021; 63: 102458.
[http://dx.doi.org/10.1016/j.jddst.2021.102458]

[68] Algahtani MS, Ahmad MZ, Ahmad J. Nanoemulsion loaded polymeric hydrogel for topical delivery of curcumin in psoriasis. J Drug Deliv Sci Technol 2020; 59: 101847.
[http://dx.doi.org/10.1016/j.jddst.2020.101847]

[69] Kaur A, Katiyar SS, Kushwah V, Jain S. Nanoemulsion loaded gel for topical co-delivery of clobitasol propionate and calcipotriol in psoriasis. Nanomedicine 2017; 13(4): 1473-82.
[http://dx.doi.org/10.1016/j.nano.2017.02.009] [PMID: 28259803]

[70] Rashid SA, Bashir S, Ullah H, *et al.* Development, characterization and optimization of methotrexate-olive oil nano-emulsion for topical application. Pak J Pharm Sci 2021; 34(1(Supplementary)): 205-15.
[PMID: 34275844]

[71] Khan R, Mirza MA, Aqil M, *et al. In Vitro* and *In Vivo* Investigation of a Dual-Targeted Nanoemulsion Gel for the Amelioration of Psoriasis. Gels 2023; 9(2): 112.
[http://dx.doi.org/10.3390/gels9020112] [PMID: 36826282]

[72] Khatoon K, Ali A, Ahmad FJ, *et al.* Novel nanoemulsion gel containing triple natural bio-actives combination of curcumin, thymoquinone, and resveratrol improves psoriasis therapy: *in vitro* and *in vivo* studies. Drug Deliv Transl Res 2021; 11(3): 1245-60.
[http://dx.doi.org/10.1007/s13346-020-00852-y] [PMID: 32965640]

[73] Algahtani MS, Ahmad MZ, Nourein IH, Ahmad J. Co-delivery of imiquimod and curcumin by nanoemugel for improved topical delivery and reduced psoriasis-like skin lesions. Biomolecules 2020; 10(7): 968.
[http://dx.doi.org/10.3390/biom10070968] [PMID: 32605030]

[74] Sahu S, Katiyar SS, Kushwah V, Jain S. Active natural oil-based nanoemulsion containing tacrolimus for synergistic antipsoriatic efficacy. Nanomedicine (Lond) 2018; 13(16): 1985-98.
[http://dx.doi.org/10.2217/nnm-2018-0135] [PMID: 30188761]

[75] Ramanunny AK, Wadhwa S, Kumar Singh S, *et al.* Topical non-aqueous nanoemulsion of Alpinia galanga extract for effective treatment in psoriasis: *In vitro* and *in vivo* evaluation. Int J Pharm 2022; 624: 121882.
[http://dx.doi.org/10.1016/j.ijpharm.2022.121882] [PMID: 35671853]

[76] Alam MS, Ali MS, Alam N, *et al.* Design and characterization of nanostructure topical gel of betamethasone dipropionate for psoriasis. J Appl Pharm Sci 2012; 2(10): 148-58.

[http://dx.doi.org/10.7324/JAPS.2012.21029]

[77] Sharma M, Chandra Sharma M, Khabiya R, *et al.* Designing of novel nanoemulsions of retinol using box Behnken design for psoriasis. Mater Today Proc 2023; 80: 420-6.
[http://dx.doi.org/10.1016/j.matpr.2022.10.191]

[78] Wang Y, Li H, Dong F, *et al.* Therapeutic effect of calcipotriol pickering nanoemulsions prepared by exopolysaccharides produced by *bacillus halotolerans* FYS strain on psoriasis. Int J Nanomedicine 2020; 15: 10371-84.
[http://dx.doi.org/10.2147/IJN.S278247] [PMID: 33376326]

[79] Pund S, Pawar S, Gangurde S, Divate D. Transcutaneous delivery of leflunomide nanoemulgel: Mechanistic investigation into physicomechanical characteristics, *in vitro* anti-psoriatic activity and *in vivo* skin irritation study. J Drug Deliv Sci Technol 2021; 66: 102951.
[http://dx.doi.org/10.1016/j.ijpharm.2015.04.015] [PMID: 25869452]

[80] Raza K, Katare OP, Setia A, Bhatia A, Singh B. Improved therapeutic performance of dithranol against psoriasis employing systematically optimized nanoemulsomes. J Microencapsul 2013; 30(3): 225-36.
[http://dx.doi.org/10.3109/02652048.2012.717115] [PMID: 23088318]

[81] Jain S, Pattewad V, Bhargavi N, *et al.* Exploring the therapeutic potential of functional excipient-based nanoemulgel of fluticasone propionate for the management of psoriasis. J Drug Deliv Sci Technol 2023; 84: 104435.
[http://dx.doi.org/10.1016/j.jddst.2023.104435]

[82] Espinoza LC, Silva-Abreu M, Calpena AC, *et al.* Nanoemulsion strategy of pioglitazone for the treatment of skin inflammatory diseases. Nanomedicine 2019; 19: 115-25.
[http://dx.doi.org/10.1016/j.nano.2019.03.017] [PMID: 31004811]

[83] Ahmed MM, Anwer MK, Fatima F, *et al.* Development of apremilast nanoemulsion-loaded chitosan gels: *In vitro* evaluations and anti-inflammatory and wound healing studies on a rat model. Gels 2022; 8(5): 253.
[http://dx.doi.org/10.3390/gels8050253] [PMID: 35621551]

CHAPTER 17

Future Prospects of Novel Carrier-Based Pharmacotherapy

Esha Vatsa[1,*], **Nidhi Chaudhary**[1] and **Shipra Gautam**[2]

[1] *School of Pharmaceutical Sciences, Jigyasa University (Formerly Himgiri Zee University), Dehradun, Uttarakhand, India*

[2] *Department of Pharmacy, Himachal institute of Pharmacy, Paonta sahib, Himachal Pradesh, India*

Abstract: Psoriasis is a serious dermal plight characterised by inflammation and hyper-proliferation of the keratinized cells of the epidermis. Because of the complicated disposition of the disease, it has a severe pessimistic impact on the patient's overall well-being. Currently, a variety of medications are available for treating psoriasis, including conventional topical therapies, UVB therapy, intrinsic or systemic immune-modulators, and biologics, which aim to alleviate symptoms and thereby improve the quality of life for patients. Conventional topical therapies, though they constitute first-line therapy, have restricted efficacy because of the mediocre drug penetration properties, deposition, and dose-related toxicity. The latest progression in topical treatments, specifically with micro-scaled medical devices like micro-needles and nanoparticle-based carriers, lipid nanoparticles offer a promising future with significantly better therapeutic potency as it has a way better skin permeation, controlled release of the drug, targeting specific pathways, such as IL-23 inhibitors like mirikizumab and RORγt inhibitors, hence contributing to better drug delivery and efficacy for psoriatic plaques. These innovative and efficient therapies may cut down the side effects and may lead to improved and better patient adherence.

Keywords: Better adherence, Better skin permeation, Dose-related toxicity, Drug delivery, Drug penetration, Efficient therapies, Immune modulators, Inflammation, Leratinized cells, Lipid nano particles, Medical devices, Micro needles, Plaques, Proliferation, Psoriasis, Therapeutic efficacy, Topical therapies.

INTRODUCTION

Psoriasis is considered a multifactorial, chronic, and inflammatory disorder that is instigated by hereditary as well as environmental aspects [1]. It shows its impact

* **Corresponding author Esha Vatsa:** School of Pharmaceutical Sciences, Jigyasa University (Formerly Himgiri Zee University), Dehradun, Uttarakhand, India; Tel: +8439543858; E-mail: esha.vatsa@hzu.edu.in

Anjali Sharma, Prerna Sharma, Roy Rillera Marzo & Ahmed A. Al Karmalawy (Eds.)

on approximately 2–3% of the whole population. The dermal papillae telangiectasia, over-maturation of keratinized cells & conscription of provocative cells over the epidermis are the major features of psoriasis [2]. Whole areas of the skin of an individual's body can also be affected by this disease [3]. Patients suffering from this disease have higher risks of developing fatty liver, the occurrence of obesity, diseases related to the heart, hyperglycaemic conditions and several kinds of syndromes related to the general metabolism of the body in comparison to normal people. These possibilities are predominantly visible in patients who are suffering from severe psoriasis. The origin of this disease is still unidentified even after the conduction of a lot of research, but in recent studies it is quite known that this disease is basically prompted by the amalgamation of hereditary (*i.e.*, family history) as well as environmental factors (*i.e.*, alcohol, tobacco, infections, medications, stress) [4 - 7].

Patients suffering from psoriasis are concomitant to stigmatization physically, which complements the augmentation of the psychology-oriented complications in their very own emotional cum socio-professional lifestyle.

According to future considerations, the effective management of psoriasis can be achieved by employing various types of therapies, including topical therapy, phototherapy, and systemic therapy, which are among the primary effective alternatives for the efficient treatment of psoriasis. Contemporarily, diversified medications are available in the market for the treatment of psoriasis, for instance, conventional topical therapies, UVB (Ultraviolet B) therapy, and intrinsic or systemic modulators of the immune system, which generally target the palliation of the signs/symptoms & hence contribute to the improvement of the quality of the patient's life. Conventional topical therapies constitute the potential to act as first-line treatment as they hold constrained efficacy due to the unexceptional drug penetration characteristics, better adherence as well as dose-related toxicity. For mild stages of Psoriasis, topical treatment is the only treatment recommended as a first-line treatment. Conversely, systemic treatment or phototherapies are considered the type of treatments that efficiently work in severe conditions of psoriasis [8]. Various types of treatment regimens currently exist, which effectively diminish the signs and symptoms of psoriasis; however, among them, not a single method works as a comprehensive treatment method that can cure the disease entirely.

Psoriasis treatment with topical therapies is considered the conventional formulation, which is also bound to several kinds of complications such as restricted penetration of the drug, reduced patient adherence compliance, and elevated frequency of dosing, *etc.* [9].

Likewise, phototherapy and systemic therapy also exhibited several adverse effects, which involve toxicity of the liver and kidneys, cancer related to the skin and the basic problem of elevated blood pressure. These are the common disputes that limit the custom usage of presently existing conventional therapies for the treatment of psoriasis [9].

In the last few years, an NDDS (Novel Drug Delivery System) based nano-formulation has been widely reconnoitred by several scientists to succeed in the development of non-toxic and effective therapy for psoriasis, which will be considered among the future prospects for the successful treatment of Psoriasis as this technique holds the potential to enhance the therapeutic efficacy and provide long-standing effects [9]. Enhancement of therapeutic efficacy and reduction of toxicity through a dose reduction yields two outstanding effects that make nano-technology-based medicine a promising medication carrier for the future. This innovative method effectively works over the site-specific administration of medicines all over the areas of the skin for the treatment of psoriatic lesions and plaques [10 - 12].

In the last few years, most of the novel anti-psoriatic drugs also come into existence and got approval for markets are MAB (Monoclonal Antibodies), which target various patho-physiological procedures which are concerned for the development and advancement of this disease. Nevertheless, this antibody-based therapy is quite expensive for individuals who fall under the category of emerging economies [13 - 15].

In the latest progression in topical treatments, specifically with micro-scaled medical devices like micro-needles and nanoparticle-based carriers, lipid nanoparticles offer a promising future with significantly better therapeutic potency as it has a way better skin permeation, controlled release of drug, and targets definite pathways. For instance, Interleukin- 23 (IL-23) inhibitors (*e.g.*, Mirikizumab) and RORγt inhibitors. These will contribute to improved drug delivery and provide effectiveness against psoriatic plaques. These kinds of novel and efficient therapies might cut down the side effects and may lead to improved and better patient adherence in the future (16).

Classification of Disease on the Basis of Severity of Psoriasis

Psoriasis can be categorised into plaque, pustular, guttate, flexural and erythrodermic forms as per its clinical manifestations. The classification of psoriasis, along with its characteristic features, is presented in Table **1**.

Table 1. Classification of psoriasis and their characteristics (5,6,7,8,17).

S. No.	Type of Psoriasis	Characteristics
1	Plaque	• Well-marinated scalp lesions • Scaly plaques • Accumulation of severe hyperkeratosis • Severe hair loss
2	Pustular	• Visible in adults primarily • Localized to definite body areas, *viz.*, hands and some areas of feet • In some cases, it is generalized and covers most areas of the body • Flushing of skin followed by the pustules development
3	Guttate	• Small, red and distinct spots over the skin areas • Lesions appear over the areas of the trunk and limbs • More than 100 lesions appear in numbers • Lesion formation over the scalp and facial regions • Not as thick as lesions of Psoriasis (Plaque) • Occurs with different types of Psoriasis (Plaque)
4	Flexural	• Different from Lesions • Erythematous • Not usually scaly • Prominent exudation
5	Erythrodermic	• Usual form of Psoriasis • Occurs in approximately 1 to 2% of individuals once or more in a lifetime • Visible in individuals having unstable plaque Psoriasis • Extreme itching and pain in the skin areas • Lesions are not present • Extreme redness and exfoliation found in the skin

Accustomed Combination of Drugs for the Treatment of Psoriasis

Sufficient number of paramount evidences supports the effectiveness of combination drug treatment over mono therapy in patients suffering from modest to the severe kinds of Psoriasis. In the systematic study of various investigations, clearance rates of mono-therapies are less than those of combination therapies.

According to the studies combination therapy is more effective and best for the treatment of psoriasis. Following are the various considerations which are followed prior to the combination treatment for psoriasis [18].

When to employ a combination treatment for the treatment of Psoriasis

- If monotherapy is not or is no longer effective.
- If we want to reduce the acute toxicity.
- Side effects are projected to be small in number.

- Improved therapeutic consequence.
- To become patient, unquestioning and satisfied.

Which combination therapy should be employed for the treatment of Psoriasis.

- Depends on disease severity.
- History relative to the use of the drug (Response and side effects).
- Reported efficacy and cost-effective.

In case of modest to severe kinds of psoriasis it might be troublesome to attain & maintain the short-term active medicament along with long-term maintenance agents which is the prime requirement of this disease. Combinational, Rational & Sequential therapies of the treatment are hence most effective and non-toxic in comparison to distinct drug treatment or mono therapy.

- Conventional combinational therapy.

More than two medicaments possess synergism or corresponding mechanism of action which are mostly utilized in these therapy only small doses, less toxic regimens of the individual drugs are used. Fewer of the broadly used combinations are PUVA (Psoralen + Ultra Violet A) + UVB (Ultra Violet B), Methotrexate + UVB (Ultra Violet B), Acitretin + UVB (Ultra Violet B) or PUVA (Psoralen + Ultra Violet A) and Cyclosporine + Methotrexate [18].

- Rational therapy.

It is another strategic mode for combining treatment medications. The patients are subjected to the treatment with mono-therapy drugs and then transferred to be treated with another mono-therapy drug to lessen the cumulative dose regimen and pre-empt noxiousness. Table **2** below represents the rational therapy treatment, which indicates the use of primary and secondary drugs for treating psoriasis.

Table 2. Rational therapy treatment [19].

Primary drugs/ agents	Secondary drugs/ agents
• Drug Acitretin • Drug Methotrexate • Ultraviolet B in the presence or absence of tar • Drug Cyclosporine • PUVA	• Drug Hydroxy- Urea • 6-Thioguanine • Drug Sulfasalazine

- Sequential therapy

It is an approach which is being considered for the maintenance of safe regimen & hence optimize initial efficacy of specific combinations by deliberate sequence. It is a three-step strategical treatment plan for curing mild psoriasis to moderate psoriasis and moderate to severe psoriasis disease [20]. Sequential therapy is divided into three phases as follows [21].

Phase 1

Month 0-1: Start maximum dermatologic dose of cyclosporine (5 mg/kg/day).

Phase 2

i). Phase 2 A

Months 2-3: Cyclosporine will be maintained at the same dose, *i.e.*, 5 mg/kg/day, and then treatment with Acitretin will start at a dosage of 25 mg, with maximum tolerance achieved by increasing the dose to 10-25 mg.

ii). Phase 2 B

Months 4-7: subsequently decrease the dose of cyclosporine *i.e.*, not more than 1 mg/kg/mol, and sustain the therapy with the drug Acitretin.

Phase 3

i). Phase 3A

After 7 months: Therapy was maintained with the drug Acitretin.

ii). Phase 3B

After 7 months: The therapy was maintained with the drug Acitretin, and if necessary, Ultraviolet B or Psoralen + Ultraviolet A can also be included.

Novel approach Nanoparticles for the treatment of Psoriasis

In the past numerous decennium, there has been a hike in the number of investigations performed on psoriasis, and researchers have investigated a plethora of biomaterials to boost and strengthen the effectiveness of medication transport for the achievement of enhanced results of treatment of Psoriasis (Plaques). Amongst all prototype bio-materials, nano-particles have been studied most profoundly, as efficacious carriers for anti-psoriatic agents [22].

Nanoparticles (NPs) extend merits like a substantial ratio of surface area to volume, facilitating their penetration in hair follicles and varied dermal passages, including the trans-cellular passages, inter-cellular lipids & the passages of follicles. The traits of nano-particles, for instance, the molecular weight, size, surface charge, and pH, impact the permeation of the drug into the skin.

For the management of psoriasis, numerous lipid-dependent NPs have been popularly explored, which include NLC (Nano-structured Lipid Carriers), transfersomes, liposomes, Niosomes, ethosomes, and SLN (Solid Lipid Nanoparticles). Lipid-reliant nano-particles have the potential to permeate through the extracellular matrix of the stratum corneum layer of the skin. Case in point, NLCs stocked with Anti-Psoriatic drugs like the drug Methotrexate, which exhibits remarkable outcomes in facilitating the permeation of the drug. Metallic nano pharmaceuticals like gold and silver have exhibited promising improvements in drug delivery and immune- restorative effects in psoriatic skin [22].

Consequently, it is definitive that the nano pharmaceutical carrier network prepared from the polymers is a combination of nano drugs which may be either natural (chitosan) or synthetic Poly (lactide-co-glycolic acid) (PLGA) in origin and might be biodegradable or non-biodegradable in the nature; furthermore, nano pharmaceutical carrier drugs are manufactured from lipids may be nano-particulate or nano vesicular networks of either natural or synthetic lipids which are of bio degradable and non-bio degradable tendencies, whereas nano drugs carrier network synthesised from inorganic materials are of metallic or non-metallic origin, for example, gold and silver [22, 23].

The futuristic nano-technology mediated methods of drug delivery system for psoriasis are summarised below.

Lipid-based Nano carriers

i. **Liposomes** are minute, double layered vesicles encompassing an aqueous core. They are constituted to frame either a monolayer *i.e.*, uni-lamellar or poly-layered *i.e.*, multi-lamellar vesicles, relying on the count of lipid layers needed to encompass the core. Liposomes embrace water-adoring drugs inside an aqueous core, whereas a lipid adoring drugs in the lipid bilayer. And hence portraying as depot to cause the prolonged release of the medicament, elevating the penetration of non-ionic and phospholipid molecules by the mechanism of diffusion into the skin layer.

   Extensive studies have proven that formulated methotrexate incorporated oleic acid liposomes for treating psoriasis exhibited elevated penetration potential across the derma because of the suppleness or elasticity and increased penetration traits rendered by the existence of oleic acid, likewise the permeability and stability of fusidic acid liposomes for the probable treatment of chronic plaque psoriatic condition was found to be truly promising and they tend to decrease the clinical manifestations of psoriasis by altering the causative bacterial microbe responsible for disease progression [24].

ii. **Solid-lipid nanoparticles** prepared using methods like hot or cold homogenization, solvent evaporation, or high shear homogenization comprise an inside core composed of a physiological fluid, which in turn is enveloped by a covering layer of surface active agents. Being fabricated using physiological fluids they extend merits like potential to incorporate a large drug, offering broad surface area and high association of phases at interphases. SLNs are of profound use in the treatment of skin ailments like psoriatic disorder. Being prepared from physiological fluids, they offer lesser risk of toxicity. Reportedly, SLNs elevate skin moisturization by 30-31% post-b--fortnight period of therapy. Studies have proven that targeted and extended release of Fluocinolone acetonide (FA) was observed by fabricating it into SLNs. A remarkable portion of FA was discovered on the epidermis of skin when treated with SLNs suspension as compared to the treatment with plain FA [24].

iii. **Nanostructured Lipid Carriers (NLCS)** are improved versions of SLNs designed to combat demerits associated with NLC, for instance, the amount of loaded drug and release of the drug. NLCs remain curated with the introduction of the liquid form of lipids into the Solid system using the methods like micro-emulsification, homogenization (at high pressures), and solvent displacement. Established evidence has demonstrated that curcumin NLCs incorporated into cellulose nitro fibre films led to increase in the curcumin penetration into the psoriatic skin and caused a significant decrease in psoriasis lesions. These NLC films also demonstrate skin moisturisation effects, which are of great benefit for treating psoriasis. Likewise, the combinational nanocarriers, for instance, lipid carriers loaded with oleic acid and cilomilast, showcased amplified effectiveness in the curing of psoriasis lesions by inhibiting multiplication and neutrophil infiltration. Likewise, there is considerable evidence from various investigations that is sufficient to explain the role of NLCs as an emerging futuristic pharmacotherapy for the treatment of psoriasis [24].

iv. **Nanoemulsions/ Nano suspensions** extend several merits like better dermal permeation, prolonged drug release, better thermal stability, improved bioavailability, improved skin hydration, and hence better skin moisturisation and lesser skin irritation over the topical delivery of drugs. They are of immense help in facilitating the delivery of poorly water-soluble drugs, as it deals with suspension of drugs into oil droplets, and then stabilised them with the creation of the skinny emulsifier film all over the place of these oil droplets. Nanoemulsions incorporating Methotrexate in Chaulmoogra oil, Clobetasol propionate and calcipotriol nanoemulsions, pioglitazone nanoemulsions, and nanoparticle suspensions of Cyclosporin A (CyA) are among the extensively investigated formulations that have demonstrated significant therapeutic potential in the treatment of psoriasis [24].

v. **Transfersomes** are vesicular structures that offer numerous pros, for instance, being immensely flexible and deformable, their amphipathic behaviour, being able to release the encapsulated drug in a better manner, being capable of passing through the minute pores, crossing various barriers and hence exhibiting improved skin delivery make them superior to conventional liposomes and hence putting them into the category of progressive drug of choice for treatment of psoriasis [24].

vi. **Emulsomes and Cerosomes** are colloidal carriers composed of an abundance of phospholipids. Emulsomes comprise the incorporation of a solid or semi-solid core, into which a lipophilic medicament is loaded. These have the advantage of being able to be incorporated into oil-in-water emulsions and render extended release of drugs with greater tolerance, for instance, dianthrol nanoemulsions. Likewise, cerosomes are ceramide-loaded surface-active dependent vesicular phospholipid systems that are loaded with a potent anti-psoriasis medicament, for instance, tazarotene. Ceramide is believed to increase the containment of tazarotene, lowering its release and elevating its accumulation within the skin, hence associating it with superior therapeutic consequences as compared to the traditional topical products [24].

Polymer-based nanocarriers

Polymer-based nanocarriers entail nanospheres, nanocapsules, and dendrimers.

i. **Nanospheres** are constructed by persistently dispersing active medicament within the polymeric matrix.

ii. **Nanocapsules** consist of the drug encircled within a shell made up of a suitable polymer, which prevents the core pharmaceutical activity from environmental degradation and hence are introduced to the dermal membrane as hydrogels and emulgels. Nanoparticles of curcumin incorporated in silk-fibroin hydrogel enhanced the curcumin transmittance through the layer of skin (stratum corneum) and also prolonged the drug effect.

iii. Possessing a highly branched structure, **dendrimers** comprise 3 operational parts: explicitly a core, one internal structure with divisions, and one external structure that bears functional groups, imparting better absorption potential, alteration of the release kinetics, biocompatibility, and high reactivity.

Dianthrol micro sponge gel dendrimers have been formulated that are believed to have reduced adverse effects associated with dianthrol, for instance, irritation, burning sensation, and necrosis at the site of application [24].

Novel Approach Target Therapy for the Treatment of Psoriasis

In order to overcome the shortcomings of conventional pharmacotherapy, the novel approach of targeting the drug to specified targets has proven to be of greater benefit in the treatment of psoriasis. Targeted drug delivery requires a lower dose, and hence eventually reduces the probability of systemic adverse effects. Additionally, topical applications of medications restrict the release of the drug, lead to degradation of the drug, and exhibit poor efficacy due to the presence of a barrier of the stratum corneum layer. In contrast, the targeted formulation has the advantage of prolonging the duration of action, lesser dosing frequency, and overall improved and better patient compliance. Targeting the receptors of psoriasis may comprise two approaches, specifically a passive or an active approach. If the accumulation of drugs is done in a particular site of a target considering its biophysical properties, then it is called passive targeting. On the other hand, active targeting, which is considered synonymous with molecular or biological targeting, utilizes physical forces such as electroporation, sonoporation, and magnetism and conjugation of target ligands to target cells to create a pharmaco-therapeutic effects at the affected site.

Targeted pharmacotherapy in the management of psoriasis is a favourable scheme to deliver the loaded therapeutic medication to specified cells in the dermal layer, which emerges from various inflammatory and immune responses occurring in psoriatic skin. Targeting dopaminergic receptors, serotonergic receptors, microRNAs, and CD44 receptors constitutes the preeminent investigated targets for bringing a revolutionary development in the treatment of psoriasis [25].

CONCLUDING REMARKS

Inspite of the enormous multitude of mainstream and conventional alternatives available for the pharmacological management of psoriasis, patients even now have unfulfilled remedial requirements because of the inadequacy of patient contentment and compliance with the therapy. Consequently, there arises an utter requirement to investigate novel therapeutic and pharmacological standpoints for the management of psoriasis. Vigilance towards the extensive and global acceptance of biological and pharmacological investigations is required for establishing medications with enhanced efficacy and contentment. Globally available and widely accepted nano carriers carry the medicament at higher dosages and cure various kinds of psoriasis with marginal aftermaths must be investigated with precedence. A superior understanding of inflammatory pathways engaged in the pathological process and advanced discoveries may result in the effective clinical management of psoriasis.

REFERENCES

[1] Pradhan M, Alexander A, Singh MR, *et al.* Understanding the prospective of nano-formulations towards the treatment of psoriasis. Biomed Pharmacother 2018; 107: 447-63. [http://dx.doi.org/10.1016/j.biopha.2018.07.156] [PMID: 30103117]

[2] Asumalahti K, Ameen M, Suomela S, *et al.* Genetic analysis of PSORS1 distinguishes guttate psoriasis and palmoplantar pustulosis. J Invest Dermatol 2003; 120(4): 627-32. [http://dx.doi.org/10.1046/j.1523-1747.2003.12094.x] [PMID: 12648227]

[3] Raychaudhuri SK, Maverakis E, Raychaudhuri SP. Diagnosis and classification of psoriasis. Autoimmun Rev 2014; 13(4-5): 490-5. [http://dx.doi.org/10.1016/j.autrev.2014.01.008] [PMID: 24434359]

[4] Garg M, Garg P, Mishra D, *et al.* Psoriasis: Treatment with Calcipotriol. Ind J Pha Sci 2005; 67: 283-91.

[5] Sala M, Elaissari A, Fessi H. Advances in psoriasis physiopathology and treatments: Up to date of mechanistic insights and perspectives of novel therapies based on innovative skin drug delivery systems (ISDDS). J Control Release 2016; 239: 182-202. [http://dx.doi.org/10.1016/j.jconrel.2016.07.003] [PMID: 27381248]

[6] Takeshita J, Grewal S, Langan SM, *et al.* Psoriasis and comorbid diseases. J Am Acad Dermatol 2017; 76(3): 377-90. [http://dx.doi.org/10.1016/j.jaad.2016.07.064] [PMID: 28212759]

[7] Zangeneh FZ, Shooshtary FS. London, UK: Psoriasis-Types, Causes and Medication. In Tech 2013; pp. 1-37.

[8] Roberson EDO, Bowcock AM. Psoriasis genetics: breaking the barrier. Trends Genet 2010; 26(9): 415-23. [http://dx.doi.org/10.1016/j.tig.2010.06.006]

[9] Pinto MF, Moura CC, Nunes C, Segundo MA, Costa Lima SA, Reis S. A new topical formulation for psoriasis: Development of methotrexate-loaded nanostructured lipid carriers. Int J Pharm 2014; 477(1-2): 519-26. [http://dx.doi.org/10.1016/j.ijpharm.2014.10.067] [PMID: 25445970]

[10] Mascarenhas-Melo F, Carvalho A, Gonçalves MBS, Paiva-Santos AC, Veiga F. Nanocarriers for the topical treatment of psoriasis - pathophysiology, conventional treatments, nanotechnology, regulatory and toxicology. Eur J Pharm Biopharm 2022; 176: 95-107. [http://dx.doi.org/10.1016/j.ejpb.2022.05.012] [PMID: 35605927]

[11] Yadav N, Aggarwal R, Targhotra M, Sahoo PK, Chauhan MK. Natural and nanotechnology based treatment: An alternative approach to psoriasis. Curr Nanomed 2021; 11(1): 21-39. [http://dx.doi.org/10.2174/2468187310999201022192318]

[12] Henseler T, Christophers E. Psoriasis of early and late onset: Characterization of two types of psoriasis vulgaris. J Am Acad Dermatol 1985; 13(3): 450-6. [http://dx.doi.org/10.1016/S0190-9622(85)70188-0] [PMID: 4056119]

[13] Mohd Nordin UU, Ahmad N, Salim N, Mohd Yusof NS. Lipid-based nanoparticles for psoriasis treatment: a review on conventional treatments, recent works, and future prospects. RSC Advances 2021; 11(46): 29080-101. [http://dx.doi.org/10.1039/D1RA06087B] [PMID: 35478537]

[14] Griffiths CEM, Barker JNWN. Pathogenesis and clinical features of psoriasis. Lancet 2007;

370(9583): 263-71.
[http://dx.doi.org/10.1016/S0140-6736(07)61128-3] [PMID: 17658397]

[15] Pradhan M, Singh D, Singh MR. Novel colloidal carriers for psoriasis: Current issues, mechanistic insight and novel delivery approaches. J Control Release 2013; 170(3): 380-95.
[http://dx.doi.org/10.1016/j.jconrel.2013.05.020] [PMID: 23770117]

[16] Lynde CW, Poulin Y, Vender R, Bourcier M, Khalil S. Interleukin 17A: Toward a new understanding of psoriasis pathogenesis. J Am Acad Dermatol 2014; 71(1): 141-50.
[http://dx.doi.org/10.1016/j.jaad.2013.12.036]

[17] Naldi L, Gambini D. The clinical spectrum of psoriasis. Clin Dermatol 2007; 25(6): 510-8.
[http://dx.doi.org/10.1016/j.clindermatol.2007.08.003] [PMID: 18021886]

[18] Menter MA, See JA, Amend WJ, *et al.* Proceedings of the psoriasis combination and rotational therapy. J Ame Acad Derm 1996; 34: 315-21.

[19] Weinstein GD, White GM. An approach to the treatment of moderate to severe psoriasis with rotational therapy. J Am Acad Dermatol 1993; 28(3): 454-9.
[http://dx.doi.org/10.1016/0190-9622(93)70067-4] [PMID: 8445062]

[20] Koo J. Systemic sequential therapy of psoriasis: A new paradigm for improved therapeutic results. J Am Acad Dermatol 1999; 41(3): S25-8.
[http://dx.doi.org/10.1016/S0190-9622(99)70363-4] [PMID: 10459144]

[21] Saurat JH. Side effects of systemic retinoids and their clinical management. J Am Acad Dermatol 1992; 27(6): S23-8.
[http://dx.doi.org/10.1016/S0190-9622(08)80256-3] [PMID: 1460121]

[22] Lee HJ, Kim M. Challenges and future trends in the treatment of psoriasis. Int J Mol Sci 2023; 24(17): 13313.
[http://dx.doi.org/10.3390/ijms241713313] [PMID: 37686119]

[23] Dadwal N, Kurmi BD, Singh D, Singh A. Recent advancements in novel formulations of anti-psoriatic agents for effective delivery: clinical importance and patent survey. Recent Pat Nanotechnol 2024; 18(3): 259-77.
[http://dx.doi.org/10.2174/1872210517666230601124620] [PMID: 37264655]

[24] Bakshil H, Nagpal M, Singh M, *et al.* Treatment of psoriasis: A comprehensive review of entire therapies. Curr Dr Safe 2020; p. 15.

[25] Ahmad MZ, Mohammed AA, Algahtani MS, Mishra A, Ahmad J. Nanoscale topical pharmacotherapy in management of psoriasis: Contemporary research and scope. J Funct Biomater 2022; 14(1): 19.
[http://dx.doi.org/10.3390/jfb14010019] [PMID: 36662067]

CHAPTER 18

Psoriasis in the Modern World: Lifestyle, Diet and Holistic Approaches

Geeta Mahlawat[1], **Tarun Virmani**[2,*], **Ashwani Sharma**[3], **Girish Kumar**[2], **Reshu Virmani**[1], **Prachi Saini**[1] and **Kanika Mangla**[1]

[1] *School of Pharmaceutical Sciences, MVN University, Palwal, Haryana, India*

[2] *Amity Institute of Pharmacy, Amity University, Greater Noida Campus, Uttar Pradesh, India*

[3] *Department of Pharmaceutics, Delhi Institute of Pharmaceutical Sciences and Research, Delhi Pharmaceutical Sciences and Research University, New Delhi, India*

Abstract: Psoriasis, a chronic autoimmune skin condition that affects millions of people worldwide, is becoming more common because of modern lifestyle variables like stress, unhealthy eating habits, and pollution in the environment. This chapter explores the intricate relationship between illness and modern living, focusing on the management of psoriasis through dietary changes, lifestyle adjustments, and holistic approaches. It explores the effects of processed foods, inflammatory triggers, and gut health, emphasizing the value of nutritional methods and anti-inflammatory diets. The chapter also looks at alternative medicines like Ayurveda and Traditional Chinese Medicine and stress-reduction methods like yoga and mindfulness. This chapter offers a thorough manual for anyone looking for a natural, well-rounded approach to managing psoriasis in today's fast-paced world by fusing scientific knowledge with useful suggestions.

Keywords: Dietary changes, Lifestyle, Pollution, Psoriasis, Stress.

INTRODUCTION

Overview of Psoriasis

Psoriasis is an immune-mediated, persistent skin condition. Nearly 125 million people globally and about 3% of the US population suffer from psoriasis, a chronic skin condition [1]. The occurrence of psoriasis varies across nations and can manifest at any stage of life [2], suggesting that ethnicity, genetic makeup, and environmental factors influence the onset of the condition. The pathophysiology of psoriasis is largely influenced by genetic factors [3]. The

* **Corresponding author Tarun Virmani:** Amity Institute of Pharmacy, Amity University, Greater Noida Campus, Uttar Pradesh, India; E-mail: tarun2feb@gmail.com

Anjali Sharma, Prerna Sharma, Roy Rillera Marzo & Ahmed A. Al Karmalawy (Eds.)

World Health Organization [WHO] approved resolution WHA 67.9 in 2014, which urges international cooperation to combat stigma and promote awareness of psoriasis as a major non-communicable disease. In order to raise awareness of the disease's effects on public health, the resolution asked WHO to compile a global report on psoriasis [4]. For this study, a new, comprehensive systematic review of the global epidemiology of psoriasis was carried out. Through the use of a strict, methodical approach, the review sought to analyze all available data regarding the global epidemiology of psoriasis [5]. The immunological and genetic factors underlying the pathogenesis of psoriasis are well understood. This greater knowledge has led to the development of certain recently approved biological treatments for psoriasis, but it has also contributed to the development of others [6]. For example, the important role that tumor necrosis factor plays in the pathogenesis of the disease has been brought to light by the notable efficacy of medications that block the cytokine. Additionally, facts that psoriasis is not limited to skin conditions are mounting [7]. Studies on the epidemiology of psoriasis patients have revealed a higher standardized death rate, especially when it comes to heart disease and cancer. Comorbidities in psychology and psychiatry that are clinically significant are also frequent and may benefit from therapeutic intervention [8]. The immune system plays a role in psoriasis, as evidenced by the disease's therapeutic response to immunosuppressive drugs, the presence of clonal T-Cell Receptor [TCR] rearrangements in psoriatic skin, and the disease's transmission through bone marrow transplantation in humans and by purified T-cells in mice with prepsoriatic human skin [9]. The chemical mechanisms that trigger this immunological activation state remain unclear. According to recent comprehensive genomic sequencing of the MHC Class I region, HLA-Cw6 itself is most likely the functional mutation predisposing to psoriasis rather than a flag for some other nearby disease gene [10].

Types of Psoriasis

- Psoriasis Vulgaris

Chronic plaque psoriasis accounts for approximately 90% of psoriasis cases. The traditional clinical signs are erythematous, painful, well-defined plaques with silvery scales covering them. Large amounts of skin may be covered by the plaques when they combine. Common locations include the trunk, limb extensor surfaces, and scalp [10, 11].

- Reverse Psoriasis

Clinically characterized by somewhat erosive erythematous plaques and patches, inverse psoriasis, also known as flexural psoriasis, affects intertriginous sites [12].

• Guttate Psoriasis

One variety is guttate psoriasis, which presents as tiny erythematous plaques that appear suddenly. It typically affects kids or teenagers, and tonsil infections caused by group A streptococci are a common cause. Plaque psoriasis is a condition that approximately one-third of adults with guttate psoriasis may have during their lifetime [13, 14].

• Pustular psoriasis

Several sterile pustules that coalesce are the hallmark of pustular psoriasis. Both localized and widespread pustulosis are possible. It has been possible to identify two unique localized phenotypes: acrodermatitis continua of Hallopeau and psoriasis pustulosapalmoplantaris [PPP]. PPP only includes the palms and soles of the hands and feet, whereas ACS is more widely distributed at the tips of the fingers and toes and impacts the nail system [2].

Causes and Triggers

Mechanical Stress

This phenomenon, known as the Koebner phenomenon, occurs when skin lesions develop in non-affected areas of psoriasis patients following injury [15]. Recent reports have indicated that exposure to ultraviolet B radiation, radiotherapy, and even mild skin irritation might cause new psoriasis lesions [16 - 18]. However, psoriatic lesions are not always visible in the skin that is not affected following trauma [19, 20]. The manner in which the Koebner phenomenon develops can be influenced by the kind, location, intensity, and degree of trauma [21]. Moreover, the psoriatic keratinocytes' secreted NGF has functional activity. It is noteworthy that keratinocytes of psoriasis sufferers produce more NGF. This study indicates that NGF is involved in the pathophysiology of psoriasis and that the early stages of psoriasis lesions are responsive to NGF's regulatory role and receptor system. Psoriasis is one of the autoimmune inflammatory skin conditions that is mediated by TRM [22]. Resident memory T cells [TRM] are a non-circulating memory T cell subpopulation that endures over time in peripheral tissues.

Surprisingly, psoriasis patients' non-lesioned skin may develop and sustain psoriasis lesions due to skin-resident pathogenic T cells.

Air Pollutants and Exposure to the Sun

Air pollutants, including polycyclic aromatic hydrocarbons, volatile organic compounds, oxides, particulate matter, ozone, heavy metals, and UV radiation, cause oxidative stress in the skin, which is one of the main impacts of increased air pollution on human skin over time [23]. Air contaminants that impact the pathogenesis of psoriasis include cadmium. Blood cadmium levels were greater in patients with severe psoriasis than in the general population [24]. According to this research, cadmium exposure in the environment may weaken immunity, and micro environmental disturbances may make psoriasis more likely to deteriorate. Two subtypes of UV radiation are identified that reach the Earth's surface: UVA radiation over 95% [315–400 nm] and UVB radiation between 1% and 5% [280–315 nm]. Psoriasis has been widely treated by phototherapy [25]. Currently, psoralen UVA [PUVA], with preference for resistant psoriatic plaques, is utilized as the second-line therapy for psoriasis, whereas excimer laser [308 nm] and narrowband UVB [311 nm] are employed as the first-line therapies.

Drugs

Drug-related psoriasis occurs when psoriasis starts and gets worse when using specific medicines. Identifying drug-related causes of psoriasis is challenging due to the varying latency period between medication start and psoriatic skin lesions onset. Erythrodermic psoriasis, palmoplantar psoriasis, plaque psoriasis, scalp psoriasis, nail psoriasis, and pustular psoriasis are among the symptoms [26]. Histopathological findings of eosinophilic infiltrates and lichenoid reaction can help diagnose drug-related psoriasis. Drug ingestion can worsen pre-existing psoriasis, induce psoriatic lesions, or precipitate the disease in patients without a family history or predisposed individuals [3].

Vaccinations

Because psoriasis patients are treated with immunomodulatory or immunosuppressive medications, they are more likely to become infected [27]. Therefore, it is advised to get vaccinated against certain illnesses [28, 29]. But psoriasis can frequently be brought on by and made worse by immunization. Numerous studies support the connection between receiving an influenza vaccination and aggravation of psoriasis [30]. Psoriasis may also develop as a result of influenza vaccination [31]. The main purpose of the live attenuated strain of Mycobacterium bovis used in the Bacillus Calmette–Guérin [BCG] vaccination is to prevent tuberculosis [32]. After receiving the BCG vaccine, psoriasis may develop [33, 34]. Additionally, BCG has been applied locally as immunotherapy for bladder cancer, and reports have indicated that BCG immunotherapy has caused erythrodermicpustular psoriasis in one case [35].

Infections

Psoriasis is linked to streptococcal infection, with guttate psoriasis being the most common type. Symptoms can recur with streptococcal infection recurrence, making tonsillectomy a potential treatment option [36]. Staphylococcus aureus is also associated with psoriasis development, with dysregulated skin microbiomes found in 60% of patients with psoriasis. Candida species, a part of the normal human microbiota, are highly detected in patients with psoriasis, particularly in the oral mucosa milieu. The most prevalent disease-causing Candida species, Candida albicans, may be involved in the pathophysiology of psoriasis and enhance antifungal immunity [37].

Lifestyles

Alcohol and smoking are associated with psoriasis, and people who smoke or have smoked in the past are more likely to have the condition. Smoking increases the risk of developing psoriasis and is strongly associated with pustular lesions. Alcohol consumption is also a risk factor, but there is not enough evidence to establish its role. Alcohol misuse raises mortality rates and is correlated with the severity of psoriasis and the effectiveness of treatment. Psoriasis can be managed with dietary changes, such as taking supplements of antioxidants, folic acid, vitamin D, and polyunsaturated fatty acids [38].

Imtrinsic Factors

Obesity

Obesity and metabolic syndrome are common in psoriasis patients, and they are closely linked to the development and aggravation of the disorder. Obesity is more prevalent in psoriasis patients and has been linked to severe psoriasis [39]. Obesity is defined as the expansion of white adipose tissue, which produces pro-inflammatory adipokines such as leptin, TNF-α, adiponectin, and IL-6. Blocking these pathways can improve the psoriasis inflammatory cycle, but not insulin sensitivity in type 2 diabetes patients [40].

Diabetes Mellitus

Diabetes Mellitus (DM) prevalence is influenced by ethnic origin and lifestyle factors, but may be similar across diverse patient populations. Psoriasis is linked to diabetes mellitus and is a sign of a higher risk of type 2 DM. Obesity is a risk factor for psoriasis, contributing to the onset and exacerbation of type 2 DM. However, the pathophysiology of psoriasis may not be directly influenced by type 2 DM.

Dyslipidemia

Psoriasis is linked to obesity, with excess adipose tissue potentially contributing to dyslipidemia. Dyslipidemia is prevalent in 62.85% of patients, often hypertriglyceridemia with a lowered HDL value. Oral systemic medications can also result in dyslipidemia, with retinoids being the most effective cause [41].

Hypertension

According to a meta-analysis, hypertension is more common in psoriasis patients, with severe psoriasis being linked to a higher incidence. A multicenter observational study found that 26% of psoriasis patients had hypertension.

Mental Stress

Psoriasis, which is frequently made worse by high levels of stress, is frequently brought on by mental stress, which is a sensation of pressure and tension. However, there is a complicated relationship between mental stress and psoriasis; a systematic analysis found a high correlation between stress and the start and aggravation of psoriasis. According to a prospective study, greater illness severity and itching were independently correlated with cognitive and behavioral patterns of worrying and scratching. Causes and Risk factors for psoriasis are well explained in Fig. (**1**).

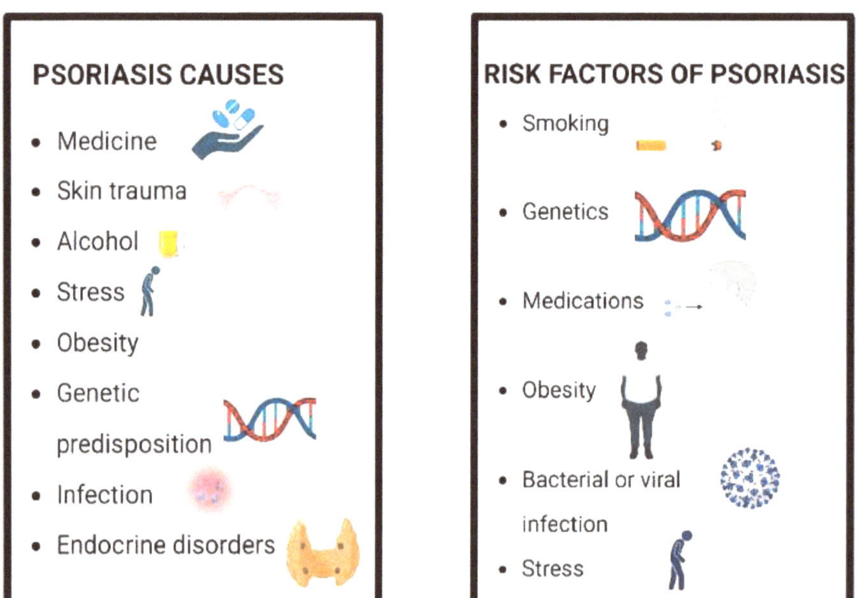

Fig. (1). Causes and risk factors of psoriasis.

Pathophysiology

Prolonged inflammation that causes unchecked keratinocyte growth and defective differentiation is the defining feature of psoriasis. Acanthosis, or epidermal hyperplasia, is evident in the histology of the psoriatic plaque and is layered atop inflammatory infiltrates made up of T cells, neutrophils, dermal dendritic cells, and macrophages (Fig. **4**). Another notable characteristic is neovascularization. Plaque psoriasis and the other clinical variants share certain inflammatory mechanisms, but they also show distinct variances that explain the variations in phenotype [42]. In Fig. (**2**), the pathophysiology of Psoriasis is well explained.

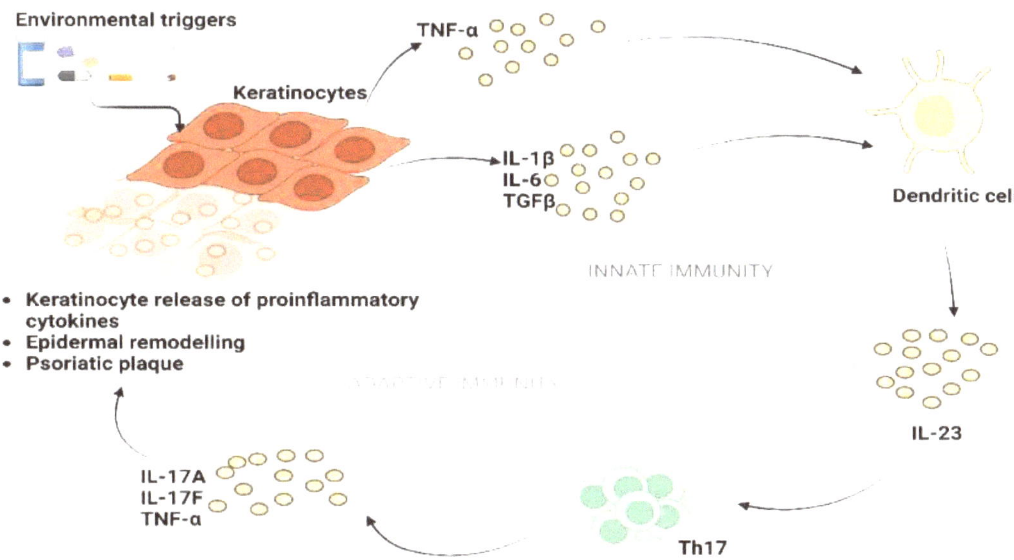

Fig. (2). Pathophysiology of psoriasis.

MEDICAL APPROACHES

Conventional Treatments [Topical Treatments, Phototherapy, Systemic Medications and Biological]

Topical corticosteroids, tars, anthralin, vitamin D analogs, tabarotene, and salicylic acid are among the treatments for skin psoriasis [43]. While many patients respond well to topical therapies, about 20% require additional systemic medications. The long-term use of all of them is limited due to the significant risk of major adverse effects, including hepatotoxicity and nephrotoxicity [methotrexate, cyclosporine], teratogenicity [oral retinoids], and skin cancer [photo/chemotherapy] [44]. The American Academy of Dermatology [AAD] released a consensus statement on psoriasis treatments recently. Rotational therapy is used to treat severe psoriasis, with an emphasis on often switching treatments to minimize adverse effects. The degree of the sickness, the efficacy of the medications, the patient's quality of life, and the simplicity of the treatment all influence the choices made. According to guidelines, if UVB treatment is ineffective, PUVA, methotrexate, cyclosporine, or acitretin should be used next [45]. Methotrexate and cyclosporine were shown to be equally effective in treating moderate to severe psoriasis, according to a recently published randomized controlled experiment. Many of the same disease-modifying antirheumatic medications that have proven effective in the treatment of rheumatoid arthritis, such as methotrexate, sulfasalazine, and cyclosporine, are administered systemically to treat severe cases of psoriatic arthritis that do not respond to nonsteroidal anti-inflammatory drugs, present with polyarticular joint involvement, or show destructive progression. When one or two joints are affected, flare-ups of psoriatic arthritis have been treated with intra-articular injections of corticosteroids. It is usually not recommended to provide corticosteroids systemically, as stopping them could make psoriasis skin lesions worse [46]. Current therapies for psoriasis are limited by potential side effects and patient dissatisfaction. Only 26% of patients are satisfied with their current treatment, and 44% prefer systemic therapy over topical treatment. A recent survey revealed that only 27% of patients express high satisfaction. Conventional drugs available for the treatment of Psoriasis are given in Table **1**. Current treatments are time-consuming, ineffective, and patients experience side effects, affecting their quality of life. Various conventional drugs available for the treatment of psoriasis are well explained in Fig. (**3**).

Table 1. Various conventional drugs available for the treatment of psoriasis.

Drug	Route of Administration	Mechanism
Methotrexate	s.c./oral	Dihydrofolate reductase inhibition blocks purine biosynthesis and induction of lymphocytes [47]
Cyclosporine	Oral	Calcineurin inhibition leading to reduced IL-2 [48]
Acitretin	Oral	Normalization of keratinocyte proliferation /differentiation through retinoid receptor binding [49]
Fumarate	Oral	Intracellular glutathione, modulation of Nrf2, NF-Kb, and HIF -1α, promoting a shift from –inflammatory Th1/Th17 response to an anti-inflammatory [50]
Apremilast	Oral	PDE4 inhibitor increases in transcellular cAMP levels in immune and non-immune cell types modulate inflammation [51]
Adalimumab	s.c.	Human monoclonal antibody against TNF-α [52]
Infliximab	i.v.	Chimeric IgG1 monoclonal antibody that binds to soluble and transmembrane forms of TNF-α [53]

(Table 1) cont.....

Drug	Route of Administration	Mechanism
Etanercept	s.c.	Dimeric human fusion protein mimicking TNF –αR [54]
Certolizumab	s.c.	A fab portion of humanized monoclonal antibody against TNF-α conjugated to polyethylene glycol [55]
Secukinumab	s.c.	Human IgG1k MONOCLONAL ANTIBODY against IL-17A [56]
Brodalumab	s.c.	Human monoclonal IgG2 antibody directed at the IL-17RA [52]
Risankizumab	s.c.	Humanized IgG1 monoclonal antibody that inhibits interleukin-23 by specifically targeting the p19 subunit [57]

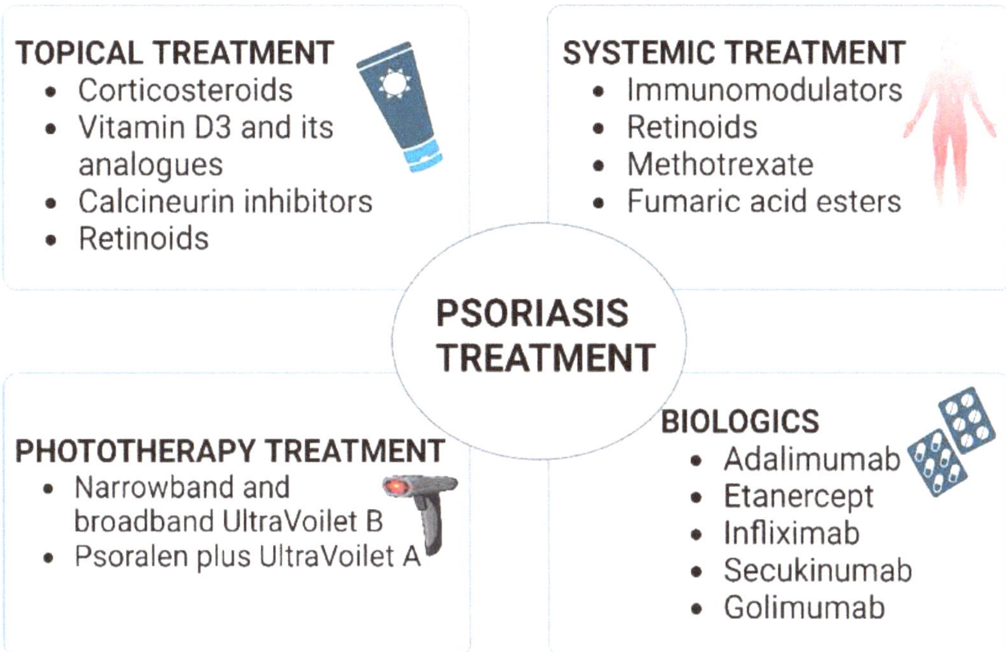

Fig. (3). Various conventional drugs available for the treatment of psoriasis.

Topical Therapy

Adherence to topical therapy regimens is poor, with only half of the patients following their treatment regimen. Improvement can be achieved by considering cosmetic acceptability, local side effects, formulation, and practicalities. Nurses with dermatological training can play a crucial role in this. Nurse-led outpatient treatment centers provide psychological support and facilitate combining topical therapy with phototherapy. Topical corticosteroids are widely used due to their effectiveness and rapid onset of action [43].

Systemic Therapies and Phototherapy

Strong, recent data supporting the effectiveness of photochemotherapy [psoralen with ultraviolet A light, PUVA] and ultraviolet B light, as well as the majority of systemic psoriasis treatments, originate from randomized controlled trials; however, there are not many comparison studies that look at the relative safety and effectiveness of the various therapies. Those that have not addressed crucial clinical problems, including how long remission lasts after treatment ends, or if continuous or intermittent use maintains efficacy. Drug vacations, combination therapy, and the rotational or sequential use of systemic medication are methods to lessen the toxicity of long-term treatment [45]. Ethotrexate is an immunosuppressive medication that lowers cell division and inflammation. One oral retinoid that helps minimize flaking and restore skin cell development is called Actinretin. Cyclosporine: It is an immunosuppressive medication that reduces inflammation and the immune response.Phosphodiesterase-4 inhibitors: These medications work by blocking a certain enzyme to lessen inflammation and cell division.

Biological Therapy

Agents used in biological therapy obstruct key molecular pathways in the psoriasis development. In the last five years, they have been well-liked as effective substitute treatments for psoriasis. At the moment, they are divided into two primary categories: drugs that target T cells or antigen-presenting cells [efalizumab] and drugs that target the cytokine tumour necrosis factor [etanercept, infliximab, adalimumab] [41]. High demand has resulted from widespread patient unhappiness with traditional therapies, even if parenteral administration is required [intravenously every eight weeks for infliximab, self-administered subcutaneous injections twice weekly, weekly, or every two weeks for the others]. Due to the relative paucity of information regarding long-term safety and efficacy, their current place in the framework of typical systemic therapy is limited [58].

Potential Side Effects

These are medications that you apply topically, including on your scalp. One of these can be sufficient to manage your psoriasis if it is mild to moderate. You might combine one with other therapies in more serious cases [59].

Anthralin: This medication inhibits the growth of skin cells and aids in the removal of scales. Skin irritation is the most typical adverse effect. In addition, it has the ability to discolor hard objects, clothing, and even your flesh. It's recommended to wash it off after a short period of time if you can [60]. This thick, black coal byproduct helps reduce inflammation, aid with scaling and itching, improve the appearance of your skin, and slow down the creation of new skin cells. However, it can also dry out, irritate, and increase your skin's sensitivity to sunlight.

Corticosteroids: These potent medications are very helpful and reduce inflammation. However, prolonged usage of these is not advised. In addition to potentially making your skin thinner, ingesting them may also result in stomach ulcers, bone thinning, early cataract development, and other health problems [40].

Roflumilast [Zoryve]: This once-daily topical treatment for plaque psoriasis relieves symptoms without the use of steroids. It can result in adverse symptoms, including hives and breathing difficulties, which are similar to allergic reactions.

Salicylic acid: This aids in the removal of skin debris. It could aggravate your skin as well. Applying it to your scalp for an extended length of time may cause your hair to become weak and eventually fall out [26].

A topical cream called Tapinarof [Vtama] is used to treat plaque psoriasis. It can be used continuously and is free of steroids.

Tazarotene: Formulated with vitamin A, this cream is a retinoid. It may cause skin irritation and increase skin sensitivity to sunlight. Because it increases the likelihood of having a child with specific birth abnormalities, it is not advised for women who are pregnant or intend to get pregnant [61].

Vitamin D: Vitamin D-containing topical therapies, such as calcitriol and calcipotriene, may cause skin irritation.

Skin cancer risk increases and mild burns are common adverse effects. Additionally, it may increase your sensitivity to sunlight. Short-term side effects of photochemotherapy, which involves a medication that improves the effectiveness of the UV light, also include nausea, itching, and red skin [62].

Methotrexate [Otrexup [PF], Rasuvo, Trexall, Xatmep]: This medication, which is often administered as a shot or pill, reduces inflammation and decreases the proliferation of skin cells. Among its possible adverse effects are: Feeling stressed, appetite decline, and upset stomach [47]. Methotrexate can result in more severe side effects, such as liver damage and blood cell abnormalities if you take it for an extended period of time.

Cyclosporine: This medication suppresses your immune system [Gengraf, Neoral, Sandimmune]. This may raise your chance of contracting an infection or developing other illnesses, such as cancer. It can develop high blood pressure or renal damage.

LIFESTYLE MODIFICATIONS

Stress Management

Psoriasis is a persistent skin disorder that can affect social, psychological, occupational, and physical functioning. Social stigma, low self-esteem, anxiety, and depression are linked to psoriasis, which reduces quality of life and creates stress [63]. Psoriasis and psychosocial stress interact in a reciprocal manner that has the potential to spiral out of control [64]. Psoriasis care that works requires not just normal pharmaceutical treatment and phototherapy, but also taking the patient's emotional health into account [65]. Despite evidence of high levels of psychological distress and a significant impact on quality of life, people with psoriasis have extremely little access to psychological care [66]. The ANS, the immune system, and the hypothalamic-pituitary-adrenal [HPA] axis are all involved in the physiological reaction brought on by stress. Adrenaline and noradrenaline are released from the adrenal medulla *via* the vagus nerve during the initial phase of the ANS's activation, which occurs seconds after the stressor is identified. After 20 to 30 minutes, the second phase is characterised by the hypothalamus's release of corticotrophin-releasing hormone [HPA], which is then activated. Next, the adrenal cortex secretes glucocorticoids [GC] for several hours, which affect the immune system, adipose tissue, and the gonadal axis [67].To prevent the organism from becoming exhausted, the HP axis's negative feedback regulates the release of GC [68]. Prolonged stress inhibits the HP axis's negative feedback, which raises CRH and GC levels. Stress causes the skin's dendritic cells to become active, which then releases neuromediators and catecholamines through the skin's nerve endings. This process exacerbates dermatological problems [69]. It looks like the skin functions similarly to the HPA axis. Skin cells and the immune system produce CRH. Acute stress-induced release of CRH from the skin increases vascular permeability and activates mast cells [43]. A crucial etiopathogenic function for the release of CRH in the development of cutaneous inflammatory illness [44].

Psoriasis is characterised by a decrease in GC secretion and an increase in catecholamine synthesis, both of which have an impact on the HP axis. It has been proposed that stress causes mast cell degranulation, which releases pro-inflammatory cytokines and exacerbates psoriasis *via* activating CRH [70], [45]. Increased CRH-R1 receptor expression has been shown by Cervigen Cemil *et al.* in psoriasis plaques, suggesting that this receptor may contribute to the etiopathogenesis of the condition. TNF-alpha, interferon-alpha, interleukins 1 and 6, and other cytokines released during psoriasis decrease serotonin synthesis and increase the generation of CRH, which increases stress and explains depressive illnesses and a tendency to stress [71, 72]. A research comparing baseline and post-stress cortisol levels in 10 psoriasis patients and 10 healthy people did not find differences in baseline cortisol levels. However, individuals with psoriasis had greater salivary cortisol levels, which may indicate the involvement of the HPA axis. Brunoni *et al.* found a clear relationship between evening cortisol levels and the PASI score, which measures the severity of psoriasis.The lack of a group of controls in this study makes the findings faulty. It is suspected that stress also acts by altering the epidermal barrier's permeability, which keeps the inflammatory skin reaction going. Additionally, stress hinders the healing of skin wounds. It has been proposed that stress may promote keratinocyte proliferation by amplifying the inhibition of epidermal lipid production. Moreover, it raises the synthesis of substance P, which causes a rise in lymphocyte activation, inflammation, and keratinocyte proliferation [46]. The effect of stress on Psoriasis is well explained in Fig. (**4**).

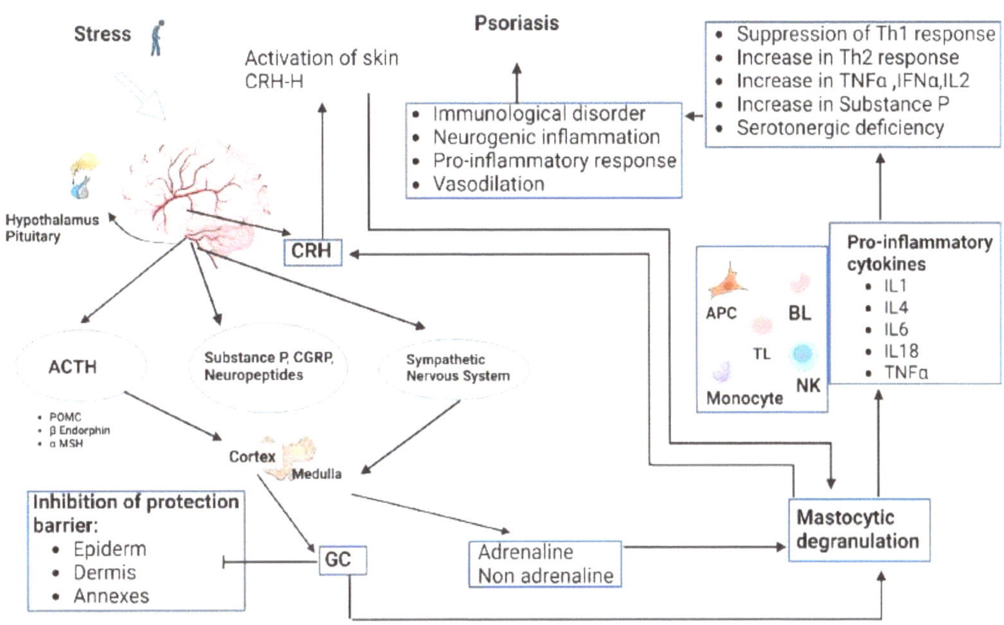

Fig. (4). Effect of stress on psoriasis.

Importance of Regular Exercise

It is recommended by the Centers for Disease Control and Prevention [CDC] that Americans engage in moderate-intensity aerobic exercise for 150 minutes each week. But as of 2018, just 53.3% of American people truly complied with these recommendations. Determining the extent and degree of exercise for those with psoriasis is crucial, as the condition is recognised to pose a danger for cardiovascular ailments. Overall, observational studies on the amount of exercise done by people with psoriasis reveal that these people exercise less frequently and less intensively than people without the condition [73]. As an instance, an experimental investigation using stress testing on 50 psoriasis patients and 32 healthy controls revealed that the psoriasis patients had a considerably poorer heart rate recovery index, which was connected with the length [$p < 0.001$] and severity [$p < 0.001$] of the condition. This study did have a significant disadvantage, though, in that it may not have been suitable to infer a direct association between the illness condition and the two groups' levels of physical fitness [74]. A research that compared patients with mild psoriasis to healthy controls assessed a range of physical measures, including body fat percentage, maximal aerobic capacity, pulmonary function tests, and body fat measurement. This study suggests that psoriasis does not significantly affect fitness since there was no change in any of these parameters between individuals with the condition and those who were healthy. Psoriasis did not appear to have an influence on exercise activities in a study of 66 patients with the skin condition and 52 controls with other skin conditions [vitiligo, atopic dermatitis, *etc.*]. There was no significant difference in the composite exercise ratings between the two groups [77]. Regular exercise is crucial for people with psoriasis to maintain a healthy weight, reduce the risk of health problems like type 2 diabetes and cardiovascular disease, and relieve stress and improve mood. Exercise also produces endorphins, which reduce anxiety, increase energy, and reduce pain. Psoriasis patients have an increased risk of developing heart disease, stroke, depression, and other diseases. Exercise is an effective way to combat these risks. However, it's important to be cautious when exercising, as the intensity or frequency may need to be adjusted based on the condition. Exercise can also decrease inflammation and alleviate psoriasis symptoms. A plant-based diet, incorporating fresh fruits, vegetables, whole grains, lean protein, and healthy fats like omega-3 fatty acids, can help lose weight. A diet planner can help maintain a balanced diet while avoiding high-sugar, refined carbohydrates, and salty foods. Exercise can relieve stress and improve circulation, which can support the liver and kidneys, reducing the chances of developing psoriasis and related illnesses. Obesity increases the risk of developing psoriasis, as fat cells release chemicals that cause the condition. Managing weight can help reduce the risk of heart problems and respiratory illnesses.

Adequate Sleep and its Impact on Psoriasis

Psoriasis is a long-term autoimmune disorder characterized by an accumulation of skin cells on the skin's outer layer. The quality of your life can be impacted by psoriasis symptoms such as inflammation, discomfort, and itching, which can also have an impact on how well you sleep. Many psoriasis sufferers find that their illness affects their ability to sleep. According to several studies, 85% or more of individuals with psoriasis may experience sleep-related problems. Psoriasis-related weariness can throw off regular sleep-wake cycles, and people with the condition may have discomfort that keeps them up at night. Psoriasis sufferers are also more prone to develop depression, sleep apnea, psoriatic arthritis, and other medical disorders that might impair their ability to get a good night's sleep [76]. As psoriasis symptoms grow, there seems to be a correlation with the chance of sleep issues. The National Psoriasis Foundation study found that persons with moderate psoriasis symptoms had a 59% higher chance [odds ratio 1.59] of having trouble sleeping compared to those without psoriasis. Individuals with severe symptoms of psoriasis had a 140% [odds ratio 2.40] increased risk of experiencing sleep disturbances. Many aspects of your physical and emotional health, including your psoriasis, can be impacted by inadequate sleep. According to the previously cited Danish study, psoriasis was more common in those who had sleep apnea. They also had a higher likelihood of having psoriatic arthritis or severe symptoms. These findings imply that the symptoms of psoriasis and sleep quality can be correlated in both directions. That is to say, psoriasis symptoms may potentially be exacerbated by sleep issues. A consistent sleep routine is essential for preparing the body for sleep, including going to bed and waking up at the same time every day, including weekends. A calming night-time routine, such as reading before bed, can help wind down the body and avoid stimulating lights. Regular exercise, such as 30 minutes of physical activity a day for at least 5 days a week, can help manage psoriasis better. Sunlight is essential for regulating the body's circadian rhythm and melatonin production, promoting a good night's sleep. A 2021 study found that exposure to daytime light was linked to less frequent tiredness, easier waking up, fewer insomnia symptoms, and an earlier chronotype. People with psoriasis should take extra precautions to protect their skin during sun exposure, using mineral-based sunscreens with an SPF of 30 or higher. A diet high in saturated fats, trans fatty acids, and refined carbohydrates can increase inflammation, leading to psoriasis symptoms and sleep problems. A Mediterranean-style diet rich in fruits, vegetables, grains, legumes, nuts, and olive oil may help manage symptoms in people with psoriasis. A French study involving nearly 36,000 participants found that greater adherence to a Mediterranean diet was linked to less severe psoriasis symptoms and improved sleep in young adults [77].

DIETARY CONSIDERATION

Anti-Inflammatory Diet

The disorder psoriasis is also immune-mediated. In other words, it triggers inflammation brought on by an overreactive immune system. Therefore, controlling the condition's symptoms may be aided by an anti-inflammatory diet.

Foods from the following categories should typically be a part of an anti-inflammatory diet for psoriasis: Seaweed, salmon and other seafood, nuts and seeds, plant oils, and some fortified foods, like some milk or egg brands, are examples of omega-3 foods. Fruit, vegetables, and whole low-glycaemic grains are examples of high-fiber foods. Vitamins and antioxidants: These can be found in meat, eggs, cheese, beans, mushrooms, and a variety of coloured vegetables.

Olive oil: The main source of protein for the Mediterranean diet is olive oil. Research indicates that the use of olive oil may help reduce inflammation. Olive oil is a monounsaturated fatty acid that has been shown to reduce LDL cholesterol, or the "bad kind" of cholesterol, and the risk of heart disease.

Dietary fiber: One of the items that has the most impact on managing and preventing inflammation is still dietary fibre. A healthy gut flora, cholesterol management, blood sugar regulation, and a healthy weight are further benefits of fibre. Prebiotics, such as fibre, encourage the development of good bacteria in the gastrointestinal microbiome. A balanced gut microbiota is linked to a lower risk of inflammation and chronic illness.

Antioxidants: Antioxidants are compounds that slow down or stop cell deterioration. Phytochemicals and flavonoids, two important elements of an anti-inflammatory diet, are frequently linked to antioxidants. Plant-based diets contain components called phytochemicals and flavonoids that reduce inflammation and combat the damage caused by free radicals. Consuming a diverse range of fresh fruits, veggies, and whole grains is a simple method to guarantee that you are obtaining adequate amounts of flavonoids, phytochemicals, and antioxidants.

Omega-3-fatty acids: Eicosapentaenoic acid [EPA], docosahexaenoic acid [DHA] and Alpha-linolenic acid [ALA] are the three different forms of omega-3 fatty acids. No, the body is unable to produce ALA. Canola oil, flaxseed, soybeans, and chia seeds all contain ALA. Flaxseed and chia seeds can be added to smoothies and muesli to increase the amount of omega-3 fatty acids in your diet.

Foods to avoid: Inflammation in psoriasis can be attributed to various foods, including alcohol, saturated fats, refined grains, and sugars. A survey by the National Psoriasis Foundation found that 13.8% of people with psoriasis reported that sugar worsened their symptoms. Heavy alcohol consumption has been linked to more severe psoriasis, with 13.6% of respondents reporting that alcohol exacerbates their symptoms. Saturated fat and trans fats are two main contributors to inflammation, found in red meat, processed meat, and full-fat dairy products. Trans fats are found in baked goods, fried foods, and some packaged foods. It is important to read nutrition labels and avoid products with hydrogenated oils or high fructose corn syrup. Refined grains and added sugar also contribute to inflammation, causing blood sugar levels to spike, leading to increased insulin production.

Hydration and Supplements

Hydration

Treatment for psoriasis should involve moisturising and emollienting the skin on a regular basis, identifying and avoiding the Koebner phenomenon triggers [excoriation, maceration], and avoiding infection foci [*Streptococcus pyogenes*]. It has been demonstrated that moisturisers greatly enhance psoriasis sufferers' skin problems and quality of life. Given that dry skin is widespread and exacerbates the irritation of skin diseases, they are an invaluable first-line therapy. When emollients, topical corticosteroids, coal tar, anthralin [dithranol], or calcipotriol are used as treatments, the majority of patients show positive results. The most often recommended medications are emollients, which offer momentary irritability alleviation and some anti-inflammatory qualities. Dry skin can affect people such as the physically healthy and is a frequent ailment that has a significant influence on patients' lives. Psoriasis, atopic dermatitis, and ichthyosis patients may find dry skin especially bothersome. Dry skin is also commonly associated with compromised skin barrier function [78]. Emollients are essential for treating various skin conditions, including psoriasis, ichthyoses, xeroderma, and disorders of keratinization, atopic dermatitis, psoriasis, and photodamaged skin. They soften the skin, improve its resistance to further damage, minimize the risk of complications, and allow for more rapid recovery. Water-in-oil emollients are useful in treating chronic plaque-type psoriasis and exert a steroid-sparing effect. They work from the top down, infusing moisture into the skin. Moisturizers are primarily composed of water [65–85%], which functions as a hydrophilic moisturizing ingredient. Once-daily application of both besolvent and hydrophilic moisturizing ingredients is shown to be significantly more effective than components that help restore skin moisture content. Emollient once-daily application of betamethasone dipropionate cream alone contains more oil and less water than other creams. Oil baths with emollients have also been shown to be a useful component of maintenance therapy in dry skin conditions, atopic eczema, psoriasis, and inflammatory dermatitis. When used alone in patients with psoriasis, emollients have a significant impact on many skin disorders. Emollients and hydrating agents have also been shown to inhibit the Koebner response, which can help relieve the clinical development of psoriatic lesions at the site of an injury. In psoriasis, the use of moisturizers containing 10% urea was shown to be effective in the treatment strategy. Moisturizers have an efficient hydrating and lipid-replenishing effect, exerting a steroid-sparing effect in patients with atopic dermatitis on the skin. They are essential to minimize the risk of skin dermatitis and psoriasis.

Supplements

Supplements are a common addition to the diets of many psoriasis sufferers.

Fish oil: It has been claimed that cold water fish oils, which are high in eicosapentaenoic acid [EPA] and docosahexaenoic acid [DHA], and omega-3 polyunsaturated fatty acids, might be used to treat psoriasis. It appears that fish oil has also been researched in conjunction with other treatments. In a double-blind, placebo-controlled research, the use of fish oil with UVB treatment compared to placebo olive oil with UVB produced a statistically significant improvement in psoriasis in 18 individuals with severe stable plaque psoriasis [79]. A study was conducted on thirty patients with mild-to-moderate plaque psoriasis and they were divided into groups based on whether they received Oravex [2.8 g EPA, 0.4 mg DHA] or tacalcitol, a synthetic vitamin D3 analogue, or both. After eight weeks, the PASI score of the Oravex group was significantly higher [$p<0.0001$] than that of the control group [80].When fish oil was combined with oral etretinate instead of etretinate alone, psoriasis showed greater clinical improvement in 40 individuals with chronic persistent plaque psoriasis, according to another research [81].

Vitamin D: There have been reports of psoriasis and vitamin D insufficiency. A single-center open trial by Perez *et al.* assessed the safety and efficacy of oral 1,25-dihydroxyvitamin D3 for psoriasis treatment. The study found that 88% of patients experienced some level of improvement, with a decrease in mean PASI scores. Five additional open-label uncontrolled studies found moderate or greater improvement in psoriasis in at least 50% of subjects. However, the only randomized, placebo-controlled trial reported a slight improvement in psoriatic arthritis. Possible side effects include hypercalcemia, hypercalciuria, kidney stones, and bone demineralization. Some studies reported an increase in blood calcium and vitamin D levels after starting oral supplementation. Kidney stones, hypercalciuria, and hypercalcemia are possible adverse effects of oral vitamin D therapy. Demineralization of the bones can also result from a prolonged excess of vitamin D. After beginning oral supplementation, several studies observed elevated blood levels of calcium and vitamin D or increased calcium in urine, but no patient encountered negative clinical side effects [82].

Selenium: Selenium, an essential element with anti-proliferative and immune regulatory properties, has been linked to increased psoriasis disease severity in patients for over three years. Several trials have assessed the role of selenium supplementation in psoriasis treatment. A double-blind placebo-controlled clinical study found that supplementation with antioxidants showed significant clinical improvement in psoriasis and a decline in oxidative stress. However, a double-blind, parallel group study showed that selenium supplementation plus narrowband UVB was not superior to placebo plus narrowband UVB for psoriasis treatment. Another case-control study found that both groups achieved almost complete remission, but the selenium group had higher PASI score and TNF level. A small prospective study involving seven patients showed that 6 weeks of 400 μg daily selenium increased the number of dermal CD4+ cells but did not result in any clinical improvement [83].

HOLISTIC APPROACHES

Herbal Remedies

Psoriasis is a skin disorder that causes red, itchy, and scaly spots. While there is no cure, herbal medicines may help to reduce symptoms. Before attempting new treatments, it is critical to consult with a healthcare practitioner.

Aloevera

Aloe vera is a thick evergreen satisfying plant that is widely used as a conventional cure to heal multiple diseases, especially skin disorders. This plant's gel is frequently used in cosmetics, medicines, and dietary supplements [84]. Aloe vera extract includes numerous potentially beneficial chemicals, such as, polysaccharides, nutrients, salicylic acid, and numerous antioxidants such as carotenoids and flavonoids. Some of these elements can help to slow the progression of psoriasis by lowering skin irritation and inflammation [85].

Artemisia Capillaris

Artemisia capillaris has traditionally been used as a herbal treatment in East Asia to treat pyrexia and liver diseases. This species contains chlorogenic acids, coumarins, and active flavonoid compounds that may be useful in the treatment of cancer, hepatitis, malaria, obesity, and pathogenic infection [86]. In the case of psoriasis, extract from Artemisia capillaris has the capacity to decrease keratinocyte development and cause death.

Curcumin

Curcumin, a component of turmeric, has been used as a medicine in Southeast Asia for generations. It possesses antioxidant, anti-inflammatory, antibacterial, and cancer-fighting properties [87]. Curcumin has been revealed to be a medical ingredient, and a daily dose of up to 8 g is both secure and not harmful to people

[88]. According to molecular docking studies, curcumin may fight psoriasis by docking at TNF receptor-binding sites, altering or preventing signal transmission, and potentially lowering inflammation caused by this cytokine [89]. Oral curcumin is well tolerated by psoriasis patients in clinical trials, although the low response rate suggests placebo effects or disease reversal. To definitely show or refute its efficacy, large, placebo-controlled trials are required [90].

Feverfew

Tanacetum parthenium is derived from feverfew. The herbs suppress platelet aggregation and 5-hydroxytryptamine release from platelets. It is a member of the Asteraceae family. This plant is used to treat arthritis, psoriasis, allergic reactions, and skin problems [91].

Acupuncture and alternative therapies

Acupuncture, as one of the complementary and alternative nonpharmacological therapies, has long been used in China to treat psoriasis, pruritus, and dermatitis [92]. It presents little risk of side effects and undesirable reactions. According to the review, acupuncture can relieve itching by increasing microcirculation in the local lesion area, which promotes the extinction of inflammation and the absorption of metabolites. Acupuncture can boost the body's immune function, increase meridian function, and cure skin lesions, hence preventing the progression to chronic recurrent seizures, according to the study.

In comparison to conventional drugs, the meta-analysis found that acupuncture may have a potential advantage in the treatment of psychosocial abnormalities such as anxiety and depression [93]. It is also linked to a lower recurrence rate of psoriasis. However, the effects of acupuncture in the treatment of psoriasis are still inconclusive, particularly in the treatment of psychosocial abnormalities caused by psoriasis. The majority of the findings come from observational studies or case reports [94]. The methodological quality of published Randomised Controlled Trials [RCT] is weak, particularly in blinding. As a result, we devised a randomised controlled trial with a placebo control to assess the effects of acupuncture for psoriasis on typical clinical symptoms and psychosocial abnormalities [95].

Essential oil

Essential Oils [EOs] are naturally obtained and synthesised from diverse plant components such as flowers, buds, stems, twigs, fruits, seeds, roots, barks, and leaves [96]. They are volatile, aromatic oily liquids that are widely utilised around the world in pharmaceutical, food, and cosmetic sectors, as well as for their therapeutic purposes as antibacterial, antifungal, anticarcinogenic, antimutagenic, antioxidant, anti-inflammatory, and antiviral agents [97]. The effect of essential oil on Psoriasis treatment is well explained by Table **2**.

Table 2. Effect of essential oil on psoriasis treatment.

S. No.	Sources of Essential Oil	uses	References
1	Sandalwood	Anti-aging properties, Antioxidant-rich and beneficial to dry skin It helps with tanning, dry skin, and chapped skin. Anti-inflammatory and anti-microbial properties	[98]
2	Rose	Unclogs pores on the skin, smoothes fine wrinkles, promotes radiant skin, and deeply conditions the strands. Helps with depression and eczema.	[27]
3	Tea tree	Reduces acne, scrubs the skin, fights dandruff, and hydrates dry hair.	[28]
4	Jasmine	It has an antispasmodic and seductive fragrance. Overcome melancholy, cold temperatures, and allergies	[29]
5	Orange	Fighting pimples, improves bright skin, builds up hair roots, and avoids constipation and poor digestion.	[30]
6	peppermint	Sunburn medication, production of collagen stimulation, and dermatitis treatment	[99]

MIND-BODY CONNECTION

Mental Health and Psoriasis

Depression prevalence estimates range from 9 to 55% of patients with psoriasis, depending on the screening method utilised [31]. One meta-analysis and systematic review assessed clinical depression rates at 28% when using surveys, 12% when using International Classification of Diseases codes, 19% when using the Diagnostic and Statistical Manual of Mental Disorders IV, and 9% when using antidepressants [32]. In this study, psoriasis patients had significantly more depressive symptoms [standardised mean differences 1.16; 95% confidence interval [CI] 0.67-1.66], and population-based studies showed that they were at least 1.5 times more likely to experience depression [odds ratio [OR] 1.57; 95% CI 1.40-1.76] and used more antidepressant medication than controls [OR 4.24, 95% CI 1.53-11.76].

Furthermore, in a study of 607 psoriasis patients, 9.9% [95% CI: 7.5-12.3%] tested positive for MDD utilising the PHQ-9 [33], 42% had severe symptoms, and 25% fulfilled the threshold for immediate mental health specialist referral.

Surprisingly, 71% of the patients in the cohort were diagnosed with severe depression for the first time. 39% of MDD patients had a Dermatology Life Quality Index [DLQI] score of 10, indicating a low to medium impact of psoriasis on quality of life. As a result, employing the DLQI alone may miss key depressive symptoms found by the PHQ-9 [34].

Mindfulness Techniques

Mindfulness methods, which promote relaxation, reduce stress, and improve general well-being, can help with the management of psoriasis, a chronic skin condition that worsens with stress.

Meditation

Particularly helpful is mindfulness meditation, which emphasizes paying attention to your physical, mental, and emotional experiences in the present moment without passing judgment. According to a review that appeared in the Journal of Integrative and Complementary Medicine in January 2022, young adults' depression was somewhat alleviated by mindfulness meditation [35]. Additionally, a meta-analysis that was published in the Journal of Affective Disorders in January 2021 indicated that mindfulness meditation applications had the potential to enhance mental health and well-being [100].

According to additional studies, people with chronic diseases can find relief from stress and physical problems by practicing meditation. Similarly, meditation was found to be a good way to lower cortisol levels in individuals who were at risk of having elevated amounts of this stress hormone, according to a 2021 study published in Health Psychology Review [101].

Cognitive Behavioral Therapy

In cognitive behavioural therapy, or CBT, patients work with a qualified therapist to examine the relationships between your thoughts, feelings, and behaviours. The purpose of cognitive behavioural therapy [CBT] is to identify harmful thought patterns that contribute to stress and provide techniques for altering them [102]. According to the American Psychological Association, CBT, which gained popularity in the 1970s, has been shown to be successful in treating a variety of mood disorders and in lowering anxiety and depression [103]. Additionally, a September 2020 study published in the Journal of Dermatological Treatment indicated that it not only helps people with chronic illnesses like psoriasis feel better about themselves, but it also helps reduce stress [2].

Aromatherapy

Aromatherapy is a Complementary and Alternative Medicine [CAM] modality that uses plant-derived essential oils to promote relaxation, heal, and enhance general health [36]. The aromas can be added to bathwater to improve a soak in the tub, applied by mixing them with massage oil, or diffused into the air. In spite of how a smell is absorbed, it is believed to function by chemically communicating with the brain's mood and emotion centres. There is a good deal of evidence that it functions well in a variety of settings. For instance, a review indicated that several smells reduced anxiety during pregnancy and labour, which was published in April 2021 in Clinical Obstetrics & Gynaecology. Lavender, petitgrain [bitter orange], and bergamot were particularly potent [104].

Hence, it seems sensible that these same oils could help anyone who is stressed out, even psoriasis sufferers. To be safe, consult your physician before using any oil in this manner, or simply use smelling as a stress-relieving method [37].

PRACTICAL DAILY LIVING TIPS

Choosing Psoriasis-Friendly Products

Choosing items that are suitable for psoriasis is essential for controlling symptoms and averting flare-ups, which are typified by red, scaly, and itchy skin areas.Products with a lot of aroma should be avoided since they might aggravate sensitive skin and cause flare-ups of psoriasis. The hypoallergenic or fragrance-free alternatives instead [2].

Soap-free or moisturizing cleansers that are gentle on the skin, and use mild, fragrance-free cleansers that don't strip the skin of its natural oils, are recommended. It is advised to use hypoallergenic, fragrance-free moisturizers, staying away from harsh chemicals [105], use dye-free hair care products, wear loose-fitting, breathable clothing made of natural fibres like cotton, and protect your skin from sunburn by using broad-spectrum, SPF-30 sunscreen. Before applying new products, especially on sensitive skin, do a patch test on a small area of skin [106]. For individualised guidance on the best products to use depending on your skin type and the severity of your psoriasis, speak with a dermatologist. Product reactions might differ from person to person, therefore, testing new things is vital [107].

Clothing and Sun Protection

When you're trying to control the symptoms of your psoriasis and avoid flare-ups, wear loose, comfy clothes made of natural materials like cotton. Put on long sleeves and trousers to be extra safe. Wearing clothing with a high UPF rating can shield you from the sun. Put on sunglasses and wide-brimmed hats to protect your face and scalp from the sun.

To keep the body cooler, wear light colours and stay away from tight elastic bands. Use a high-SPF broad-spectrum sunscreen and reapply it every two hours. To minimise direct exposure, seek shade, especially during the hottest parts of the day [38]. For individualised guidance on sun protection and wardrobe selections, speak with a dermatologist. Effective psoriasis management requires finding a balance between sun protection and limited sunlight exposure [108].

CONCLUSION

Psoriasis management in the modern world involves lifestyle, nutrition, holistic techniques, and traditional medical therapies. This chronic autoimmune condition's rising incidence emphasizes how stress, the environment, and unhealthy eating habits can affect skin health. People can improve their general health and symptom control by implementing holistic therapies like Ayurveda and Traditional Chinese Medicine, increasing physical exercise and mindfulness to manage stress, and implementing anti-inflammatory diets. The best outcomes for psoriasis management come from a customized, integrative strategy that combines medication with lifestyle changes. A move toward natural and preventive methods is even more crucial as studies reveal the complex relationships among immunity, gastrointestinal health, and skin inflammation. Ultimately, in today's hectic, stress-filled world, equipping people with information and useful tools can help them manage their psoriasis and lead healthier lives.

REFERNCES

[1] Armstrong AW, Read C. Pathophysiology, clinical presentation, and treatment of psoriasis. JAMA 2020; 323(19): 1945-60.
[http://dx.doi.org/10.1001/jama.2020.4006] [PMID: 32427307]

[2] Rendon A, Schäkel K. Psoriasis pathogenesis and treatment. Int J Mol Sci 2019; 20(6): 1475.
[http://dx.doi.org/10.3390/ijms20061475] [PMID: 30909615]

[3] Kamiya K, Kishimoto M, Sugai J, Komine M, Ohtsuki M. Risk factors for the development of psoriasis. Int J Mol Sci 2019; 20(18): 4347.
[http://dx.doi.org/10.3390/ijms20184347] [PMID: 31491865]

[4] Virmani T, Gupta J. Pharmaceutical application of microspheres: an approach for the treatment of various diseases. Int J Pharm Sci Res 2017; 8(8): 3253-60.

[5] Michalek IM, Loring B, John SM. A systematic review of worldwide epidemiology of psoriasis. J Eur Acad Dermatol Venereol 2017; 31(2): 205-12.
[http://dx.doi.org/10.1111/jdv.13854] [PMID: 27573025]

[6] Sanduja M, Gupta J, Virmani T. Recent advancements in Uracil and 5-Fluorouracil hybrids as potential anticancer agents: A review. J Appl Pharm Sci 2020; 10(2): 129-46.
[http://dx.doi.org/10.7324/JAPS.2020.102019]

[7] Sharma A, Virmani T, Pathak V, *et al.* Artificial intelligence-based data-driven strategy to accelerate research, development, and clinical trials of COVID vaccine. BioMed Res Int 2022; 2022(1): 7205241.
[http://dx.doi.org/10.1155/2022/7205241] [PMID: 35845955]

[8] Smith CH, Barker JNWN. Psoriasis and its management. BMJ 2006; 333(7564): 380-4.
[http://dx.doi.org/10.1136/bmj.333.7564.380] [PMID: 16916825]

[9] Grover M, Behl T, Sehgal A, *et al. In vitro* phytochemical screening, cytotoxicity studies of *Curcuma longa* extracts with isolation and characterisation of their isolated compounds. Molecules 2021; 26(24): 7509.
[http://dx.doi.org/10.3390/molecules26247509] [PMID: 34946592]

[10] Gudjonsson JE, Elder JT. Psoriasis: epidemiology. Clin Dermatol 2007; 25(6): 535-46.
[http://dx.doi.org/10.1016/j.clindermatol.2007.08.007] [PMID: 18021890]

[11] Menter A, Griffiths CEM. Current and future management of psoriasis. Lancet 2007; 370(9583): 272-84.
[http://dx.doi.org/10.1016/S0140-6736(07)61129-5] [PMID: 17658398]

[12] Sharma A, Tiwari RK, Kaushik A, Tyagi LK, Shankar K, Virmani T, *et al.* Standardisation of *Carissa carandas* Linn: A drug used in Indian system of medicine as per WHO Guidelines. Cont J Pharm Sci 2007; 1(1): 9-14.

[13] Greaves MW, Weinstein GD. Treatment of psoriasis. N Engl J Med 1995; 332(9): 581-9.
[http://dx.doi.org/10.1056/NEJM199503023320907] [PMID: 7838193]

[14] Lowes MA, Suárez-Fariñas M, Krueger JG. Immunology of psoriasis. Annu Rev Immunol 2014; 32(1): 227-55.
[http://dx.doi.org/10.1146/annurev-immunol-032713-120225] [PMID: 24655295]

[15] Virmani T, Kumar G, Virmani R, Sharma A, Pathak K. Nanocarrier-based approaches to combat chronic obstructive pulmonary disease. Nanomedicine (Lond) 2022; 17(24): 1833-54.
[http://dx.doi.org/10.2217/nnm-2021-0403] [PMID: 35856251]

[16] Nevitt GJ, Hutchinson PE. Psoriasis in the community: prevalence, severity and patients' beliefs and attitudes towards the disease. Br J Dermatol 1996; 135(4): 533-7.
[http://dx.doi.org/10.1046/j.1365-2133.1996.d01-1035.x] [PMID: 8915141]

[17] Johnson MT, Roberts J. Skin conditions and related need for medical care among persons 1-74 years. United States, 1971-1974. Vital Health Stat 11 1978; (212): i-v, 1-72.
[PMID: 741665]

[18] Gelfand JM, Stern RS, Nijsten T, *et al.* The prevalence of psoriasis in African Americans: Results from a population-based study. J Am Acad Dermatol 2005; 52(1): 23-6.
[http://dx.doi.org/10.1016/j.jaad.2004.07.045] [PMID: 15627076]

[19] Gladman DD. Natural history of psoriatic arthritis. Baillieres Clin Rheumatol 1994; 8(2): 379-94.
[http://dx.doi.org/10.1016/S0950-3579(94)80024-3] [PMID: 8076393]

[20] Williams R, Chen YF, Endres R, *et al.* Molecular variation at the HLA-A, B, C, DRB1, DQA1, and DQB1 loci in full heritage American Indians in Arizona: private haplotypes and their evolution. Tissue Antigens 2009; 74(6): 520-33.
[http://dx.doi.org/10.1111/j.1399-0039.2009.01381.x] [PMID: 19845915]

[21] Virmani R, Virmani T, Singh C, Sorout G, Gupta J. Hidden potential of natural herb *Carissa carandas* (Karonda). Res Pharm Health Sci 2017; 3: 294-302.

[22] Shbeeb M, Uramoto KM, Gibson LE, O'Fallon WM, Gabriel SE. The epidemiology of psoriatic arthritis in Olmsted County, Minnesota, USA, 1982-1991. J Rheumatol 2000; 27(5): 1247-50.
[PMID: 10813295]

[23] Kumar G, Virmani T, Pathak K, Alhalmi A. A revolutionary blueprint for mitigation of hypertension

via nanoemulsion. BioMed Res Int 2022; 2022(1): 4109874.
[http://dx.doi.org/10.1155/2022/4109874] [PMID: 35463984]

[24] Grover M, Behl T, Virmani T, Bhatia S, Al-Harrasi A, Aleya L. Chrysopogon zizanioides—a review on its pharmacognosy, chemical composition and pharmacological activities. Environ Sci Pollut Res Int 2021; 28(33): 44667-92.
[http://dx.doi.org/10.1007/s11356-021-15145-1] [PMID: 34215988]

[25] Kumar G, Virmani T, Pathak K, Kamaly OA, Saleh A. Central composite design implemented azilsartan medoxomil loaded nanoemulsion to improve its aqueous solubility and intestinal permeability: *In vitro* and *ex vivo* evaluation. Pharmaceuticals (Basel) 2022; 15(11): 1343.
[http://dx.doi.org/10.3390/ph15111343] [PMID: 36355515]

[26] Grover M, Behl T, Virmani T, *et al.* Exploration of cytotoxic potential of longifolene/junipene isolated from *Chrysopogon zizanioides.* Molecules 2022; 27(18): 5764.
[http://dx.doi.org/10.3390/molecules27185764] [PMID: 36144491]

[27] Dawid-Pać R. Medicinal plants used in treatment of inflammatory skin diseases. Postepy Dermatol Alergol 2013; 3(3): 170-7.
[http://dx.doi.org/10.5114/pdia.2013.35620] [PMID: 24278070]

[28] Carson CF, Hammer KA, Riley TV. Melaleuca alternifolia (Tea Tree) oil: a review of antimicrobial and other medicinal properties. Clin Microbiol Rev 2006; 19(1): 50-62.
[http://dx.doi.org/10.1128/CMR.19.1.50-62.2006] [PMID: 16418522]

[29] Rath CC, Devi S, Dash SK, Mishra RK. Antibacterial potential assessment of jasmine essential oil against <i> E. coli</i>. Indian J Pharm Sci 2008; 70(2): 238-41.
[http://dx.doi.org/10.4103/0250-474X.41465] [PMID: 20046722]

[30] Ould Yerou K, Ibri K, Bouhadi D, Hariri A, Meddah B, Tir Touil A. The use of orange (<i>Citrus sinensis</i>) peel as antimicrobial and anti-oxidant agents. Rev Sci Fondam Appl 2017; 9(3): 1351.
[http://dx.doi.org/10.4314/jfas.v9i3.7]

[31] Dommasch ED, Li T, Okereke OI, Li Y, Qureshi AA, Cho E. Risk of depression in women with psoriasis: a cohort study. Br J Dermatol 2015; 173(4): 975-80.
[http://dx.doi.org/10.1111/bjd.14032] [PMID: 26186277]

[32] Dowlatshahi EA, Wakkee M, Arends LR, Nijsten T. The prevalence and odds of depressive symptoms and clinical depression in psoriasis patients: a systematic review and meta-analysis. J Invest Dermatol 2014; 134(6): 1542-51.
[http://dx.doi.org/10.1038/jid.2013.508] [PMID: 24284419]

[33] Lamb RC, Matcham F, Turner MA, *et al.* Screening for anxiety and depression in people with psoriasis: a cross-sectional study in a tertiary referral setting. Br J Dermatol 2017; 176(4): 1028-34.
[http://dx.doi.org/10.1111/bjd.14833] [PMID: 27363600]

[34] Kleyn CE, Talbot PS, Mehta NN, Sampogna F, Bundy C, Ashcroft DM, *et al.* Psoriasis and mental health workshop report: Exploring the links between psychosocial factors, psoriasis, neuroinflammation and cardiovascular disease risk. Acta Derm Venereol. 2020 Jan 7; 100(1): 5639.

[35] Jiménez-Picón N, Romero-Martín M, Ponce-Blandón JA, Ramirez-Baena L, Palomo-Lara JC, Gómez-Salgado J. The relationship between mindfulness and emotional intelligence as a protective factor for healthcare professionals: Systematic review. Int J Environ Res Public Health 2021; 18(10): 5491.
[http://dx.doi.org/10.3390/ijerph18105491] [PMID: 34065519]

[36] Hedigan F, Sheridan H, Sasse A. Benefit of inhalation aromatherapy as a complementary treatment for stress and anxiety in a clinical setting – A systematic review. Complement Ther Clin Pract 2023; 52: 101750.
[http://dx.doi.org/10.1016/j.ctcp.2023.101750] [PMID: 37031643]

[37] Burns J. Common herbs for stress: The science and strategy of a botanical medicine approach to self-care. J Interprof Educ Pract 2023; 30: 100592.

[http://dx.doi.org/10.1016/j.xjep.2022.100592] [PMID: 36530213]

[38] Schalka S, Steiner D, Ravelli FN, *et al.* Brazilian consensus on photoprotection. An Bras Dermatol 2014; 89(6 suppl 1) (Suppl. 1): 1-74. [http://dx.doi.org/10.1590/abd1806-4841.20143971] [PMID: 25761256]

[39] Virmani T, Parvez N, Yadav S, Pathak K. Solid inclusion complexes of class II imidazole derivative with β–cyclodextrin. Continental Journal of Pharmaceutical Sciences 2007; 1: 1-8.

[40] Kumar G, Virmani T, Sharma A, Pathak K. Codelivery of phytochemicals with conventional anticancer drugs in form of nanocarriers. Pharmaceutics 2023; 15(3): 889. [http://dx.doi.org/10.3390/pharmaceutics15030889] [PMID: 36986748]

[41] Gupta V, Virmani T, Singh V. A Comparative diagnostic account of the roots of Boerhavia diffusa Linn. From four different geographical regions in India. Journal of Community Pharmacy Practice (JCPP) 2799-1199. 2022; 2(03): 1–6.

[42] Zill JM, Dirmaier J, Augustin M, *et al.* Psychosocial distress of patients with psoriasis: Protocol for an assessment of care needs and the development of a supportive intervention. JMIR Res Protoc 2018; 7(2): e22. [http://dx.doi.org/10.2196/resprot.8490] [PMID: 29415875]

[43] Singh LK, Pang X, Alexacos N, Letourneau R, Theoharides TC. Acute immobilization stress triggers skin mast cell degranulation *via* corticotropin releasing hormone, neurotensin, and substance P: A link to neurogenic skin disorders. Brain Behav Immun 1999; 13(3): 225-39. [http://dx.doi.org/10.1006/brbi.1998.0541] [PMID: 10469524]

[44] Kane MO, Murphy EP, Kirby B. The role of corticotropin-releasing hormone in immune-mediated cutaneous inflammatory disease. Exp Dermatol 2006; 15(3): 143-53. [http://dx.doi.org/10.1111/j.1600-0625.2006.00382.x] [PMID: 16480421]

[45] Harvima IT, Nilsson G, Suttle MM, Naukkarinen A. Is there a role for mast cells in psoriasis? Arch Dermatol Res 2008; 300(9): 461-78. [http://dx.doi.org/10.1007/s00403-008-0874-x] [PMID: 18719932]

[46] Farber EM, Nickoloff BJ, Recht B, Fraki JE. Stress, symmetry, and psoriasis: Possible role of neuropeptides. J Am Acad Dermatol 1986; 14(2): 305-11. [http://dx.doi.org/10.1016/S0190-9622(86)70034-0] [PMID: 2419375]

[47] Friedman B, Cronstein B. Methotrexate mechanism in treatment of rheumatoid arthritis. Joint Bone Spine 2019; 86(3): 301-7. [http://dx.doi.org/10.1016/j.jbspin.2018.07.004] [PMID: 30081197]

[48] Whitehouse G, Gray E, Mastoridis S, *et al.* IL-2 therapy restores regulatory T-cell dysfunction induced by calcineurin inhibitors. Proc Natl Acad Sci USA 2017; 114(27): 7083-8. [http://dx.doi.org/10.1073/pnas.1620835114] [PMID: 28584086]

[49] Törmä H. Regulation of keratin expression by retinoids. Dermatoendocrinol 2011; 3(3): 136-40. [http://dx.doi.org/10.4161/derm.15026] [PMID: 22110773]

[50] Sciacovelli M, Gonçalves E, Johnson TI, *et al.* Fumarate is an epigenetic modifier that elicits epithelial-to-mesenchymal transition. Nature 2016; 537(7621): 544-7. [http://dx.doi.org/10.1038/nature19353] [PMID: 27580029]

[51] Li H, Zuo J, Tang W. Phosphodiesterase-4 inhibitors for the treatment of inflammatory diseases. Front Pharmacol 2018; 9: 1048. [http://dx.doi.org/10.3389/fphar.2018.01048] [PMID: 30386231]

[52] Jeon C, Sekhon S, Yan D, Afifi L, Nakamura M, Bhutani T. Monoclonal antibodies inhibiting IL-12, -23, and -17 for the treatment of psoriasis. Hum Vaccin Immunother 2017; 13(10): 2247-59. [http://dx.doi.org/10.1080/21645515.2017.1356498] [PMID: 28825875]

[53] Jang D, Lee AH, Shin HY, *et al.* The role of tumor necrosis factor alpha (TNF-α) in autoimmune

disease and current TNF-α inhibitors in therapeutics. Int J Mol Sci 2021; 22(5): 2719. [http://dx.doi.org/10.3390/ijms22052719] [PMID: 33800290]

[54] Bauer S, Adrian N, Williamson B, *et al.* Targeted bioactivity of membrane-anchored TNF by an antibody-derived TNF fusion protein. J Immunol 2004; 172(6): 3930-9. [http://dx.doi.org/10.4049/jimmunol.172.6.3930] [PMID: 15004201]

[55] Goel N, Stephens S. Certolizumab Pegol. MAbs 2010; 2(2): 137-47. [http://dx.doi.org/10.4161/mabs.2.2.11271] [PMID: 20190560]

[56] Godse K. Secukinumab – first in class interleukin-17A inhibitor for the treatment of psoriasis. Indian J Dermatol 2017; 62(2): 195-9. [http://dx.doi.org/10.4103/ijd.IJD_233_16] [PMID: 28400641]

[57] Blair HA. Risankizumab: A review in moderate to severe plaque psoriasis. Drugs 2020; 80(12): 1235-45. [http://dx.doi.org/10.1007/s40265-020-01357-1] [PMID: 32632826]

[58] Garakani A, Murrough JW, Freire RC, *et al.* Pharmacotherapy of anxiety disorders: Current and emerging treatment options. Front Psychiatry 2020; 11: 595584. [http://dx.doi.org/10.3389/fpsyt.2020.595584] [PMID: 33424664]

[59] Schlager JG, Rosumeck S, Werner RN, *et al.* Topical treatments for scalp psoriasis. Cochrane Database Syst Rev 2016; 2(2): CD009687. [PMID: 26915340]

[60] Singh S, Virmani T, Kohli K. Phytochemicals and medicinal uses of red raspberry -. Review 2020; 5: 48-52.

[61] Bozzo P, Chua-Gocheco A, Einarson A. Safety of skin care products during pregnancy. Can Fam Physician 2011; 57(6): 665-7. [PMID: 21673209]

[62] George E, Baranwal N, Kang J, Qureshi A, Drucker A, Cho E. Photosensitizing medications and skin cancer: A comprehensive review. Cancers (Basel) 2021; 13(10): 2344. [http://dx.doi.org/10.3390/cancers13102344] [PMID: 34066301]

[63] Parisi R, Symmons DPM, Griffiths CEM, Ashcroft DM. Global epidemiology of psoriasis: a systematic review of incidence and prevalence. J Invest Dermatol 2013; 133(2): 377-85. [http://dx.doi.org/10.1038/jid.2012.339] [PMID: 23014338]

[64] Kimball AB, Jacobson C, Weiss S, Vreeland MG, Wu Y. The psychosocial burden of psoriasis. Am J Clin Dermatol 2005; 6(6): 383-92. [http://dx.doi.org/10.2165/00128071-200506060-00005] [PMID: 16343026]

[65] Hunter HJA, Griffiths CEM, Kleyn CE. Does psychosocial stress play a role in the exacerbation of psoriasis? Br J Dermatol 2013; 169(5): 965-74. [http://dx.doi.org/10.1111/bjd.12478] [PMID: 23796214]

[66] Al'Abadie MS, Kent GG, Gawkrodger DJ. The relationship between stress and the onset and exacerbation of psoriasis and other skin conditions. Br J Dermatol 1994; 130(2): 199-203. [http://dx.doi.org/10.1111/j.1365-2133.1994.tb02900.x] [PMID: 8123572]

[67] Gupta MA, Gupta AK. The Psoriasis Life Stress Inventory: a preliminary index of psoriasis-related stress. Acta Derm Venereol 1995; 75(3): 240-3. [http://dx.doi.org/10.2340/0001555575240243] [PMID: 7653188]

[68] Delévaux I, Chamoux A, Aumaître O. Stress et auto-immunité. Rev Med Interne 2013; 34(8): 487-92. [http://dx.doi.org/10.1016/j.revmed.2012.10.366] [PMID: 23182292]

[69] Saint-Mezard P, Chavagnac C, Bosset S, *et al.* Psychological stress exerts an adjuvant effect on skin dendritic cell functions *in vivo*. J Immunol 2003; 171(8): 4073-80. [http://dx.doi.org/10.4049/jimmunol.171.8.4073] [PMID: 14530328]

[70] Evers AWM, Verhoeven EWM, Kraaimaat FW, *et al.* How stress gets under the skin: cortisol and stress reactivity in psoriasis. Br J Dermatol 2010; 163(5): 986-91. [http://dx.doi.org/10.1111/j.1365-2133.2010.09984.x] [PMID: 20716227]

[71] Cemil BÇ, Canpolat F, Yılmazer D, Eskioğlu F, Alper M. The association of PASI scores with CRH-R1 expression in patients with psoriasis. Arch Dermatol Res 2012; 304(2): 127-32. [http://dx.doi.org/10.1007/s00403-012-1218-4] [PMID: 22350180]

[72] García-Bueno B, Caso JR, Leza JC. Stress as a neuroinflammatory condition in brain: Damaging and protective mechanisms. Neurosci Biobehav Rev 2008; 32(6): 1136-51. [http://dx.doi.org/10.1016/j.neubiorev.2008.04.001] [PMID: 18468686]

[73] Duchnik E, Kruk J, Tuchowska A, Marchlewicz M. The impact of diet and physical activity on psoriasis: A narrative review of the current evidence. Nutrients 2023; 15(4): 840. [http://dx.doi.org/10.3390/nu15040840] [PMID: 36839198]

[74] Yeroushalmi S, Hakimi M, Chung M, Bartholomew E, Bhutani T, Liao W. Psoriasis and Exercise: A Review. Psoriasis (Auckl). 2022 Jul 2;12:189-197. [http://dx.doi.org/10.2147/PTT.S349791] [PMID: 35813078] [PMCID: PMC9258800]

[75] Demirel R, Genc A, Ucok K, *et al.* Do patients with mild to moderate psoriasis really have a sedentary lifestyle? Int J Dermatol 2013; 52(9): 1129-34. [http://dx.doi.org/10.1111/ijd.12042] [PMID: 23879519]

[76] CHELLI C, MISERY L, TAIEB J, TAIEB C. Sleep disorders and psoriasis: An update. Acta Derm Venereol 2022; 102: 1991.

[77] Gupta MA, Simpson FC, Gupta AK. Psoriasis and sleep disorders: A systematic review. Sleep Med Rev 2016; 29: 63-75. [http://dx.doi.org/10.1016/j.smrv.2015.09.003] [PMID: 26624228]

[78] Lodén M. Role of topical emollients and moisturizers in the treatment of dry skin barrier disorders. Am J Clin Dermatol 2003; 4(11): 771-88. [http://dx.doi.org/10.2165/00128071-200304110-00005] [PMID: 14572299]

[79] Gupta AK, Ellis CN, Tellner DC, Anderson TF, Voorhees JJ. Double-blind, placebo-controlled study to evaluate the efficacy of fish oil and low-dose UVB in the treatment of psoriasis. Br J Dermatol 1989; 120(6): 801-7. [http://dx.doi.org/10.1111/j.1365-2133.1989.tb01378.x] [PMID: 2667615]

[80] Márquez-Balbás G, Sánchez-Regaña M, Millet U. Study on the use of omega-3 fatty acids as a therapeutic supplement in treatment of psoriasis. Clin Cosmet Investig Dermatol 2011; 4: 73-7. [http://dx.doi.org/10.2147/CCID.S17220] [PMID: 21760742]

[81] Danno K, Sugie N. Combination therapy with low-dose etretinate and eicosapentaenoic acid for psoriasis vulgaris. J Dermatol 1998; 25(11): 703-5. [http://dx.doi.org/10.1111/j.1346-8138.1998.tb02487.x] [PMID: 9863281]

[82] Huckins D, Felson DT, Holick M. Treatment of psoriatic arthritis with oral 1,25-dihydroxyvitamin D_3 : a pilot study. Arthritis Rheum 1990; 33(11): 1723-7. [http://dx.doi.org/10.1002/art.1780331117] [PMID: 2242069]

[83] Harvima RJ, Jägerroos H, Kajander EO, *et al.* Screening of effects of selenomethionine/enriched yeast supplementation on various immunological and chemical parameters of skin and blood in psoriatic patients. Acta Derm Venereol 1993; 73(2): 88-91. [http://dx.doi.org/10.2340/000155557388891] [PMID: 8103273]

[84] Sánchez M, González-Burgos E, Iglesias I, Gómez-Serranillos MP. Pharmacological Update Properties of *Aloe Vera* and its Major Active Constituents. Molecules 2020; 25(6): 1324. [http://dx.doi.org/10.3390/molecules25061324] [PMID: 32183224]

[85] Radha MH, Laxmipriya NP. Evaluation of biological properties and clinical effectiveness of *Aloe*

vera: A systematic review. J Tradit Complement Med 2015; 5(1): 21-6.
[http://dx.doi.org/10.1016/j.jtcme.2014.10.006] [PMID: 26151005]

[86] Ha H, Lee H, Seo CS, *et al.* Artemisia capillaris inhibits atopic dermatitis-like skin lesions in Dermatophagoides farinae-sensitized Nc/Nga mice. BMC Complement Altern Med 2014; 14(1): 100.
[http://dx.doi.org/10.1186/1472-6882-14-100] [PMID: 24624888]

[87] Prasad S, Gupta SC, Tyagi AK, Aggarwal BB. Curcumin, a component of golden spice: From bedside to bench and back. Biotechnol Adv 2014; 32(6): 1053-64.
[http://dx.doi.org/10.1016/j.biotechadv.2014.04.004] [PMID: 24793420]

[88] Kanai M, Yoshimura K, Asada M, *et al.* A phase I/II study of gemcitabine-based chemotherapy plus curcumin for patients with gemcitabine-resistant pancreatic cancer. Cancer Chemother Pharmacol 2011; 68(1): 157-64.
[http://dx.doi.org/10.1007/s00280-010-1470-2] [PMID: 20859741]

[89] Saeed MEM, Yücer R, Dawood M, *et al.* *In silico* and *in vitro* screening of 50 curcumin compounds as EGFR and NF-κB inhibitors. Int J Mol Sci 2022; 23(7): 3966.
[http://dx.doi.org/10.3390/ijms23073966] [PMID: 35409325]

[90] Kurd SK, Smith N, VanVoorhees A, *et al.* Oral curcumin in the treatment of moderate to severe psoriasis vulgaris: A prospective clinical trial. J Am Acad Dermatol 2008; 58(4): 625-31.
[http://dx.doi.org/10.1016/j.jaad.2007.12.035] [PMID: 18249471]

[91] Sondhi S, Singh N, Jindal S. Natural remedies used in the treatment of psoriasis: A short review. Asian Journal of Pharmaceutical Research 2021; 11(1): 43-5.
[http://dx.doi.org/10.5958/2231-5691.2021.00009.5]

[92] Yu C, Zhang P, Lv ZT, *et al.* Efficacy of acupuncture in itch: A systematic review and meta-analysis of clinical randomized controlled trials. Evid Based Complement Alternat Med 2015; 2015: 1-5.
[http://dx.doi.org/10.1155/2015/208690] [PMID: 26064156]

[93] Armour M, Smith C, Wang LQ, *et al.* Acupuncture for depression: A systematic review and meta-analysis. J Clin Med 2019; 8(8): 1140.
[http://dx.doi.org/10.3390/jcm8081140] [PMID: 31370200]

[94] Garbicz J, Całyniuk B, Górski M, *et al.* Nutritional therapy in persons suffering from psoriasis. Nutrients 2021; 14(1): 119.
[http://dx.doi.org/10.3390/nu14010119] [PMID: 35010995]

[95] Jing M, Shi L, Zhang Y, *et al.* Efficacy and safety of acupuncture therapy for psoriasis: an overview of systematic reviews. Ann Palliat Med 2021; 10(10): 10804-20.
[http://dx.doi.org/10.21037/apm-21-2523] [PMID: 34763442]

[96] Manion CR, Widder RM. Essentials of essential oils. Am J Health Syst Pharm 2017; 74(9): e153-62.
[http://dx.doi.org/10.2146/ajhp151043] [PMID: 28438819]

[97] Sharmeen J, Mahomoodally F, Zengin G, Maggi F. Essential oils as natural sources of fragrance compounds for cosmetics and cosmeceuticals. Molecules 2021; 26(3): 666.
[http://dx.doi.org/10.3390/molecules26030666] [PMID: 33514008]

[98] Michalak M. Plant-derived antioxidants: Significance in skin health and the ageing process. Int J Mol Sci 2022; 23(2): 585.
[http://dx.doi.org/10.3390/ijms23020585] [PMID: 35054770]

[99] Chumpitazi BP, Kearns GL, Shulman RJ. Review article: the physiological effects and safety of peppermint oil and its efficacy in irritable bowel syndrome and other functional disorders. Aliment Pharmacol Ther 2018; 47(6): 738-52.
[http://dx.doi.org/10.1111/apt.14519] [PMID: 29372567]

[100] Gál É, Ştefan S, Cristea IA. The efficacy of mindfulness meditation apps in enhancing users' well-being and mental health related outcomes: a meta-analysis of randomized controlled trials. J Affect Disord 2021; 279: 131-42.

[http://dx.doi.org/10.1016/j.jad.2020.09.134] [PMID: 33049431]

[101] Turakitwanakan W, Mekseepralard C, Busarakumtragul P. Effects of mindfulness meditation on serum cortisol of medical students. J Med Assoc Thai 2013; 96 (Suppl. 1): S90-5. [PMID: 23724462]

[102] Nakao M, Shirotsuki K, Sugaya N. Cognitive–behavioral therapy for management of mental health and stress-related disorders: Recent advances in techniques and technologies. Biopsychosoc Med 2021; 15(1): 16. [http://dx.doi.org/10.1186/s13030-021-00219-w] [PMID: 34602086]

[103] Hofmann SG, Asnaani A, Vonk IJJ, Sawyer AT, Fang A. The efficacy of cognitive behavioral therapy: A review of meta-analyses. Cognit Ther Res 2012; 36(5): 427-40. [http://dx.doi.org/10.1007/s10608-012-9476-1] [PMID: 23459093]

[104] Bertone A, Dekker R. Aromatherapy in Obstetrics: A Critical Review of the Literature. Clinical Obstetrics & Gynecology. 2021 Apr 29;Publish Ahead of Print. [http://dx.doi.org/10.1097/GRF.0000000000000622]

[105] Mijaljica D, Spada F, Harrison IP. Skin Cleansing without or with Compromise: Soaps and Syndets. Molecules 2022; 27(6): 2010. [http://dx.doi.org/10.3390/molecules27062010] [PMID: 35335373]

[106] Xie W, Pakdel E, Liu D, Sun L, Wang X. Waste hair-derived natural melanin/TiO2 hybrids as highly efficient and stable UV-shielding fillers for polyurethane films. ACS Sustain Chem& Eng 2019; 8.

[107] Kim WB, Jerome D, Yeung J. Diagnosis and management of psoriasis. Can Fam Physician 2017; 63(4): 278-85. [PMID: 28404701]

[108] Ting WW, Vest CD, Sontheimer R. Practical and experimental consideration of sun protection in dermatology. Int J Dermatol 2003; 42(7): 505-13. [http://dx.doi.org/10.1046/j.1365-4362.2003.01867.x] [PMID: 12839597]

SUBJECT INDEX

A

Acanthosis 7, 89, 109, 175, 244, 337
Acrodermatitis continua 5, 107, 333
Adalimumab 22, 23, 34, 55, 62, 77, 244, 299, 338, 340
Adaptive immunity 1, 19, 175, 236, 241, 296, 332
Age distribution 14, 15, 51
Amphotericin b 285
Angiogenesis 18, 51, 109, 242
Anthralin 57, 136, 251, 297, 301, 310, 340, 347
Antimicrobial peptides 49, 296, 297
Apoptosis 8, 92, 123, 243, 298
Apremilast 24, 34, 75, 194, 276, 298, 311, 324, 338
Aquasomes 278
Artemisia capillaris 90, 349
Autoimmunity 286, 345

B

B-cells 20, 132
Biosimilars 277
Brodalumab 23, 34, 339
Bubble electrospinning 183

C

Caffeine 179, 188, 189
Calcipotriene 33, 157, 238, 275, 295, 307, 347
Capsaicin 92, 242, 243, 295
Cerosomes 327
Cerium oxide 212, 213, 217, 218, 220
Chitosan 196, 201, 218, 311, 325
Clobetasol 23, 57, 134, 181, 188, 189, 201, 251, 267, 295, 306, 307, 311, 327
Coal tar 33, 135, 195, 245, 294, 297, 301, 340, 347

D

Dendrimers 57, 104, 121, 132, 163, 164, 196, 200, 278, 279, 327
Diagnosis 8, 49, 123, 175, 213, 305, 332
Diclofenac potassium 250, 252
Dyslipidemia 49, 336

E

Efalizumab 340
Epidemiology 3, 14, 15, 125, 278, 295, 332, 360
Erythrodermic psoriasis 5, 30, 106, 134, 152, 274, 334
Etiology 58, 132, 151, 241, 295, 360
Etanercept 34, 77, 194, 299, 339, 340

F

Feverfew 350
Fish oil 303, 306, 308, 348
Flexural psoriasis 5, 81, 108, 133, 332
Fluorescein 240, 265
Fumaric acid esters 75, 194, 298, 338
Fusidic acid 326

G

Guttate psoriasis 4, 30, 82, 106, 133, 152, 274, 333, 335

H

Holistic 331, 349, 354
Human Leukocyte Antigens 15, 17, 59, 123, 193, 278, 339, 360

Anjali Sharma, Prerna Sharma, Roy Rillera Marzo & Ahmed A. Al Karmalawy (Eds.)

Hyperkeratosis 7, 51, 137, 153, 175, 244, 272, 360
Hypericum perforatum 90, 93
Hypotension 240

I

Immunomodulation 144, 215, 301, 338, 340, 350
Infliximab 34, 77, 194, 299, 339, 340
Innate immunity 1, 19, 175, 241, 296, 332
Inverse psoriasis 5, 80, 108, 133, 136, 274, 332
Iron oxide 212, 213
Ixekizumab 34, 339

K

Koebner phenomenon 1, 4, 240, 333, 347

L

Leflunomide 310, 312
Lornoxicam 285
Lycopene 95

M

Mangiferin 250, 252
Matricaria chamomilla 79
Micro- 57, 104, 132, 160, 164, 196, 200, 247, 248, 278, 279 326,
  emulsions 57, 160, 247, 278, 279, 326
  spheres 57, 104, 132, 164, 196, 200, 248, 279
Monoclonal antibodies 22, 77, 118, 194, 244, 299, 339, 340
Mycophenolate mofetil 75

N

Nanocapsules 132, 165, 200, 248, 279, 327
Naringenin 94
Naringin 94

O

Omega-3-fatty acids 336, 346

P

Palmoplantar 5, 51, 107, 132, 134, 152, 276, 333, 334
PASI 93, 142, 143, 243, 249, 251, 277, 339, 343, 348
PEGylation 117, 118, 124, 157, 197, 325
Pentoxifylline 57, 141, 143
Pioglitazone 311, 312
Psoralea corylifolia 91
Psoriasis 20, 132

Q

Quercetin 93

R

Rehmannia glutinosa 90
Resveratrol 92, 251, 308, 312
Roflumilast 24, 341
Rottlerin 93
Rutin 9

S

Salicylic acid 33, 136, 195, 245, 295, 297, 301, 340, 341, 347
Salvia miltiorrhiza 90
Scalp psoriasis 56, 108, 135, 136, 300, 334
Secukinumab 23, 34, 339, 340
Selenium 213, 217, 218, 219, 220, 348, 349
Smilax china 80

T

Tacrolimus 136, 195, 197, 199, 245, 251, 275, 308, 309, 326, 330
Tazarotene 33, 135, 245, 327, 341
Th 18, 20, 21, 123, 132, 162, 175, 242, 244, 296, 332
  1 cells 20, 132, 175, 242, 244, 296, 332

17 cells 18, 20, 21, 123, 132, 162, 175, 242, 244, 296, 332
Thymoquinone 243, 251, 308, 312
Transgenic model 111, 155, 332
Triamcinolone 33, 388, 391
Turmeric oil 295, 305, 306, 311

U

Ustekinumab 34, 77, 194, 299

V

Vaccinations 334, 347
Vascular endothelial growth factor 109, 244
Vasodilation 243, 342

X

Xenotransplantation model 111, 155, 332

www.ingramcontent.com/pod-product-compliance
Lightning Source LLC
LaVergne TN
LVHW072012300926
849160LV00002B/5
9798898812751